I0065843

A Practical Guide to Veterinary Medicine

A Practical Guide to Veterinary Medicine

Edited by Mel Roth

SYRAWOOD
PUBLISHING HOUSE

New York

Published by Syrawood Publishing House,
750 Third Avenue, 9ᵗʰ Floor,
New York, NY 10017, USA
www.syrawoodpublishinghouse.com

A Practical Guide to Veterinary Medicine
Edited by Mel Roth

© 2018 Syrawood Publishing House

International Standard Book Number: 978-1-68286-577-4 (Hardback)

This book contains information obtained from authentic and highly regarded sources. Copyright for all individual chapters remain with the respective authors as indicated. All chapters are published with permission under the Creative Commons Attribution License or equivalent. A wide variety of references are listed. Permission and sources are indicated; for detailed attributions, please refer to the permissions page and list of contributors. Reasonable efforts have been made to publish reliable data and information, but the authors, editors and publisher cannot assume any responsibility for the validity of all materials or the consequences of their use.

Trademark Notice: Registered trademark of products or corporate names are used only for explanation and identification without intent to infringe.

Cataloging-in-Publication Data

A practical guide to veterinary medicine / edited by Mel Roth.
    p. cm.
Includes bibliographical references and index.
ISBN 978-1-68286-577-4
1. Veterinary medicine. 2. Animals--Diseases. 3. Animal health. I. Roth, Mel.
SF745 .P73 2018
636.089--dc23

TABLE OF CONTENTS

PREFACE

Veterinary medicine is the branch of medicine, which deals with the prevention and cure of diseases and disorders causing ill health in animals and birds. It includes sub-branches like veterinary dentistry, animal physiotherapy, etc. This book provides significant information about the discipline of veterinary medicine to help develop a good understanding of the subject and its related fields. It elaborates the different concepts and applications of the area. The text traces the progress of this field and highlights some of its key concepts and applications. It is a valuable compilation of topics, ranging from the basic to the most complex advancements in the field of veterinary medicine. It is meant for students who are looking for an elaborate reference text on the subject.

This book is a result of research of several months to collate the most relevant data in the field.

When I was approached with the idea of this book and the proposal to edit it, I was overwhelmed. It gave me an opportunity to reach out to all those who share a common interest with me in this field. I had 3 main parameters for editing this text:

1. Accuracy – The data and information provided in this book should be up-to-date and valuable to the readers.

2. Structure – The data must be presented in a structured format for easy understanding and better grasping of the readers.

3. Universal Approach – This book not only targets students but also experts and innovators in the field, thus my aim was to present topics which are of use to all.

Thus, it took me a couple of months to finish the editing of this book.

I would like to make a special mention of my publisher who considered me worthy of this opportunity and also supported me throughout the editing process. I would also like to thank the editing team at the back-end who extended their help whenever required.

Editor

Apocrine Sweat Gland Ductal Adenoma with Sebaceous Differentiation in a Dog

Masaki Michishita, Junki Yasui, Rei Nakahira, Hisashi Yoshimura, and Kimimasa Takahashi

Department of Veterinary Pathology, Nippon Veterinary and Life Science University,
1-7-1 Musashino, Kyounan-cho, Tokyo 180-8602, Japan

Correspondence should be addressed to Masaki Michishita; michishita@nvlu.ac.jp

Academic Editors: N.-Y. Park and R. L. Santos

A 7-year-old male, Border Collie, developed a firm mass, measuring approximately 1 cm in diameter, in the left buccal skin. Histologically, the mass was composed of ductal structures lined by bilayered luminal epithelial and basaloid tumor cells along with a few nests of sebaceous cells. Immunohistochemical staining revealed that the luminal epithelial tumor cells were positive for cytokeratin (CK, CAM5.2) and CK19 but not for CK14 or p63. In contrast, the basaloid tumor cells were positive for CK14, p63, and αSMA but not for CK19 or CAM5.2. CK8 expression was observed in both luminal epithelial and basaloid tumor cells. The tumor cells with sebaceous differentiation were positive for CK14 but not for the other markers. This is the first case of an apocrine sweat gland ductal adenoma with sebaceous differentiation occurring in the buccal skin of a dog.

1. Introduction

Apocrine sweat gland tumors are rather common in dogs and tend to occur on the head, neck, and limb. Approximately 70% of canine apocrine sweat gland tumors are benign in nature [1]. Benign tumors of the apocrine sweat gland are classified as apocrine adenomas, complex and mixed apocrine adenomas, or apocrine ductal adenomas [2]. Apocrine ductal adenomas in dogs are uncommon benign neoplasms and accounted for only 0.3% of canine skin tumors in a large survey [1]. In dogs, sebaceous differentiation has been described in five cases of mammary gland tumors [3–6]. However, to the authors' knowledge, a nonmammary-associated apocrine tumor with sebaceous differentiation in dog has not been previously reported.

2. Case Report

A 7-year-old male, Border Collie, developed a firm mass in the left buccal skin, which was surgically removed and submitted to the Department of Veterinary Pathology, Nippon Veterinary and Life Science University (Tokyo, Japan), for histopathological examination. Grossly, the mass was approximately 1 cm in diameter, and a cut surface of the mass appeared homogeneously greyish-white in color. A physical examination including complete blood count and a routine serum biochemical profile revealed no further abnormalities. Detailed radiographic and X-ray examinations did not reveal any mass suggestive of a tumor in the thoracic and abdominal cavities. No tumor recurrence or metastasis was noted after 9 months of surgical excision. Additional therapy was not performed.

The excised mass was fixed in 10% neutral buffered formalin, embedded in paraffin wax, cut into 4 μm sections, and stained with hematoxylin and eosin (HE), periodic acid-Schiff (PAS), alcian blue, and oil red O stains. Serial sections were subjected to immunohistochemical (IHC) staining using a labeled streptavidin-biotin peroxidase technique with mouse monoclonal antibodies against low molecular weight cytokeratin (CK; clone CAM5.2, prediluted, BD Biosciences, Franklin Lakes, NJ, USA), CK8 (clone Ks 8.7, 1:50, Progen Biotechnik GmbH, Heidelberg, Germany), CK14 (clone LC002, 1:50, BioGenex Laboratories Inc., San Ramon, CA, USA), α-smooth muscle actin (αSMA; clone 1A4, 1:400,

DAKO, Glostrup, Denmark), CK19 (clone 170.2.14, 1 : 100, Boehringer Mannheim, Germany), and p63 (clone 4A4, 1 : 400, NeoMarkers Inc., Fremont, CA, USA). All tissue sections were pretreated with citrate buffer (pH 6.0) and incubated at 121°C for 15 min. The reaction to each antigen was visualized by the addition of 3,3′-diaminobenzidine tetrahydrochloride chromogen and counterstained with hematoxylin.

Histologically, the mass was well demarcated and encapsulated. It consisted of various nodules and proliferating nests mainly composed of bilayered ductal structures with an inner layer of cuboidal to columnar luminal epithelial tumor cells and an outer layer of basaloid tumor cells separated by a thin fibrous stroma (Figure 1). The inner layer of luminal epithelial cells had clear cytoplasm and small hyperchromatic nuclei. The outer layer of basaloid tumor cells had scant eosinophilic cytoplasm and slightly larger euchromatic nuclei. Mitotic activity was moderate. Within the tumor, there were a few nests of large foamy cells similar to the sebaceous cells surrounded by basaloid cells (Figure 2). The nuclei of these cells were centrally located with finely vacuolated cytoplasm and were negative for PAS and alcian blue staining but positive for lipids by oil red O staining (Figure 2 inset). No squamous differentiation or keratinization was observed within the tumor. Furthermore, no necrosis, invasion, or emboli of the tumor cells was observed.

As shown in Table 1, immunohistochemical staining revealed that the luminal epithelial tumor cells were positive for CK19 (Figure 3) and CAM5.2 but not for CK14, αSMA, and p63. In contrast, basaloid tumor cells were positive for CK14 (Figure 4), p63 (Figure 5), and αSMA but not for CK19 and CAM5.2. CK8 expression was observed in both luminal epithelial and basaloid tumor cells (Figure 6). The tumor cells showing sebaceous differentiation were positive for CK14 but not for the other markers.

3. Discussion

On the basis of the histological and immunohistochemical findings, the tumor was diagnosed as an apocrine sweat gland ductal adenoma with sebaceous differentiation. According to the World Health Organization classification of epithelial and melanocytic tumors of the skin of domestic animals, benign tumors of the apocrine sweat gland are classified as apocrine adenomas, complex and mixed apocrine adenomas, or apocrine ductal adenomas [2]. In dogs, sebaceous differentiation has been described in four cases of mammary gland tumors: two complex adenomas [3, 4] and two carcinomas [5, 6] and a case of salivary gland tumor [7], whereas one has not been previously described in apocrine sweat glands. The present report describes a case of apocrine sweat gland ductal adenoma with sebaceous differentiation occurring in the buccal skin of Border Collie.

CK19 and CAM5.2 are useful markers of luminal cell markers, while CK14, p63, and αSMA are markers of basal/myoepithelial cells in dogs [1, 8–11]. CK8 expression has been observed in both luminal and basaloid cells in canine apocrine gland tumors [12]. In contrast, CK14 was expressed

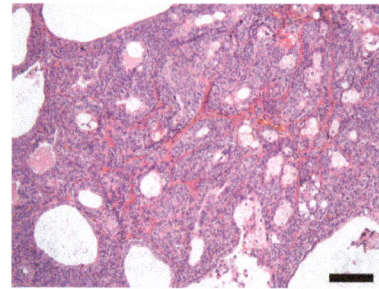

FIGURE 1: Histopathological appearance of the buccal mass. The mass is composed of the ductal structures lined by the bilayered luminal epithelial and basaloid tumor cells. Hematoxylin and eosin (HE). Bar = 100 μm.

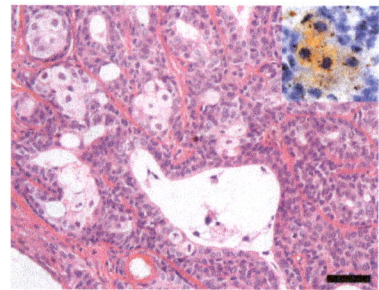

FIGURE 2: Sebaceous differentiation observed within the apocrine ductal adenoma. Sebaceous cells are characterized by abundant, clear, and vacuolated cytoplasm and a centrally located nucleus surrounded by basaloid cells in the apocrine ductal adenoma. HE. Bar = 50 μm. Inset: a frozen section stained with oil red O revealing the lipid droplets within the cytoplasm of sebaceous cells.

TABLE 1: Summary of immunohistochemical findings.

Tumor cell type	CAM5.2	CK8	CK14	CK19	p63	αSMA
Luminal cells	+	+	−	+	−	−
Basaloid cells	−	+	+	−	+	+
Sebaceous-like cells	−	−	+	−	−	−

in the normal sebaceous gland and myoepithelial cells of apocrine and mammary glands [3, 4, 10]. αSMA expression was observed in the myoepithelial cells but not in the basaloid cells in apocrine gland tumors [10]. In canine apocrine carcinoma, p63+SMA+, p63+SMA−, and CK8+p63− cells were identified in myoepithelial, basaloid, and luminal cells, respectively [13]. Additionally, in concordance with previous studies, this tumor primarily consisted of two tumor cell types, luminal cells and basaloid cells, with sebaceous differentiation.

This tumor appeared to be differentiated from a sebaceous adenoma and trichoblastoma of the skin. The tumor characteristics in the present case included cellular proliferation with bilayered ductal structures with sebaceous differentiation, which is not a feature of a sebaceous tumor or trichoblastoma. Canine mammary gland tumors are often observed in squamous differentiation [3, 4]. Some canine apocrine sweat gland ductal adenomas have foci of squamous differentiation

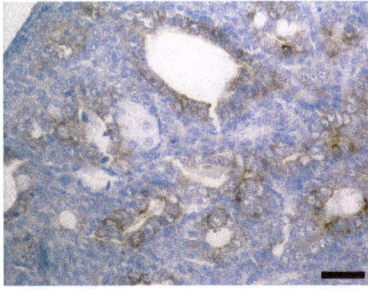

FIGURE 3: Luminal tumor cells are positive for CK19. Immunohistochemistry for CK19 with hematoxylin counterstain. Bar = 50 μm.

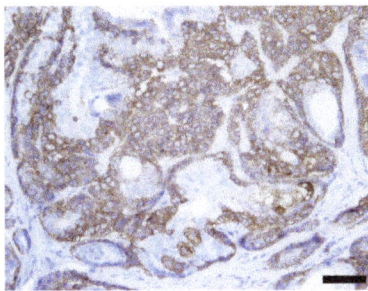

FIGURE 4: Basaloid tumor cells and cells showing sebaceous differentiation are positive for CK14. Immunohistochemistry for CK14 with hematoxylin counterstain. Bar = 50 μm.

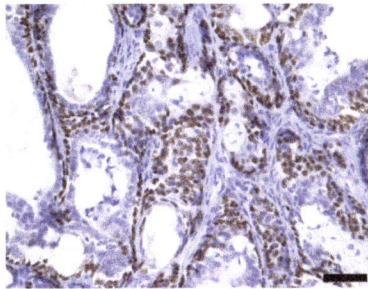

FIGURE 5: Basaloid tumor cells are positive for p63. Immunohistochemistry for p63 with hematoxylin counterstain. Bar = 50 μm.

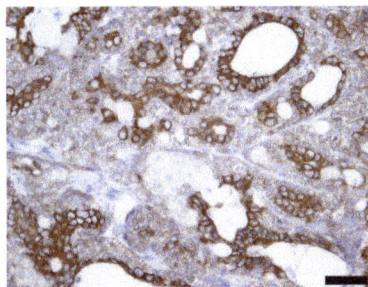

FIGURE 6: Both luminal and basaloid tumor cells are positive for CK8. Immunohistochemistry for CK8 with hematoxylin counterstain. Bar = 50 μm.

with small keratin deposits in the infundibular portion of the apocrine duct [2]. However, squamous differentiation was not observed in this case.

The origin of the sebaceous component in this tumor was unclear. However, previous studies suggested that tumor basaloid cells can differentiate into sebaceous epithelial cells and that cutaneous stem cells might give rise to sebocytes in canine mammary tumors [5, 14, 15]. Therefore, we propose that the sebaceous differentiation in this tumor may have been derived from basaloid cells or local pluripotent stem cells, similar to canine mammary gland tumors.

Conflict of Interests

The authors declare that there is no conflict of interests.

Acknowledgments

The authors would like to thank Dr. Hidemi Kitagawa for providing the follow-up information and the tumor specimen for this study and Drs. Yoko Matsuda, Toshiyuki Ishiwata, and Zenya Naito from Departments of Pathology and Integrative Oncological Pathology, Nippon Medical School, for their helpful discussions.

References

[1] M. H. Goldschmidt and F. S. Shofer, "Apocrine gland tumors," in Skin Tumors of the Dog and Cat, M. H. Goldschmidt and F. S. Shofer, Eds., pp. 85–89, Pergamon Press, Oxford, UK, 1992.

[2] M. H. Goldschmidt, R. W. Dunstan, A. A. Standnard et al., "Histological classification of epithelial and melanocytic tumors of the skin of domestic animals," in World Health Organization International Histological Classification of Tumors of Domestic Animals, F. Y. Schulman, Ed., pp. 21–32, Armed Forces Institute of Pathology (AFIP), Washington, DC, USA, 1998.

[3] K. Yasuno, Y. Takagi, R. Kobayashi et al., "Mammary adenoma with sebaceous differentiation in a dog," Journal of Veterinary Diagnostic Investigation, vol. 23, no. 4, pp. 832–835, 2011.

[4] A. G. Kurilj, M. Hohšteter, A. Beck, B. Artuković, I.-C. Šoštarić-Zuckermann, and Ž. Grabarević, "Complex mammary adenoma with sebaceous differentiation in a dog," Journal of Comparative Pathology, vol. 146, no. 2-3, pp. 165–167, 2012.

[5] S. C. Chang, J. W. Liao, M. L. Wong, Y. S. Lai, and C. I. Liu, "Mammary carcinoma with sebaceous differentiation in a dog," Veterinary Pathology, vol. 44, no. 4, pp. 525–527, 2007.

[6] F. Grandi, M. M. Colodel, R. M. Rocha, and J. L. Sequeira, "Sebaceous metaplasia in a canine mammary gland non-infiltrative carcinoma with myoepithelial component," Journal of Veterinary Diagnostic Investigation, vol. 23, no. 6, pp. 1230–1233, 2011.

[7] O. A. Smrkovski, A. K. LeBlanc, S. H. Smith, C. J. LeBlanc, W. H. Adams, and K. M. Tobias, "Carcinoma ex pleomorphic adenoma with sebaceous differentiation in the mandibular salivary gland of a dog," Veterinary Pathology, vol. 43, no. 3, pp. 374–377, 2006.

[8] A. Gama, A. Alves, F. Gartner, and F. Schmitt, "p63: a novel myoepithelial cell marker in canine mammary tissues," Veterinary Pathology, vol. 40, no. 4, pp. 412–420, 2003.

[9] A. L. Saraiva, F. Gärtner, and M. A. Pires, "Expression of p63 normal canine skin and primary cutaneous glandular carcinomas," *Veterinary Journal*, vol. 177, no. 1, pp. 136–140, 2008.

[10] K. Yasuno, S. Nishiyama, F. Suetsugu, K. Ogihara, H. Madarame, and K. Shirota, "Cutaneous clear cell adnexal carcinoma in a dog: special reference to cytokeratin expression," *Journal of Veterinary Medical Science*, vol. 71, no. 11, pp. 1513–1517, 2009.

[11] A. Gama, A. Alves, and F. Schmitt, "Expression and prognostic significance of CK19 in canine malignant mammary tumours," *Veterinary Journal*, vol. 184, no. 1, pp. 45–51, 2010.

[12] K. Kato, K. Uchida, K. Nibe, and S. Tateyama, "Immunohistochemical studies on cytokeratin 8 and 18 expressions in canine cutaneous adnexus and their tumors," *Journal of Veterinary Medical Science*, vol. 69, no. 3, pp. 233–239, 2007.

[13] A. Shiraki, Y. Hojo, T. Tsuchiya et al., "Complex apocrine carcinoma with dominant myoepithelial proliferation in a dog," *Journal of Veterinary Medical Sciences*, vol. 74, no. 6, pp. 801–804, 2012.

[14] F. A. Tavassoli and H. J. Norris, "Mammary adenoid cystic carcinoma with sebaceous differentiation. A morphologic study of the cell types," *Archives of Pathology and Laboratory Medicine*, vol. 110, no. 11, pp. 1045–1053, 1986.

[15] Y. F. Jiao, S. Nakamura, T. Oikawa, T. Sugai, and N. Uesugi, "Sebaceous gland metaplasia in intraductal papilloma of the breast," *Virchows Archiv*, vol. 438, no. 5, pp. 505–508, 2001.

Caudal Elbow Luxation in a Dog Managed by Temporary Transarticular External Skeletal Fixation

K. Hamilton, S. Langley-Hobbs, C. Warren-Smith, and K. Parsons

Langford Veterinary Services, University of Bristol, Langford BS40 5DU, UK

Correspondence should be addressed to K. Hamilton; k.hamilton@bristol.ac.uk

Academic Editor: Sheila C. Rahal

This case report details a caudal unilateral traumatic elbow luxation in a 4-year-old male neutered Labrador following a road traffic trauma. This is a highly unusual injury in the dog. The pathogenesis and successful treatment by closed reduction followed by stabilisation with a temporary transarticular external skeletal fixator are discussed. The dog was assessed at 4 weeks and 6 months after surgery. Findings at 6 months after treatment demonstrated a normal gait with no pain or crepitation. A mild amount of soft tissue thickening around the elbow was noted. The range of motion of the elbow was limited to 45 degrees of flexion and 150 degrees of extension. This is the first case of a traumatic caudal luxation of the elbow in a dog described in the English veterinary literature and the first report of successful management of an elbow luxation in a dog by closed reduction and temporary transarticular fixation.

1. Introduction

The elbow consists of the humeroradial, humeroulnar, and proximal radioulnar joints. The elbow joint is regarded as a stable joint as a result of the combination of strong surrounding muscular and ligamentous structures and the presence of the anconeal process which interlocks into the olecranon fossa when the elbow is extended beyond 45 degrees [1–3]. Due to these anatomical features and the nature of the forces that the elbow is most commonly subjected to during trauma, fracture of the distal humerus or proximal radius and ulna is more common than elbow joint luxation in the dog [2–6]. The majority of luxations reported in dogs occur due to road traffic accidents [7, 8]. In over ninety percent of elbow luxations the radius and ulna dislocate laterally relative to the humerus [1–4, 6, 7].

Traumatic elbow luxation in dogs can be managed by either closed or open reduction. Early closed reduction of the elbow has a good prognosis for return to normal function [1, 2]. However, open reduction is indicated if there is marked instability following closed reduction, if there are fractures (avulsion or articular associated with the elbow joint), or if a chronic luxation is present [3]. The goals of an open procedure, in addition to reduction of the luxation, are to assess the articular surfaces and to reconstruct or replace the collateral support structures. Joint immobilization is indicated following both open and closed elbow reduction techniques [2, 3, 9, 10].

This case report details a caudal unilateral traumatic elbow luxation which is highly unusual in a dog. The pathogenesis and successful treatment by closed reduction followed by stabilisation with a temporary transarticular external skeletal fixator are discussed.

2. Case Presentation

A 4-year-old male neutered Labrador weighing 28.4 kg was referred following a road traffic trauma that had occurred several hours earlier that day. First aid involving administration of analgesia and intravenous fluids had been initiated by the referring clinic. Luxation of the left elbow and multiple pelvic fractures had been identified via radiographs taken prior to referral.

On presentation the dog was quiet, alert, and responsive. He was nonambulatory. His mucous membranes were pale and cardiopulmonary auscultation revealed slightly decreased bronchovesicular sounds. Superficial skin abrasions were noted over the right carpus, over the tarsi bilaterally, and over the craniolateral aspect of the left thigh. Marked bruising was evident over the caudal abdomen and inguinal region. Neurological assessment of the left pelvic limb was indicative of a sciatic nerve deficit; pain sensation was present and the patellar reflex was intact, but there was a reduced withdrawal response. Neurological examination of the left forelimb was unremarkable; pain sensation and a withdrawal response were within normal limits and voluntary motor function in this limb was noted. Pain was elicited on palpation and manipulation of the left elbow and pelvis. Thoracic radiographs demonstrated changes consistent with mild pulmonary contusions. A urinary catheter was placed to assist management of the dog and analgesia was provided by administration of methadone (Dechra, Sansaw Business Park, Hadnall, Shrewsbury, Shropshire, UK) 0.2 mg/kg via intravenous injection every 4 hours.

The following day the dog was premedicated with 0.02 mg/kg acepromazine (Novartis, Frimley Business Park, Frimley, Camberley, Surrey, UK) and 0.2 mg/kg methadone (Dechra, Sansaw Business park, Hadnall, Shrewsbury, Shropshire, UK) via intravenous injection. General anaesthesia was induced with propofol (Abbott Animal Health, Abbott House, Vanwall Business Park, Vanwall Road, Maidenhead, Berkshire, UK) total dose 1.4 mg/kg and maintained with isoflurane (Novartis; Frimley Business Park, Frimley, Camberley, Surrey, UK) in oxygen. Examination at that time revealed that the left thoracic limb appeared shorter than the right and it was maintained in a flexed position. The tip of the olecranon was felt to be displaced caudally relative to the distal humeral epicondyle. Marked swelling, crepitus, and instability of the left elbow joint were evident on palpation and manipulation.

Computed tomography (CT) was performed using a 5th generation helical multislice scanner (Somatom Emotion 16; Siemens Healthcare, Erlangen, Germany) of both elbows, the pelvis, and left femur. CT imaging of the left thoracic limb demonstrated a caudal luxation of the left humeroradial and humeroulnar joints (Figures 1 and 2). The left medial coronoid of the ulna appeared sclerotic and a small fragment was visible at the coronoid consistent with medial coronoid disease. Additionally, pelvic CT revealed comminuted fractures of the right ischium and pubis, separation of the pubic symphysis, and a comminuted left ilial fracture. The right sacroiliac joint was displaced laterally.

The left thoracic limb was suspended from a drip stand for ten minutes prior to attempting closed reduction. The dog's body weight was used to distract the joint. Reduction was achieved by applying further manual traction and gentle supination to the antebrachium (with the elbow in a moderately flexed position) to distract the coronoid process of the ulna from the olecranon fossa. Pressure was applied to the caudal aspect of the olecranon with the other hand. A clunk was felt when reduction of the joint was achieved. Manipulation of the joint after reduction demonstrated a normal range of flexion and extension. Stability was assessed with Campbell's test [11]. Pronation of greater than 60 degrees was

achievable with the elbow and carpus in 90 degrees of flexion and exceeded the angles achievable in the contralateral limb. This finding was suggestive of rupture of the medial collateral ligaments. Further manipulation of the elbow caused it to reluxate caudally. Closed reduction of the left elbow was easily repeatable.

As the left elbow was unstable after closed reduction and the dog had further orthopaedic injuries affecting other limbs, surgical stabilisation of the luxated elbow was indicated. Stabilisation was achieved with application of a type I transarticular external skeletal fixator (SK ESF System; IMEX Veterinary, Inc., Longview, TX, USA). Four, positive profile end threaded 2.5 mm pins were placed laterally into the radius and four 3.2 mm positive profile pins were placed laterally into the humerus. The holes were predrilled with a 2.0 mm drill bit prior to insertion of the 2.5 mm pins and with a 2.5 mm drill bit prior to insertion of the 3.2 mm pins. Pins were connected to a connecting bar with medium SK clamps. The connecting bars of the radial and humeral component of the external skeletal fixator were connected with an IMEX angular hinge. The hinge was locked to prevent motion. Postoperative radiographs confirmed satisfactory pin positioning. Following imaging a triangulating connecting bar was added to the construct spanning from the proximal aspect of the humeral connecting bar to the distal aspect of the radial connecting bar with two SK clamps. Analgesia was provided with topical transdermal fentanyl ("RECUVYRA", Elanco Animal Health, Eli Lilly and Company Limited, Lilly House, Priestley Road, Basingstoke, Hampshire, UK). Pin insertion sites were covered with a protective bandage that was changed daily for three days before being removed.

The dog was taken to surgery 24 hours later to reduce and stabilise the right sacroiliac luxation with a single 3.5 mm/45 mm Synthes cortical screw (Synthes Ltd., Veterinary Division, 20 Tewin Road, Welwyn Garden City, Hertfordshire, UK) sacroiliac lag screw. The left ilial shaft fracture was stabilised with two polyaxial locking cuttable plates (VetLOX reconstruction plates 3.5 mm and 2.7 mm) (VetLOX Freelance Surgical Ltd., Havyat Business Park, Havyat Road, Wrington, Somerset, UK).

Postoperatively the dog was ambulatory on all four legs with sling support. The dog received daily physiotherapy for the pelvic limb injuries. The dog was discharged from the hospital 12 days postoperatively by which time it was ambulatory on all limbs without assistance. The hinge of the transarticular external skeletal fixator was maintained in a fixed position until removal of the frame.

The dog was reexamined four weeks after application of the transarticular external fixator for the luxated left elbow. At this time the dog was bearing weight well on both forelimbs. Some circumduction of the left forelimb was evident during limb protraction, enabling limb usage with immobilisation of the elbow. A moderate amount of serous discharge was noted to be associated with the most proximal pin tract in the humerus. The frame remained stable. A sciatic neuropraxia was still apparent in the left hind limb, with postural deficits and a reduced withdrawal reflex still evident associated with this limb. Pain sensation and motor function, however, remained intact. The radiographs taken

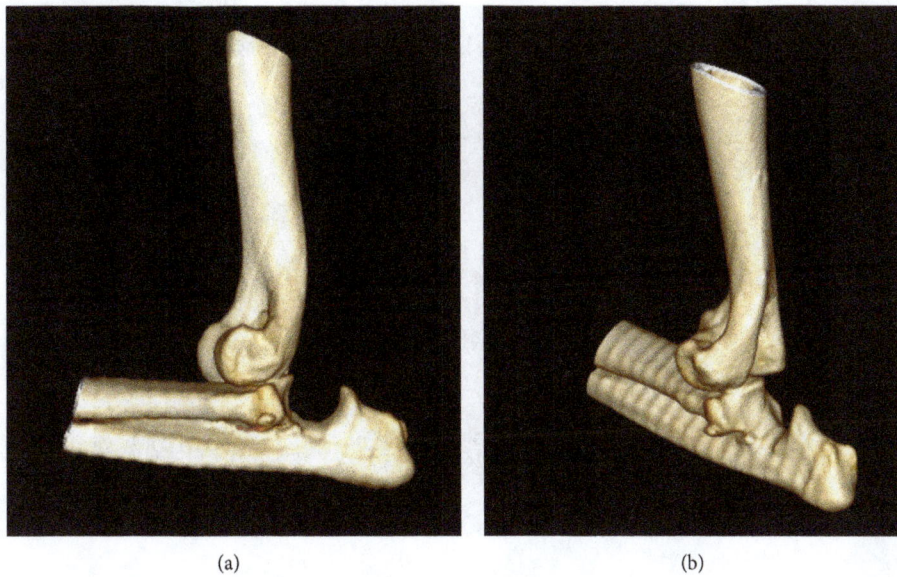

FIGURE 1: (a) CT 3D reconstruction of left elbow viewed from lateral aspect demonstrating caudal luxation of the humeroradial and humeroulnar joint. (b) CT 3D reconstruction of left elbow viewed from caudolateral aspect demonstrating caudal luxation of the humeroradial and humeroulnar joint.

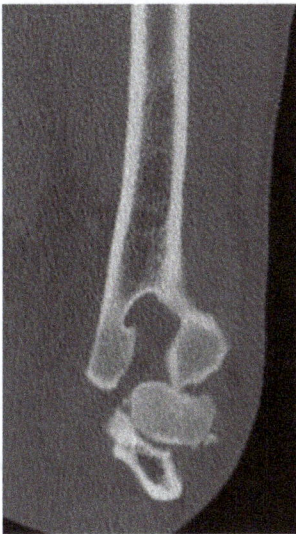

FIGURE 2: Transverse bone algorithm [B60] image of left elbow at the level of the coronoid before reduction demonstrating caudal luxation of the humeroradial and humeroulnar joint. Two well-defined smoothly marginated mineral opacities were also noted; measuring approximately 3 mm and 1 mm, respectively, on the caudal lateral aspect of the radius at the level of the medial coronoid process of the ulna. The medial coronoid appears sclerotic and irregularly defined.

at this time confirmed continued successful reduction of the luxated elbow and appropriate alignment (Figure 3) and the frame was removed. At that time the elbow joint range of movement was measured with an orthopaedic goniometer. The range of motion of the elbow was severely reduced. A limit of 90 degrees of flexion and 115 degrees of extension

was present. No crepitus or instability was felt and Campbell's test demonstrated stability of the medial and lateral collateral support. Radiographs of the femoral and pelvic fractures showed that there were no complications associated with the implants and there was evidence of fracture healing. Following removal of the external skeletal fixator, the dog continued to bear weight well on the left thoracic limb despite mild discomfort being elicited on palpation and manipulation of the left elbow. Left elbow passive range of motion exercises were commenced immediately following external skeletal fixator removal. These involved slow flexion and extension of the joint beyond the pain-free range of motion of the elbow to enable stretching of the tissue. The stretch was held for 10 seconds and repeated 10 times per session. The owners were instructed to perform three to four sessions daily. The owners were also advised to continue to rest the dog for a further four weeks (crate rest with ten minutes of short lead exercise three times daily). Following the four weeks of restricted activity the dog's exercise was gradually increased over a further six-week period. At repeat assessment six months after trauma the dog was not lame. Exercise was well tolerated with no requirement for medication. Range of motion of the left elbow was still slightly reduced compared to the other limb but with no pain or crepitation. A mild amount of soft tissue thickening around the elbow was noted. The range of motion of the elbow was limited to 45 degrees of flexion and 150 degrees of extension. Despite identification of medial coronoid disease from the CT imaging at the time of injury, no further treatment was specifically advised relating to this finding as the dog had been asymptomatic prior to the trauma and the pathology identified was subtle. However, if symptoms developed, further assessment would be appropriate.

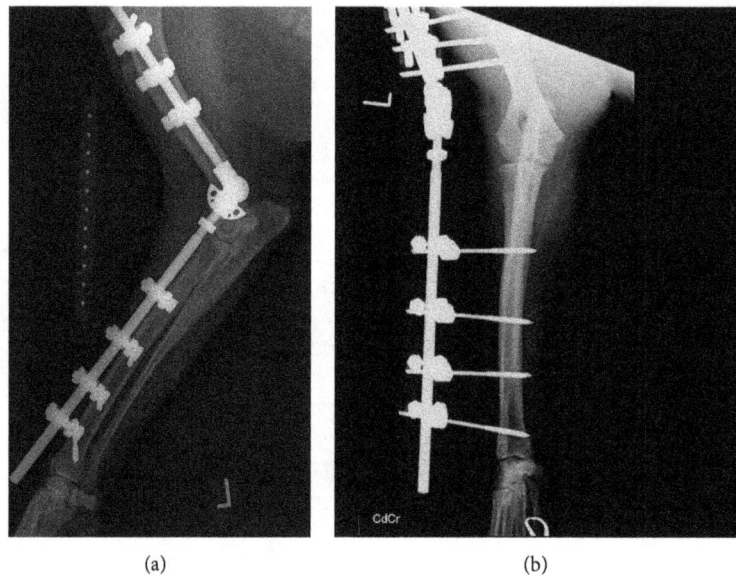

<table>
<tr><td>(a)</td><td>(b)</td></tr>
</table>

FIGURE 3: (a) Mediolateral radiograph of the left forelimb after reduction and stabilisation of left elbow. (b) Caudocranial radiograph of the left forelimb after reduction and stabilisation of left elbow.

3. Discussion

This report describes a polytrauma case in a dog with multiple injuries including a unilateral, caudal elbow luxation. This caudal elbow luxation was successfully stabilised by closed reduction and placement of a temporary transarticular external skeletal fixator. To the authors' knowledge, this is the first case of a caudal luxation of the elbow in a dog described in the English veterinary literature and the first report of management of an elbow luxation in a dog by closed reduction and temporary transarticular fixation.

Caudal luxation accounts for 90% of all elbow luxations in man [12, 13]. It is also extremely common in rabbits and is reported in cats, although lateral luxation is most common in this species [3, 14–16]. Elbow luxation in man, rabbits, and cats is usually the result of a fall or jump from a height (direct trauma) [14, 17, 18]. In man, luxation usually results from a fall onto an extended elbow resulting in compressive forces being directed onto the outstretched hand, the radius, and ulna, along with a valgus force at the elbow, resulting in the common caudolateral or caudal dislocation [14, 19–22]. In cats it is thought that the manner in which the cat lands on its paws determines the direction of luxation [18]. In rabbits, however, it is not clear whether dislocation occurs with the elbow flexed or when it is overextended during impact [23]. Rabbits have good lateral and medial stability of the elbow due to the presence of a well-developed central sagittal ridge of the humeral condyle. This anatomical feature protects the joint from lateral and medial luxation.

Traumatic elbow luxation in dogs is usually the result of road traffic accidents [7, 8]. It is hypothesised that the forces necessary to luxate the elbow in dogs occur when the body of the animal pivots around the flexed elbow during the traumatic event resulting in indirect rotational forces usually contributing to lateral elbow luxation [2, 3, 11].

There is limited lateral elbow joint stability in the flexed position because the anconeal process is not anchored in the olecranon fossa, which allows the humeral condyle to slide craniomedially over the head of the radius. In addition, the articular surface of the medial epicondyle slopes distally and the relatively large size of the trochlea of the humerus prevents medial displacement of the radius and ulna [1–4, 6, 24]. It is hypothesised in this case that at the time of trauma the forces acting through the elbow of this Labrador must have more closely resembled the forces of a fall or a jump and it is also likely that the elbow was in an extended position with the anconeal process engaged within the olecranon, increasing stability in the mediolateral plane. Best clinical results in cases of elbow luxation in dogs are obtained with an acute closed stable reduction [2–5, 7, 11]. Initial attempts of closed reduction were successful in this case; however, further manipulation and assessment identified marked instability and reluxation occurred. Use of a splint to maintain the elbow in extension was felt unlikely to provide adequate stability due to the orientation of the luxation and the dog's multiple orthopaedic injuries. Maintaining extension of the elbow is advantageous in cases of lateral and medial luxation as this optimises lateral stability by enabling interlocking of the anconeal process into the olecranon fossa. This does not however improve caudal stability, which was necessary to prevent reluxation in this case.

Treatment recommendations in man following reduction of simple caudal luxation of the elbow are immobilization with a caudal plaster cast in 90-degree flexion or an initial plaster cast followed by functional treatment in a hinged brace, sling, or pressure bandage, regardless of the degree of ligamentous and muscular damage to the elbow [25, 26]. Similarly, in rabbits use of a Velpeau sling after reduction is recommended [14]. The flexed forearm maintains the humerus in a reduced position and relieves tension on the cranial soft tissues. This was not considered in this case due to the instability identified from Campbell's test; pronation of the elbow was greater than 60 degrees, with the elbow and carpus in 90 degrees of flexion, consistent with complete transection of the medial collateral ligament. In addition fixing the elbow in a flexed position would not be optimal in this polytrauma case with multiple limb injuries as it was felt that the dog would need to bear weight on this leg following surgery due to its compromised pelvic limbs. In dogs when elbow instability remains after closed reduction and/or there is significant instability of either the medial or lateral collateral ligaments, surgical stabilisation is recommended followed by immobilisation [1, 2, 4, 24]. Reported surgical techniques in dogs include reconstruction of the collateral support structures with suture repair or humeral transcondylar and proximal radial and ulnar bone tunnels in combination with adjunct joint immobilisation to allow healing [1, 2, 4, 24]. Described methods of secondary immobilisation to protect the ligamentous repair include splints, transarticular pinning, or use of a modified external skeletal fixator [1–3, 10, 24, 27, 28]. However, application of an external skeletal fixator alone following closed elbow reduction, without primary repair of collateral ligaments or placement of prosthetic ligaments, has not been reported in dogs to the authors' knowledge. In the authors' clinical experience closed reduction and stabilisation with a transarticular external skeletal fixator can be used as a successful treatment where collateral ligament injury is evident on Campbell's test, without the need for internal stabilisation in cases of lateral elbow luxation. The duration of joint immobilisation is critical to enable enough time for soft tissue repair without promoting joint stiffness and adverse effects on joint health. Optimal periods of joint immobilisation for dogs are currently not described. However, the degree of degenerative and destructive cartilage changes increases with greater periods of immobilization. With the reintroduction of mobilization, reparative processes do occur [29, 30].

The fixator applied in this case included a hinge over the elbow joint. Rigid joint immobilisation can have adverse effects on connective tissue and can result in decreased range of motion, muscle atrophy, joint contracture, and cartilage degeneration [10, 31–35]. Consequently controlled motion after surgical repair is considered beneficial. Because the motion of the elbow joint approximates that of a simple hinge, rigid fixation of an unstable elbow with a constrained hinge aligned along the best-fit axis is possible and should be a consideration for the future. However, appropriate hinge alignment would be essential as off-axis positioning imposes abnormal joint kinematics, with resultant incongruous articulation and/or joint instability. In addition, as healing progresses to create a more constrained situation, increases in stress would be transferred to the pins and the pin-bone interface. This may account for the clinical problems of pin loosening, pin breakage, and persistent instability [36, 37]. Controlled motion across the joint was not considered at the time of frame application in this case due to the lack of published research to describe an accurate intraoperative axis detection procedure for hinge placement and the lack of availability of a fixator hardware

system that allows flexible hinge positioning, independent of the fixator pin. Consequently the fixator design did not accommodate hinge motion and the benefits of maintaining joint motion were lost. Despite maintaining the hinge in the locked position, the clinical outcome was excellent in this case and closed reduction and stabilisation of a caudal elbow luxation with a type 1 transarticular external skeletal fixator provided a successful outcome with a good clinical recovery.

We did not make any recommendations for further investigations or treatment of the medial coronoid disease identified associated with the left elbow while it remained asymptomatic. Multiple studies have made recommendations relating to the optimum treatment for medial coronoid disease, including fragment retrieval [38–40], subtotal coronoidectomy [41], cartilage debridement [40], proximal ulna osteotomy [42, 43], biceps/brachialis muscle release [44], and medical management [38, 39]. It is difficult to make a definitive treatment recommendation in a previously asymptomatic dog recovering from a major orthopaedic injury, when the majority of treatment options currently have the potential for some degree of morbidity.

Conflict of Interests

The authors declare that there is no conflict of interests regarding the publication of this paper.

References

[1] L. A. Billings, P. B. Vasseur, R. J. Todoroff, and W. Johnson, "Clinical results after reduction of traumatic elbow luxation in nine dogs and one cat," *Journal of the American Animal Hospital Association*, vol. 28, pp. 137–142, 1992.

[2] M. G. O'Brien, R. J. Boudrieau, and G. N. Clark, "Traumatic luxation of the cubital joint (elbow) in dogs: 44 cases (1978–1988)," *Journal of the American Veterinary Medical Association*, vol. 201, no. 11, pp. 1760–1765, 1992.

[3] I. G. F. Schaeffer, P. Wolvekamp, B. P. Meij, L. F. H. Theijse, and H. A. W. Hazewinkel, "Traumatic luxation of the elbow in 31 dogs," *Veterinary and Comparative Orthopaedics and Traumatology*, vol. 12, no. 2, pp. 33–39, 1999.

[4] J. R. Campbell, "Luxation and ligamentous injuries of the elbow of the dog," *The Veterinary Clinics of North America*, vol. 1, no. 3, pp. 429–440, 1971.

[5] M. A. Pass and J. G. Ferguson, "Elbow dislocation in the dog," *Journal of Small Animal Practice*, vol. 12, no. 6, pp. 327–332, 1971.

[6] C. Dassler and P. B. Vasseur, "Elbow luxation," in *Textbook of Small Animal Surgery*, D. Slatter, Ed., vol. 2, pp. 1919–1927, WB Saunders, Philadelphia, Pa, USA, 2002.

[7] K. E. Mitchell, "Traumatic elbow luxation in 14 dogs and 11 cats," *Australian Veterinary Journal*, vol. 89, no. 6, pp. 213–216, 2011.

[8] D. Savoldelli, P. M. Montavon, and P. F. Suter, "Traumatic elbow luxation in the dog and the cat: perioperative findings," *Schweizer Archiv fur Tierheilkunde*, vol. 138, no. 8, pp. 387–391, 1996.

[9] R. P. Suess Jr., E. J. Trotter, D. Konieczynski, R. J. Todhunter, D. L. Bartel, and J. A. Flanders, "Exposure and postoperative stability of three medial surgical approaches to the canine elbow," *Veterinary Surgery*, vol. 23, no. 2, pp. 87–93, 1994.

[10] Z. Schwartz and D. J. Griffon, "Nonrigid external fixation of the elbow, coxofemoral, and tarsal joints in dogs," *Compendium of Continuing Education for the Practising Veterinarian*, vol. 30, no. 12, pp. 648–653, 2008.

[11] A. Bongartz, F. Carofiglio, T. Piaia, and M. Balligand, "Traumatic partial elbow luxation in a dog," *Journal of Small Animal Practice*, vol. 49, no. 7, pp. 359–362, 2008.

[12] L. L. Lattanza and G. Keese, "Elbow instability in children," *Hand Clinics*, vol. 24, no. 1, pp. 139–152, 2008.

[13] C. R. Wheeles, Ed., *Wheeless' Textbook of Orthopaedics*, http://www.wheelessonline.com/.

[14] J. Ertelt, J. Maierl, A. Kaiser, and U. Matis, "Anatomical and pathophysiological features and treatment of elbow luxation in rabbits," *Tierarztliche Praxis Ausgabe K: Kleintiere—Heimtiere*, vol. 38, no. 4, pp. 201–210, 2010.

[15] J. de Haan, D. den Hartog, W. E. Tuinebreijer et al., "Functional treatment versus plaster for simple elbow dislocations (FuncSiE): a randomized trial," *BMC Musculoskeletal Disorders*, vol. 11, article 263, 2010.

[16] A. Von Kriegsheim, *A retrospective study of joint dislocations of the extremities of dogs and cats [Ph.D. thesis]*, 2001, http://www.diss.fu-berlin.de/diss/receive/FUDISS_thesis_000000000524.

[17] M. D. McKee, E. H. Schemitsch, M. J. Sala, and S. W. O'Driscoll, "The pathoanatomy of lateral ligamentous disruption in complex elbow instability," *Journal of Shoulder and Elbow Surgery*, vol. 12, no. 4, pp. 391–396, 2003.

[18] B. Vollmerhaus, H. Schebitz, H. Roos, L. Brunnberg, and H. Waibl, "Anatomische Grundlagen und funkionelle Betrachtungen zur Olekranonfraktur beim Hund," *Kleintierprax*, vol. 28, pp. 5–15, 1983.

[19] J. de Haan, N. W. L. Schep, R. W. Peters, W. E. Tuinebreijer, and D. den Hartog, "Simple elbow dislocations in the Netherlands: what are Dutch surgeons doing?" *Nederlands Tijdschrift voor Traumatologie*, vol. 17, no. 5, pp. 124–1127, 2009.

[20] D. Eygendaal, "Treatment of the chronic medial unstable elbow," *Acta Orthopaedica Scandinavica*, vol. 71, no. 5, pp. 475–479, 2000.

[21] T. L. Mehlhoff, P. C. Noble, J. B. Bennett, and H. S. Tullos, "Simple dislocation of the elbow in the adult. Results after closed treatment," *Journal of Bone and Joint Surgery A*, vol. 70, no. 2, pp. 244–249, 1988.

[22] G. E. Garrigues, W. H. Wray III, A. L. C. Lindenhovius, D. C. Ring, and D. S. Ruch, "Fixation of the coronoid process in elbow fracture-dislocations," *Journal of Bone and Joint Surgery A*, vol. 93, no. 20, pp. 1873–1881, 2011.

[23] D. Lorinson, *Grundlagen und Methodik der Behandlung von Frakturen und Luxationen beim Zwergkaninchen Habilitationsschrift*, Veterinärmedizinische Universität Wien, 1998.

[24] J. R. Campbell, "Nonfracture injuries to the canine elbow," *Journal of the American Veterinary Medical Association*, vol. 155, no. 5, pp. 735–744, 1969.

[25] G. Schippinger, F. Seibert, J. Steinböck, and M. Kucharczyk, "Management of simple elbow dislocations: does the period of immobilization affect the eventual results?" *Langenbeck's Archives of Surgery*, vol. 384, no. 3, pp. 294–297, 1999.

[26] K. A. Hildebrand, S. D. Patterson, and G. J. W. King, "Acute elbow dislocations: simple and complex," *Orthopedic Clinics of North America*, vol. 30, no. 1, pp. 63–79, 1999.

[27] S. C. Rahal, F. de Biasi, L. C. Vulcano, and F. J. T. Neto, "Reduction of humeroulnar congenital elbow luxation in 8 dogs by using the transarticular pin," *Canadian Veterinary Journal*, vol. 41, no. 11, pp. 849–853, 2000.

[28] M. Farrell, D. Draffan, T. Gemmill, D. Mellor, and S. Carmichael, "In vitro validation of a technique for assessment of canine and feline elbow joint collateral ligament integrity and description of a new method for collateral ligament prosthetic replacement," *Veterinary Surgery*, vol. 36, no. 6, pp. 548–556, 2007.

[29] V. I. Shevtsov and S. N. Asonova, "Ultrastructural changes of articular cartilage following joint immobilization with the Ilizarov apparatus," *Bulletin Hospital for Joint Diseases*, vol. 54, no. 2, pp. 69–75, 1995.

[30] M. A. LeRoux, H. S. Cheung, J. L. Bau, J. Y. Wang, D. S. Howell, and L. A. Setton, "Altered mechanics and histomorphometry of canine tibial cartilage following joint immobilization," *Osteoarthritis and Cartilage*, vol. 9, no. 7, pp. 633–640, 2001.

[31] F. Behrens and W. Johnson, "Unilateral external fixation. Methods to increase and reduce frame stiffness," *Clinical Orthopaedics and Related Research*, no. 241, pp. 48–56, 1989.

[32] W. H. Akeson, D. Amiel, M. F. Abel, S. R. Garfin, and S. L. Woo, "Effects of immobilization on joints," *Clinical Orthopaedics and Related Research*, vol. 219, pp. 28–37, 1987.

[33] W. H. Akeson, S. L.-Y. Woo, D. Amiel, and J. V. Matthews, "Biomechanical and biochemical changes in the periarticular connective tissue during contracture development in the immobilized rabbit knee," *Connective Tissue Research*, vol. 2, no. 4, pp. 315–323, 1974.

[34] S. Houshian, B. Gynning, and H. A. Schrøder, "Chronic flexion contracture of proximal interphalangeal joint treated with the compass hinge external fixator. A consecutive series of 27 cases," *Journal of Hand Surgery*, vol. 27, no. 4, pp. 356–358, 2002.

[35] G. M. Kerkhoffs, B. H. Rowe, W. J. Assendelft, K. Kelly, P. A. Struijs, and C. N. van Dijk, "Immobilisation and functional treatment for acute lateral ankle ligament injuries in adults," *Cochrane Database of Systematic Reviews*, no. 3, Article ID CD003762, 2002.

[36] M. B. Sommers, D. C. Fitzpatrick, K. M. Kahn, J. L. Marsh, and M. Bottlang, "Hinged external fixation of the knee: intrinsic factors influencing passive joint motion," *Journal of Orthopaedic Trauma*, vol. 18, no. 3, pp. 163–169, 2004.

[37] S. M. Madey, M. Bottlang, C. M. Steyers, J. L. Marsh, and T. D. Brown, "Hinged external fixation of the elbow: optimal axis alignment to minimize motion resistance," *Journal of Orthopaedic Trauma*, vol. 14, no. 1, pp. 41–47, 2000.

[38] N. J. Burton, M. R. Owen, L. S. Kirk, M. J. Toscano, and G. R. Colborne, "Conservative versus arthroscopic management for medial coronoid process disease in dogs: a prospective gait evaluation," *Veterinary Surgery*, vol. 40, no. 8, pp. 972–980, 2011.

[39] R. B. Evans, W. J. Gordon-Evans, and M. G. Conzemius, "Comparison of three methods for the management of fragmented medial coronoid process in the dog: a systematic review and meta-analysis," *Veterinary and Comparative Orthopaedics and Traumatology*, vol. 21, no. 2, pp. 106–109, 2008.

[40] R. H. Palmer, "Arthroscopic and open surgical treatment of MCPD/OCD," in *Proceedings of the 25th Annual Meeting of the International Elbow Working Group*, pp. 14–20, Bologna, Italy, 2010.

[41] N. Fitzpatrick, "Subtotal coronoid ostectomy (SCO) for the treatment of medial coronoid disease: a prospective study of 228 dogs (389 elbows) evaluating short and medium term outcome," in *Proceedings of the British Veterinary Orthopaedic Association*,

Autumn Scientific Meeting—Enigmas of the Canine Elbow, pp. 22–29, Chester, UK, 2006.

[42] C. A. Preston, K. S. Schulz, K. T. Taylor, P. H. Kass, C. E. Hagan, and S. M. Stover, "In vitro experimental study of the effect of radial shortening and ulnar ostectomy on contact patterns in the elbow joint of dogs," *The American Journal of Veterinary Research*, vol. 62, no. 10, pp. 1548–1556, 2001.

[43] B. M. Turner, R. H. Abercromby, J. Innes, W. M. McKee, and M. G. Ness, "Dynamic proximal ulnar osteotomy for the treatment of ununited anconeal process in 17 dogs," *Veterinary and Comparative Orthopaedics and Traumatology*, vol. 11, no. 2, pp. 76–79, 1998.

[44] N. Fitzpatrick, R. Yeadon, T. Smith, and K. Schulz, "Techniques of application and initial clinical experience with sliding humeral osteotomy for treatment of medial compartment disease of the canine elbow," *Veterinary Surgery*, vol. 38, no. 2, pp. 261–278, 2009.

3

Gastric Smooth Muscle Hamartomas Mimicking Polyps in a Dog: A Case Description and a Review of the Literature

Marian A. Taulescu,[1] Irina Amorim,[2] Fatima Gärtner,[2] Laura Fãrcaş,[1] Mircea V. Mircean,[3] and Cornel Cătoi[1]

[1] Pathology Department, Faculty of Veterinary Medicine, University of Agricultural Sciences and Veterinary Medicine, 3-5 Calea Mãnãştur Street, 400372 Cluj-Napoca, Romania
[2] Department of Pathology and Molecular Immunology of the Institute of Biomedical Sciences Abel Salazar (ICBAS), University of Porto, Rua Jorge Viterbo Ferreira Nr. 228, 4050-313 Porto, Portugal
[3] Department of Internal Medicine, Faculty of Veterinary Medicine, University of Agricultural Sciences and Veterinary Medicine, 3-5 Calea Mãnãştur Street, 400372 Cluj-Napoca, Romania

Correspondence should be addressed to Marian A. Taulescu; taulescumarian@yahoo.com

Academic Editors: N. D. Giadinis, S. Hecht, and R. L. Santos

This report presents a case of two smooth muscle hamartomas of the stomach in a 10-year-old male Boxer. The clinical history of the animal was of chronic vomiting, weight loss, and intermittent gastric distension, and it died because of chronic and congestive heart failure. Gross, histology, and immunohistochemistry (IHC) exams were performed. On necropsy, in the pyloric region of the stomach, two closely related polypoid growths between 10 and 15 mm in diameter were identified. On the cut sections, both polyps presented white to gray color, with homogenous architecture and well-defined limits. The thickness of the submucosal layer was seen to be increased to 1 cm. No other gastric alterations were identified by the necropsy exam. Histologically, both masses growth consisted of hyperplastic glands lined by foveolar epithelium, arranged in a papillary or branching pattern, and supported by a core of well-vascularised and marked smooth muscle tissue interspersed between glands. No dysplastic cells and mitotic figures were observed in these lesions. Immunohistochemistry revealed a strong cytoplasm labelling for smooth muscle actin of the bundles around the mucosal glands. To our knowledge, this is the first report of smooth muscle hamartomas mimicking multiple gastric polyps in dogs.

1. Introduction

Gastric polyps (GP) are sessile or pedunculated growths that arise from the mucosa and protrude into the gastric lumen as the result of either hyperplasia or neoplasia [1]. GP occur sporadic in dogs [2, 3], cats [4], cattle [5], and horses [6]; they are observed during gastric endoscopy or necropsy. GP are often in the pyloric region, and the affected animals usually do not show any clinical signs however. GP can produce vomiting after food intake, weight loss, and bleeding when these lesions reach a considerable size and rarely cause pyloric stenosis [2, 3]. Macroscopically, GP are described as solitary or multiple bulging sessile or pedunculated formations, with an irregular and arborescent surface [7]. In human pathology, various types of nonneoplastic gastric polyps, including

hyperplastic, inflammatory fibroid, xanthoma, hamartomatous of the Peutz-Jeghers type, juvenile, gastric polyps in Cowden disease, and gastric polyps in Cronkhite-Canada syndrome, are described [8]. In domestic animals, there is a lack of data about the histological features of the gastric polyps. Based on histological findings, two gastric polyps have been distinguished: hyperplastic and inflammatory (benign lymphoid) [1]. The pathogenesis of development of the GP in dogs is still unknown, but previous reports suggest a possible hereditary predisposition in French Bulldog [3, 9].

2. Case Description

This short communication describes an unprecedented case of gastric hamartomatous polyps in a 10-year-old male Boxer.

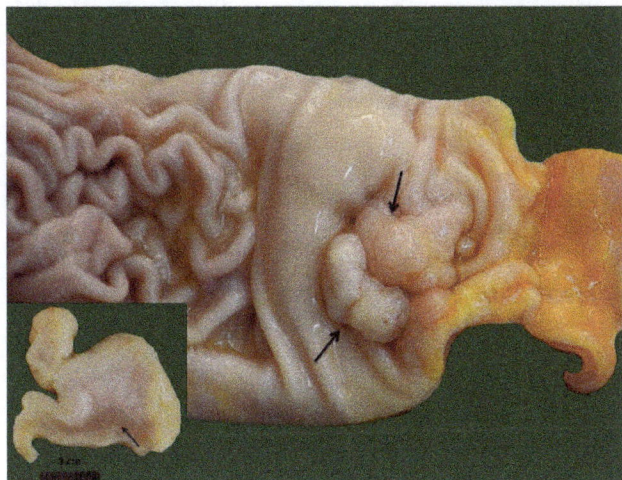

FIGURE 1: Photograph of the opened stomach showing two intra-luminal and closely related polyp-like masses, measuring approximately 15 mm in diameter that was easily seen in the pyloric region (arrows). The inset illustrates the morphological aspects of the cross-section of the polypoid mass with a white to gray and dense structure and muscular layer thickening (arrow).

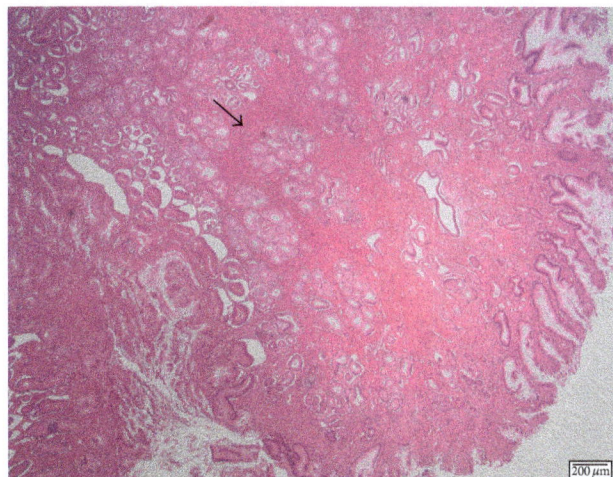

FIGURE 2: The histological exam of a section of the polypoid mass showing a branching framework consisting of numerous bands of smooth muscle cells (arrow) with intervening glandular tissue and covered by a mild to moderate foveolar hyperplasia. HE stain. Bar = 200 μm.

The animal was presented for examination with history of chronic vomiting, weight loss, and intermittent gastric distension. No endoscopy or other paraclinical investigations were made. The animal died 1 month later, due to congestive stage of heart chronic failure. During the necropsy, gastric lesions were collected, fixed in 10% buffered formalin, and submitted to histological examination. Tissues samples were routinely processed, dehydrated, and embedded in paraffin wax. Four μm consecutive sections were cut and stained with haematoxylin and eosin. Immunohistochemistry was also performed using the avidin-biotin-peroxidase complex (ABC) method, employing the monoclonal antisera muscular α-actin (clone HHF35, Dako). Negative controls for each sample were prepared by replacing the primary antibody with mouse IgG1 Negative Control (Code X0931, Dako, Denmark). Semiquantitative assessment of immunohisto-chemical intensity was performed and scored negative (−), weak (+), moderate (++), and intense (+++).

On necropsy, luminal fluid and gases accumulation and two closely related polypoid growths were identified in the pyloric region of the stomach: one pedunculated measuring 1.5 cm in diameter and another sessile and dense on palpation with 1.0 cm in diameter. On the cut sections, both polyps present white to gray color, with homogenous architecture and well-defined limits; thickening of the muscular layer was also macroscopically observed (Figure 1). No other gastric alterations were identified; however, the necropsy exam also revealed bilateral ventricular dilation, severe and chronic pulmonary edema and diffuse pulmonary anthracosis, chronic and diffuse liver congestion, cystic mucinous hyperplasia of the gallbladder mucosa, and multifocal nodular exocrine pancreatic hyperplasia.

Histologically, both gastric masses projected above the level of the surrounding mucosa into the gastric lumen. The

lesions were covered by hyperplastic foveolar epithelium with minimal branching and cystic dilatation, supported by an extensive smooth-muscle proliferation, with an elongated, arborized pattern of polyp formation (Figure 2). The deep area of the gastric polyp revealed several bands of smooth muscle cells between the gastric antral-type glands lined by well-differentiated mucinous epithelium and mild mononu-clear cells infiltration consisting of lymphocytes, plasma cells, and hystiocytes (Figure 3). Neither cytological atypia nor mitotic figures were observed in this lesion. The presence of muscle fibres in the lamina propria was further confirmed by immunohistochemistry which revealed a strong cytoplasm labelling for smooth muscle actin of the bundles around the mucosal glands (Figure 4). No histological changes were found in the adjacent mucosa of the polypoid growths. The histopathological findings along with the immunohis-tochemical results suggested a diagnosis of canine gastric hamartomatous polyp.

3. Discussion

Hamartoma is a tumor-like malformation composed of an abnormal mixture of normal tissue elements or an abnormal proportion of a single element [10]. By definition, hamar-tomas are congenital lesions, with limited propensity for growth, and normally paralleling the growth of the host; however, they may not be detected until later in life [10]. In dogs, hamartomas are more commonly found in the skin [11], but some vascular hamartomas of the cerebrum [12] and lung [13] are also documented.

The gastric hamartomatous polyp is predominantly com-posed by hyperplastic mucosal glands, smooth muscle bun-dles in the mucosal layer, and asymptomatic lesions found incidentally in fewer than 0,1% of all endoscopy examinations [14].

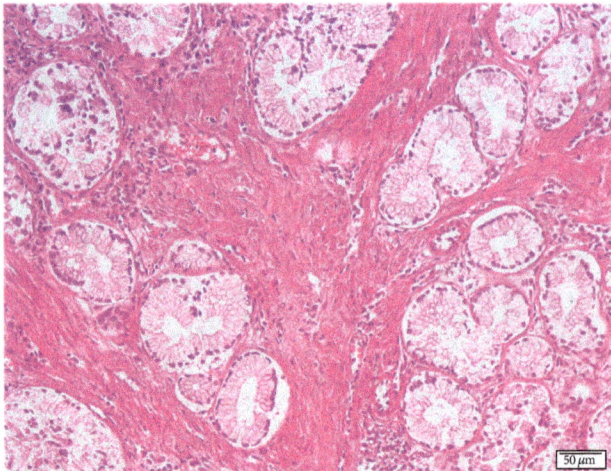

FIGURE 3: High power photomicrograph of a section of the polypoid mass showing several bands of well-differentiated smooth muscle cells between gastric antral-type glands lined by tall columnar mucinous epithelium. HE stain. Bar = 50 μm.

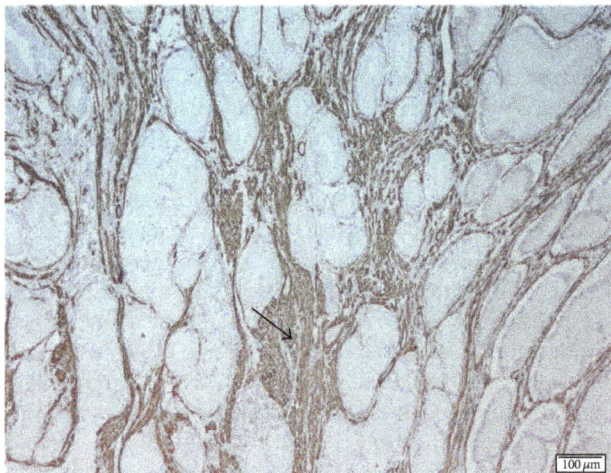

FIGURE 4: Immunohistochemistry showing hyperplastic cells with diffuse and strong positivity with smooth muscle actin (SMA) (arrow), while the gastric glands epithelium was negative. Immunoperoxidase-diaminobenzidine stain, Mayer hematoxylin counterstain. Bar = 100 μm.

To the best of our knowledge, only 28 cases of human gastric solitary hamartomatous polyps were so far documented in the literature [15]. In animals, gastric smooth muscle hamartoma has only been described in the abomasum of a calf [5] and adjacent to the lower gastroesophageal sphincter in a cat [4]. Our current case demonstrated extensive branching of the alpha actin stained smooth muscle fibers from muscularis mucosae to the mucosal layer between gastric glands and foveolae and their atrophy. These characteristics thus need to be differentiated from hyperplastic and inflammatory types. This constitutes the first report of this kind of lesion in canine stomach. In the majority of cases, these lesions are probably subdiagnosed and classified as hyperplastic gastric polyps because endoscopic biopsies are superficial and fail

to obtain the representative features of the lesion or because immunohistochemistry studies are not performed.

On the other hand, hamartomatous polyposis syndromes are a diverse group of inherited conditions grouped together because they exhibit hamartomatous rather than epithelial polyp histology. If in human pathology several reports revealed the malignant potential of the hamrtoamatous gastric polyps associated with Peutz-Jeghers syndrome, Cowden syndrome, juvenile polyposis, and PTEN hamartoma tumour syndrome [16], in dogs, a malignant transformation was found only in the hyperplastic polyps [9]. The progression of these polyps to cancer is not well understood, but a possible malignant transformation of the epithelial components was debated [17]. No changes of the epithelial cells of both foveole and glands were observed in the present case.

Brown et al. (1994) described the presence of hamartomatous polyps in the intestine of two dogs, reporting for the first time the occurrence of such lesions in domestic animals [18]. A case of colorectal hamartomatous polyposis and ganglioneuromatosis with PTEN duplication affecting a Great Dane puppy was recently documented. In this case, similar to what occurs in human Cowden syndrome, a possible mutation was investigated in the PTEN gene; however, such mutation was not proven [19].

In human medicine, a gastric hamartomatous polyp is a well-defined entity, already described and recognized by WHO. A more precise and elaborated gastric classification scheme is needed in veterinary medicine, where the histological and immunophenotypic features of a lesion should be taken together in consideration. Thus, being the third case described affecting different animal species, this entity should be included in this classification. On the other hand, an important challenge will be to determine the mechanisms involved for development of the hamartomatous gastric polyps in dogs and their correlation with a possible genetic mutation.

To our knowledge, this is the first report of smooth muscle hamartomas mimicking multiple gastric polyps in dogs. If the smooth muscle hamartomatous gastric polyps could represent a predisposing factor to the development of malignancy in dogs, a generic hypothesis remains which needs further studies for confirmation.

Authors' Contribution

Taulescu Marian and Irina Amorim contributed equally to this work.

Acknowledgments

I. Amorim (SFRH/BD/76237/2011) acknowledges FCT, the Portuguese Foundation for Science and Technology, for financial support. The Institute of Molecular Pathology and Immunology of the University of Porto (IPATIMUP) is an Associate Laboratory of the Portuguese Ministry of Science, Technology and Higher Education and is partially supported by FCT.

References

[1] K. W. Head, J. M. Cullen, R. R. Dubielzig et al., "Histological histological classification of tumors of the alimentary system of domestic animals," in *International Histological Classification of Tumors of Domestic Animals*, F. Y. Schulman, Ed., pp. 75–111, AFIP, Washington, DC, USA, 2003.

[2] A. Diana, D. G. Penninck, and J. H. Keating, "Ultrasonographic appearance of canine gastric polyps," *Veterinary Radiology and Ultrasound*, vol. 50, no. 2, pp. 201–204, 2009.

[3] S. Kuan, K. Hoffmann, and P. Tisdall, "Ultrasonographic and surgical findings of a gastric hyperplastic polyp resulting in pyloric obstruction in an 11-week-old French Bulldog," *Australian Veterinary Journal*, vol. 87, no. 6, pp. 253–255, 2009.

[4] T. J. Smith, W. I. Baltzer, C. G. Ruaux, J. R. Heidel, and P. Carney, "Gastric smooth muscle hamartoma in a cat," *Journal of Feline Medicine and Surgery*, vol. 12, no. 4, pp. 334–337, 2010.

[5] M. Yamaguchi, N. Machida, K. Mitsumori, M. Nishimura, and Y. Ito, "Smooth muscle hamartoma of the abomasum in a calf," *Journal of Comparative Pathology*, vol. 130, no. 1, pp. 66–69, 2004.

[6] C. C. Morse and D. W. Richardson, "Gastric hyperplastic polyp in a horse," *Journal of Comparative Pathology*, vol. 99, no. 3, pp. 337–342, 1988.

[7] R. P. Happe, I. Van Der Gaag, W. C. Wolvekamp Th., and J. Van Toorenburg, "Multiple polyps of the gastric mucosa in two dogs," *Journal of Small Animal Practice*, vol. 18, no. 3, pp. 179–189, 1977.

[8] Y. P. Do and G. Y. Lauwers, "Gastric polyps: classification and management," *Archives of Pathology and Laboratory Medicine*, vol. 132, no. 4, pp. 633–640, 2008.

[9] M. Gualtieri, M. G. Monzeglio, E. Scanziani, and C. Domeneghini, "Pyloric hyperplastic polyps in the French Bulldog," *European Journal of Companion animal Practice*, vol. 6, pp. 51–57, 1996.

[10] C. C. Brown, D. C. Baker, and I. K. Barker, "Alimentary system," in *Pathology of Domestic Animals*, K. V. F. Jubb, P. C. Kennedy, and N. Palmer, Eds., pp. 1–296, Saunders Elsevier, Philadelphia, Pa, USA, 2007.

[11] Y. Kim, S. Reinecke, and D. E. Malarkey, "Cutaneous angiomatosis in a young dog," *Veterinary Pathology*, vol. 42, no. 3, pp. 378–381, 2005.

[12] M. Sakurai, T. Morita, H. Kondo, T. Uemura, A. Haruna, and A. Shimada, "Cerebral vascular hamartoma with thrombosis in a dog," *Journal of Veterinary Medical Science*, vol. 73, no. 10, pp. 1367–1369, 2011.

[13] G. Chanoit, K. G. Mathews, B. W. Keene, M. T. Small, and K. Linder, "Surgical treatment of a pulmonary artery vascular hamartoma in a dog," *Journal of the American Veterinary Medical Association*, vol. 240, no. 7, pp. 858–862, 2012.

[14] K. M. Zbuk and C. Eng, "Hamartomatous polyposis syndromes," *Nature Clinical Practice Gastroenterology and Hepatology*, vol. 4, no. 9, pp. 492–502, 2007.

[15] J. S. Jin, J. K. Yu, T. Y. Tsao, and L. F. Lin, "Solitary gastric Peutz-Jeghers type stomach polyp mimicking a malignant gastric tumor," *World Journal of Gastroenterology*, vol. 18, pp. 1845–1848, 2012.

[16] A. Gammon, K. Jasperson, W. Kohlmann, and R. W. Burt, "Hamartomatous polyposis syndromes," *Best Practice and Research*, vol. 23, no. 2, pp. 219–231, 2009.

[17] J. R. Jass, "Pathology of polyposis syndromes with special reference to juvenile polyposis," in *Hereditary Colorectal Cancer*, J. Utsunomiya and H. T. Lynch, Eds., p. 343, Springer, Tokyo, Japan, 1990.

[18] P. J. Brown, S. M. Adam, P. R. Wotton, C. Gibbs, and R. H. Swan, "Hamartomatous polyps in the intestine of two dogs," *Journal of Comparative Pathology*, vol. 110, no. 1, pp. 97–102, 1994.

[19] I. Bemelmans, S. Küry, O. Albaric et al., "Colorectal hamartomatous polyposis and ganglioneuromatosis in a dog," *Veterinary Pathology*, vol. 48, no. 5, pp. 1012–1015, 2011.

4

A Case of Enzootic Nasal Adenocarcinoma in a Ewe

**Devorah Marks Stowe, Kevin L. Anderson, James S. Guy,
Keith E. Linder, and Carol B. Grindem**

North Carolina State University College of Veterinary Medicine, 1060 William Moore Drive, Raleigh, NC 27607, USA

Correspondence should be addressed to Devorah Marks Stowe, devorah_stowe@ncsu.edu

Academic Editors: J. S. Munday and S. Stuen

An approximately 2-year-old open Suffolk ewe presented to the North Carolina State University College of Veterinary Medicine Veterinary Health Complex for evaluation of a left nasal mass. An ultrasound-guided aspirate and core biopsies were performed. An epithelial neoplasia with mild mixed inflammation (neutrophils and plasma cells) was diagnosed on cytology and confirmed on histopathology. Immunohistochemistry (IHC), reverse transcriptase polymerase chain reaction (RT-PCR), and transmission electron microscopy were also performed. IHC and RT-PCR identified the presence of enzootic nasal tumor virus and confirmed the final diagnosis of enzootic nasal adenocarcinoma.

1. Case History and Presentation

An approximately 2-year-old open Suffolk ewe presented to the North Carolina State University College of Veterinary Medicine Veterinary Health Complex (NCSU-VHC) for evaluation of a left nasal mass, (Figure 1). Four months previously, the ewe started having clear nasal discharge. The following month, slight facial distortion was first observed by her owner. At that time, the ewe was not showing any signs of depression or illness and had a normal appetite and activity level. The facial distortion evolved into a left-sided fluid filled dorsal nasal mass with bilateral serosanguinous nasal discharge when pressure was applied to the mass. The ewe was subsequently referred to the NCSU-VHC where radiographs confirmed a left nasal mass with frontal sinus involvement. An ultrasound-guided aspirate of the mass was performed at that time.

2. Cytologic Findings

Direct smears and cytocentrifuged preparations of fluid from an ovine nasal mass aspirate produced highly cellular cytological samples with a thick pink background, mild-to-moderate hemodilution, and windrowing of RBCs. Large clusters of round to polygonal-shaped epithelial cells with minimal anisocytosis and anisokaryosis were present. Cell-cell junctions were noted within the clusters. The cells had round nuclei with ropey chromatin and occasional small round nucleoli and a small amount of medium blue cytoplasm. Scattered neutrophils and plasma cells were present. The cytologic interpretation and diagnosis was epithelial neoplasia (carcinoma) with mild mixed inflammation (neutrophils and plasma cells), (Figure 2).

3. Histologic, Immunohistochemical, Polymerase Chain Reaction, and Electron Microscopy Findings

The ewe returned 1 month later for a recheck examination and additional diagnostic tests. Ultrasound-guided core needle biopsies were performed and tissue was collected into neutral buffered formalin for histology and Trump's fixative for transmission electron microscopy (TEM). A well-differentiated, expansile epithelial neoplasm contained acini and tubules supported by scant fibrovascular stroma. The cells were tall cuboidal to tall columnar with distinct cell borders and a moderate amount of eosinophilic to amphophilic cytoplasm. The nuclei were round to oval and central to eccentrically located. Cells exhibited mild

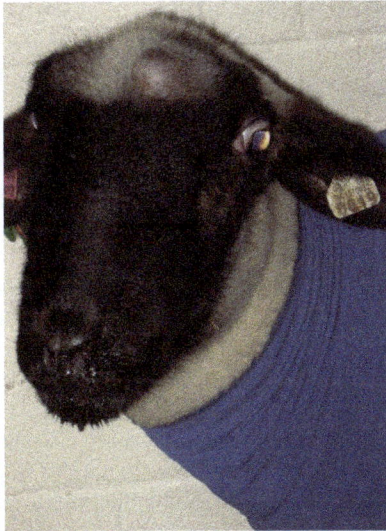

FIGURE 1: Picture of ewe on initial presentation with left-sided dorsal nasal mass.

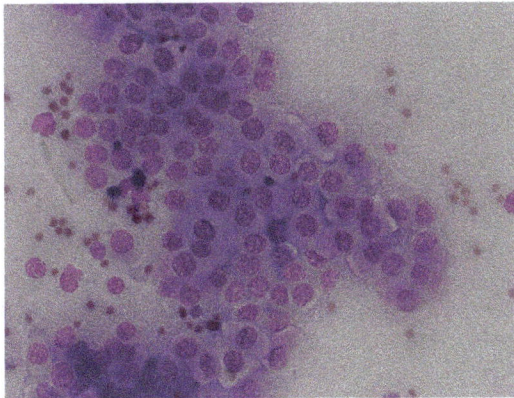

FIGURE 2: Initial cytology of nasal mass with large cluster of round to polygonal epithelial cells, Wright-Geimsa stain, 50x objective.

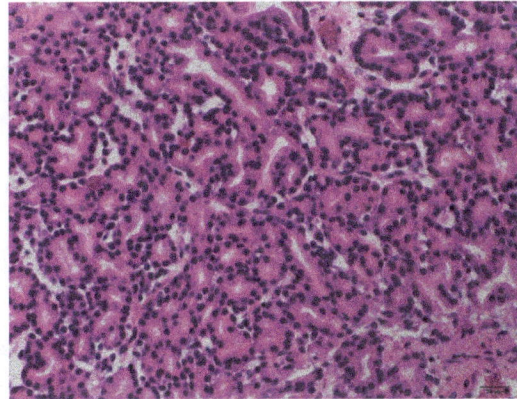

FIGURE 3: Histopathology of nasal mass, hematoxylin and eosin stain, 40x objective.

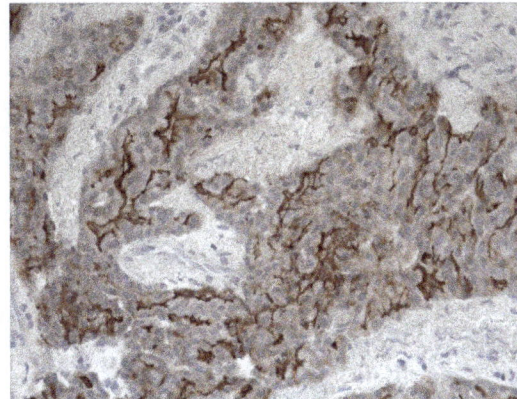

FIGURE 4: Immunohistochemistry of nasal mass using mouse monoclonal antibody against JSRV envelope protein. Note the positive apical staining.

anisocytosis and anisokaryosis. Mitotic figures were rare, less than 1 per 10 high powered fields. There were multifocal mild lymphoplasmacytic and neutrophilic infiltrates. Nasal carcinoma with mild multifocal mixed inflammation was the final diagnosis (Figure 3).

Additional diagnostic tests that were performed included immunohistochemistry (IHC), reverse transcriptase polymerase chain reaction (RT-PCR), and TEM. IHC was performed using a mouse monoclonal antibody against the Jaagsiekte sheep retrovirus (JSRV) envelope protein. This antibody cross-reacts with the enzootic nasal tumor virus (ENTV) envelope protein. Strong positive surface staining was observed (Figure 4). The same tissue was similarly stained with normal mouse serum as a negative control and there was no detectable staining.

RT-PCR was performed using oligonucleotide primers specific for ENTV and RNA extracted from tumor tissues; oligonucleotide primers previously were developed by Dr.

Sarah Wootton, University of Guelph. The RT-PCR procedure yielded a distinct product of approximately 155 base pairs, and direct nucleotide sequencing of this product indicated 88% sequence identity with ovine ENTV [1]. The 88% identity to a previous known strain of ENTV suggests that the virus identified in this case is likely a distinct strain of ENTV. TEM results were equivocal for the presence of retrovirus. Epithelial cells contained well-formed junctional complexes at apical areas. The cytology, histology, IHC, and RT-PCR all confirmed a diagnosis of enzootic nasal adenocarcinoma (ENA).

4. Necropsy Findings

The ewe did not receive treatment and remained comfortable and active for several months in an isolated area. Eventually her clinical signs worsened and she was humanely euthanized five months after presenting to NCSU-VHC which was nine months after clinical signs were first noticed. Complete necropsy revealed a large, expansile, friable mass effacing the left and right ethmoidal conchae which was mottled tan to red and measured 11.0 cm × 11.0 cm × 1.0 cm.

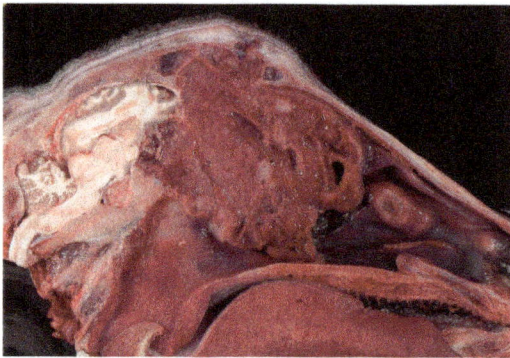

FIGURE 5: Gross image of the tumor invading the nasal cavity and compressing the cerebrum at necropsy (courtesy of Dr. Allison C. Boone).

The mass replaced approximately 50% of the left and right rostral frontal sinus, 50% of the dorsal nasal concha, and 100% of the middle nasal concha. The mass compressed but did not invade the ventral portion of the brain and extended ventrally to the vomer bone (Figure 5). Bony lysis caused an externally palpable, focal, soft depression of the frontal bone (3.0 cm × 3.0 cm and was 1.0 cm deep) with a small open draining track to the neoplasm in conjunction with local hemorrhage and edema. The lungs failed to collapse when the thoracic cavity was opened, contained rib impressions, and was mottled pink to dark red. The remaining viscera were grossly unremarkable. The lungs contained a multifocal neutrophilic and lymphoplasmacytic bronchointerstitial pneumonia with intralesional bacterial colonies and peribronchial lymphoid hyperplasia. A gram stain was applied to the lung tissue and no infectious agents were identified. A culture was not performed on the lung tissue. Histopathology performed on necropsy tissue samples confirmed the diagnosis of a nasal adenocarcinoma.

5. Discussion

Adenomas and carcinomas of the nasal cavity in sheep have the greatest prevalence in the United States, Canada, France, Germany, and Spain [2] and can be caused by *"enzootic nasal tumor virus-1"* (ENTV-1) infection, which is a betaretrovirus [2, 3]. ENTV-2 causes the same disease process in goats [3]. Individual or multiple animals in a flock can be infected. It is presumed that the disease is spread by contact with nasal secretions [2]. Clinical disease is usually present in adult sheep, but young lambs have also been affected [2]. Tumors originate from the ethmoid turbinates and can be unilateral or bilateral [2, 3]. The tumors can fill a large portion of the nasal cavity before clinical signs develop, which includes abundant seromucinous nasal discharge [2, 3]. Clinical signs are usually slowly progressive, with additional clinical signs being dyspnea, facial deformities, exophthalmia, and weight loss [4]. These neoplasms are typically invasive, predominantly low grade and rarely metastasize [3, 5]. When presented with a suspect case of ENA on cytopathology or

histopathology, additional diagnostics such as immunohistochemistry and/or polymerase chain reaction (PCR) are required to make a definitive diagnosis. Once the diagnosis is confirmed, the patient should be separated from the remainder of the flock to avoid spread of disease.

Gross evaluation, cytology, histopathology, IHC, PCR, and TEM are diagnostics that can aid in the diagnosis of ENA. Grossly the tumor is tan to white, firm, and multinodular. The tissue may also contain red-brown areas of hemorrhage or necrosis [2]. The histologic appearance is consistent with that of an adenoma or adenocarcinoma. The classic description includes cuboidal or pseudostratified nonciliated epithelial cells that form orderly tubular, papillary, or acinar arrangements. Neoplastic cells have basal round nuclei and a variable mitotic rate. Mucus secretion is usually abundant, and the fibrovascular stroma is usually scant. Neoplastic tissue and adjacent nonneoplastic tissues often contain numerous lymphocytes [2]. A viral etiology can be definitively proven by several methods. IHC can be performed using a mouse monoclonal antibody against the JSRV envelope protein which cross-reacts with the ENTV-envelope protein. The positive staining pattern is typically apical along the cell periphery. RT-PCR can detect the exogenous ENTV-1 using virus specific primers. TEM is variably reported to reveal extracellular or budding retroviral particles in 75–100% of ovine cases [2].

Cytologic differentials include well-differentiated adenopapillomas, adenomas, and adenocarcinomas which account for the majority of nasal neoplasms in sheep [6]. Nasal epithelial hyperplasia is another consideration for this lesion. It is not possible to differentiate these three neoplasms on cytology, biopsy, and histopathology, making IHC, PCR, or TEM required to identify evidence of viral infections. Nonneoplastic differentials in sheep with gross lesions causing exophthalmia, facial deformity, nasal discharge, and dyspnea include nasal fungal or bacterial granuloma, actinobacillosis, actinomycosis, and sinusitis [6]. Conidiobolomycosis is a zygomycosis characterized by granulomatous and necrotic lesions in the ethmoidal and nasopharyngeal regions that extend into the turbinate bones and can invade the brain and orbit [7]. These patients often experience exophthalmia along with nasal discharge, dyspnea, anorexia, facial distortion, and enlargement of the anterior or posterior nasal cavity [7].

Ovine pulmonary adenocarcinoma (OPA), also known as Jaagsiekte, is caused by the betaretrovirus JSRV and is another common neoplasm of the respiratory tract in sheep. JSRV induces neoplastic transformation of alveolar and bronchial secretory epithelial cells which results in pulmonary tumors [4]. The main clinical sign is difficulty in breathing which is due to pulmonary edema that may drain from the nostrils [4]. Similar to ENA, a definitive diagnosis of OPA requires further diagnostic testing: gross and histologic evaluation, immunohistochemistry using antibodies against JSRV proteins, PCR with JSRV specific primers, and/or TEM. Grossly affected animals have a thin carcass with fluid filling the trachea and nares. Lungs are enlarged, heavy, and edematous and also contain consolidated foci or diffuse areas of tumor [3]. The tumor has a solid, grey, granular surface, and exudes fluid when cut [3]. Similar to ENA, OPA is a contagious disease that is spread through contact of nasal drainage. It can infect sheep of any age, but is usually diagnosed in sheep between 2 and 4 years of age [4]. This disease has been reported in many sheep-rearing regions around the world including the United States. Infected animals can live with subclinical disease for months to years, which aids in spread of disease. Once clinical signs become severe, the sheep have a very poor prognosis.

Conflict of Interests

The authors declared no potential conflict of interests with respect to the research, authorship, and/or publication of this paper.

Acknowledgments

Dr. Sarah Wooton, Ph.D., at the University of Guelph Ontario Veterinary College developed the oligonucleotide primers to detect ENTV. The authors received funding from the North Carolina State University Veterinary Health Complex for diagnostic testing.

References

[1] S. R. Walsh, N. M. Linnerth-Petrik, A. N. Laporte, P. I. Menzies, R. A. Foster, and S. K. Wootton, "Full-length genome sequence analysis of enzootic nasal tumor virus reveals an unusually high degree of genetic stability," *Virus Research*, vol. 151, no. 1, pp. 74–87, 2010.

[2] J. L. Caswell and K. J. Williams, "Enzootic nasal tumor of sheep," in *Jubb, Kennedy, and Palmer's Pathology of Domestic Animals*, M. G. Maxie, Ed., vol. 2, pp. 620–621, Saunders Elsevier, Philadelphia, Pa, USA, 5th edition, 2007.

[3] K. A. Fox, S. K. Wootton, S. L. Quackenbush et al., "Paranasal sinus masses of rocky mountain bighorn sheep (Ovis canadensis canadensis)," *Veterinary Pathology*, vol. 48, no. 3, pp. 706–712, 2011.

[4] D. J. Griffiths, H. M. Martineau, and C. Cousens, "Pathology and pathogenesis of ovine pulmonary adenocarcinoma," *Journal of Comparative Pathology*, vol. 142, no. 4, pp. 260–283, 2010.

[5] A. Lopez, "Endemic ethmoidal tumors (enzootic nasal tumors, enzootic intranasal tumors, enzootic nasal carcinoma)," in *Pathologic Basis of Veterinary Disease*, M. D. McGavin and J. F. Zachary, Eds., p. 485, Mosby Elsevier, St. Louis, Mo, USA, 5th edition, 2012.

[6] A. R. Woolums, J. C. Baker, and J. A. Smith, "Upper respiratory tract diseases," in *Large Animal Internal Medicine*, B. P. Smith, Ed., pp. 595–593, Mosby Elsevier, St. Louis, Mo, USA, 4th edition, 2009.

[7] S. M. M. S. Silva, R. S. Castro, F. A. L. Costa et al., "Conidiobolomycosis in Sheep in Brazil," *Veterinary Pathology*, vol. 44, pp. 314–319, 2007.

5

Surgical Treatment of a Chronic Brain Abscess and Growing Skull Fracture in a Dog

Amy W. Hodshon,[1] Jill Narak,[2] Linden E. Craig,[3] and Andrea Matthews[4]

[1]*Department of Small Animal Clinical Sciences, College of Veterinary Medicine, The University of Tennessee, 2407 River Drive, Knoxville, TN 37996, USA*
[2]*Department of Clinical Sciences, Auburn University, Auburn, AL 36849, USA*
[3]*Department of Biomedical and Diagnostic Sciences, College of Veterinary Medicine, The University of Tennessee, 2407 River Drive, Knoxville, TN 37996, USA*
[4]*Antech Imaging Services, Charlottetown, PE, Canada C1A 1B6*

Correspondence should be addressed to Jill Narak; narakjc@auburn.edu

Academic Editor: Sheila C. Rahal

A 2-year-old female spayed Miniature Dachshund was presented for seizures and right prosencephalic signs. A multiloculated, ring-enhancing mass in the right cerebrum associated with dilation of the right lateral ventricle and brain herniation was seen on magnetic resonance imaging. An irregular calvarial defect with smoothly scalloped edges was seen overlying the mass on computed tomography. The mass was removed via craniectomy and was diagnosed as a chronic brain abscess caused by *Peptostreptococcus anaerobius*. The patient was maintained on antibiotics for 12 weeks. Follow-up MRI performed 14 weeks after surgery confirmed complete removal of the abscess as well as a contrast-enhancing collection of extra-axial material consistent with a chronic subdural hematoma. The neurologic abnormalities, including seizures, have improved in the 44 months since surgery. Brain abscesses in dogs can have an insidious clinical course prior to causing serious neurologic deterioration. Ventricular entrapment by an intracranial mass can contribute to acute neurologic decline. If surgically accessible, outcome following removal of a brain abscess can be excellent; aerobic and anaerobic bacterial culture should be performed in these cases. Subdural hematoma can occur following removal of a large intracranial mass. Growing skull fractures can occur in dogs but may not require specific surgical considerations.

1. Introduction

Brain abscesses are a relatively uncommon cause of neurologic disease in dogs. Surgical treatment has been reported in one dog and eight cats, each with a brain abscess suspected to be caused by a bite wound received within 14 days of presentation [1–3]. In contrast, this report describes the surgical treatment of a dog with a chronic, mature brain abscess. Additional interesting features of this case that are presented and discussed include the presence of a growing skull fracture, compartmentalized hydrocephalus of the lateral ventricle, and a suspected chronic subdural hematoma on postoperative imaging.

2. Case Presentation

A 2-year-old female spayed Miniature Dachshund was presented for a 5-day history of circling to the right and blindness in the left eye. This had been preceded by 2 weeks of lethargy and reluctance to traverse stairs for which she was receiving carprofen (unknown dose). The dog had a history of generalized seizures that had begun 7 months earlier and occurred about twice monthly; she had been receiving phenobarbital (8 mg by mouth twice daily) for the previous 6 months. The dog was obtained from a breeder at 7 months of age; she had a scar on her head at that time that according to the breeder had always been present. The owner reported that occasionally the area of the scar would swell for a period of time and then go back down.

On presentation, the patient was quiet but responsive with normal vital parameters. General physical exam was normal other than an irregular scar present over the right frontal bone; a bony defect with underlying soft, compressible tissue was palpable under the scar. On neurologic exam the dog's mentation was depressed, and she circled to the right with a normal gait. Cranial nerve exam revealed blindness in the left visual field with normal pupillary light reflexes. Postural reactions were delayed on the left side and normal on the right. Spinal reflexes were normal. Pain was elicited on palpation of the cranial cervical spine and head. These findings were consistent with a structural lesion in the right forebrain. Primary differential diagnoses included a brain abscess, other inflammatory diseases (infectious or sterile), and a neoplastic mass.

A complete blood count and serum chemistry were within normal limits. The patient was anesthetized, and magnetic resonance imaging (MRI) of the brain was performed (1.0 Tesla Magnetom Harmony, Siemens Medical Solutions, Malvern, PA). A mass lesion was seen in the right cerebrum located under a defect in the dorsal calvarium. Within the mass were several pockets of T2-hyperintense material incompletely suppressed on T2-weighted fluid attenuated inversion recovery (FLAIR) (Figures 1(a) and 1(b)). These pockets were surrounded by a T2-hypointense, T1-isointense rim. There was significant T2W hyperintensity within the right cerebral white matter, consistent with vasogenic edema. The rostral horn of the right lateral ventricle was adjacent to the caudal extent of the mass, and caudal to this the ventricle was markedly dilated and surrounded by a rim of T2W and FLAIR hyperintensity (Figure 1(c)). The cumulative mass effect was causing significant shifts in brain parenchyma, including subfalcine herniation (Figures 1(d) and 2). The cervical spinal cord was T2-hyperintense, especially dorsally starting at C2-C3, suggestive of syringohydromyelia formation. On the T2*-weighted gradient-echo sequence, there were several irregular areas of signal void associated with the mass, likely indicative of hemorrhage or mineral fragment (Figure 1(e)). The periphery of the mass strongly enhanced immediately following administration of intravenous (IV) paramagnetic contrast agent (Magnevist, Bayer Healthcare Pharmaceuticals Inc., Wayne, NJ; 0.1 mmol/kg). This enhancement clearly delineated at least three distinct pockets of T1-hypointense fluid (Figure 1(f)). No ependymal or diffuse meningeal contrast enhancement was seen.

A computed tomography (CT) scan (Philips Brilliance 40, Philips Healthcare, Andover, MA) was performed following the MRI. A large area of hypodense parenchyma in the right cerebral hemisphere causing a significant midline shift toward the left was seen (Figure 3(a)). There was a large, irregular, chevron-shaped defect in the right frontal bone with a smaller triangular-shaped bone flap overlying it; this bone flap extended cranially tangential to the convexity of the skull (Figure 3(b)). The margins of the bone flap and the underlying skull defect were smoothly scalloped. The defect did not extend into the frontal sinus. A small mineral fragment was also noted within the intracranial mass

(Figure 3(a)). Postcontrast CT was not performed. Based on examination and imaging findings, a cerebral abscess was suspected, and the patient was taken immediately to surgery.

The patient received 1 g/kg mannitol IV over about 20 minutes following MRI; perioperative antibiotics were withheld. A modified right rostrotentorial craniectomy was performed centered over the bony defect. The triangular flap of bone was removed using rongeurs and was noted to be spongier than normal bone. The cerebrum under the bony defect was covered with tenacious fibrous tissue; distinct dura mater was difficult to identify. The edges of the calvarial defect were freshened, and the dura and fibrous tissue overlying the protruding brain tissue were incised and removed.

An ultrasonic aspirator (Sonastar, Mixonix, Inc., Farmingdale, NY) was inserted to a premeasured depth to reach the contrast-enhancing mass seen on MRI; however, the mass's firm consistency precluded use of the aspirator. Gentle probing with lint-free eye spears (Eagle Labs, Rancho Cucamonga, CA) allowed movement of the intra-axial mass, which was green/brown, firm, and distinct from the surrounding brain parenchyma. The mass was gently dissected free of surrounding tissue using an ophthalmic spatula and removed. A small bone chip was embedded in the mass, and the center was cavitated and had a foul odor on cut section. Half of the removed tissue was submitted for aerobic, anaerobic, and fungal tissue culture. The remaining tissue was fixed in 10% formalin for histopathologic analysis. During removal of the mass, the right lateral ventricle was inadvertently entered, presumably at the site where the two were adjacent; the ependymal lining and choroid plexus were visible, and cerebrospinal fluid flowed into the surgical field. The ventricular tissue was gently replaced into the parenchymal defect created by removal of the mass in as normal an anatomic orientation as possible.

Following removal of the mass, 20 mg/kg enrofloxacin was given IV over one hour. Once hemostasis was achieved, the surgical site was copiously lavaged with sterile saline, and the durectomy was covered with swine intestinal submucosa (SurgiVet, Dublin, OH). Polypropylene mesh (C.R. Bard, Inc., Warwick, RI) was cut slightly larger than the craniectomy and was sutured to the surrounding periosteum. The subcutaneous tissues and skin were closed in a routine fashion.

The patient recovered from anesthesia uneventfully. Postoperative care included a fentanyl and lidocaine infusion (titrated for analgesia), enrofloxacin (20 mg/kg IV once daily), clindamycin (12 mg/kg IV twice daily), famotidine (0.5 mg/kg IV twice daily), phenobarbital (2.5 mg/kg IV twice daily), maintenance IV fluids, and standard monitoring and nursing care. The morning after surgery, the patient was sedated but was responsive and nonpainful. She was ambulatory with mild left-sided hemiparesis 24 hours following surgery (likely due to peracute disruption of the right frontoparietal lobe at the time of surgery). Postoperative complications included a seroma at the surgery site and two instances of regurgitation on the first day of oral feeding (48 hours after surgery); these were treated with intermittent warm compresses and metoclopramide (0.25 mg/kg orally every 6 hours), respectively. A five-day course of anti-inflammatory prednisone (0.25 mg/kg orally twice daily) was

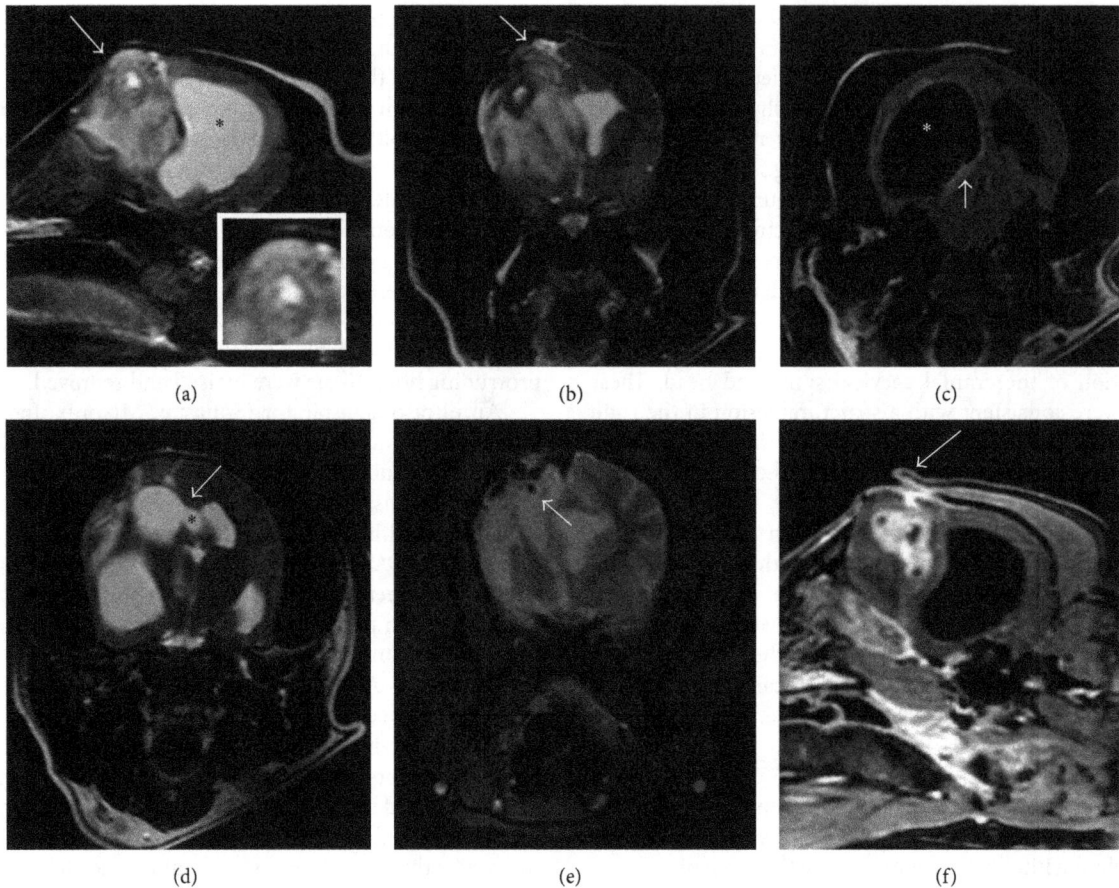

FIGURE 1: Preoperative magnetic resonance (MR) images of the head. (a) T2-weighted right parasagittal image. There is a predominantly T2-hyperintense mass in the right cerebrum underlying a calvarial defect (arrow) and significant dilation of the right lateral ventricle (asterisk). Inset: note the multiple rims of alternating intensity surrounding the T2-hyperintense center, not suppressed on a T2-weighted FLAIR sequence. (b) T2-weighted transverse image at the level of the optic chiasm. The mass is causing midline shift toward the left and brain herniation through the calvarial defect (arrow). (c) T2-weighted FLAIR transverse image at the level of the midbrain. There is hyperintensity immediately surrounding the markedly dilated right lateral ventricle (asterisk) and descending transtentorial herniation of the right parahippocampal gyrus (arrow). (d) T2-weighted transverse image at the level of the caudal thalamus. There is subfalcine herniation of the right cingulate gyrus (arrow) and part of the right lateral ventricle (asterisk). (e) T2*-weighted transverse image at the level of the optic chiasm. There are several irregular areas of signal void, one (arrow) that corresponds with the bone fragment seen on CT imaging. (f) Postcontrast T1-weighted gradient-recalled echo right parasagittal image. There are three pockets of T1-hypointense material surrounded by a strongly contrast-enhancing rim. Note the elevated bone flap that incompletely spans the calvarial defect (arrow).

initiated four days after surgery. No seizures were observed during the 5 days the patient was hospitalized. At the time of discharge the neurologic exam was similar to that on presentation. Oral clindamycin (12 mg/kg twice daily) and enrofloxacin (20 mg/kg once daily) were continued at home as well as the maintenance dose of phenobarbital.

Anaerobic culture of tissue obtained at surgery yielded growth of *Peptostreptococcus anaerobius*. Aerobic bacterial and fungal cultures were negative. Microscopically, the central cavity of the mass contained a linear fragment of necrotic bone (Figure 4(a)) and innumerable Gram-positive bacterial cocci (Figure 4(b)). The tissue immediately surrounding the cavity contained abundant neutrophils and fewer macrophages; the inflammation became more lymphoplasmacytic with fibroblasts and large bands of fibrosis at the periphery (Figure 4(c)). The most peripheral neuropil

in the submitted sample had diffuse gliosis and perivascular cuffs of lymphocytes and plasma cells (Figure 4(d)).

The patient returned two weeks after surgery for a recheck exam, and the owners reported marked improvement in her attitude at home. She continued to circle to the right and was blind in her left visual field. She had not had any seizures since surgery. Postural reactions on the left were improved though still not normal, and cervical pain was no longer present. At this point enrofloxacin was discontinued based on the identification of an anaerobic organism, and metronidazole therapy (10 mg/kg by mouth twice daily) was instituted.

Peptostreptococcus isolates were submitted to the University of Illinois Veterinary Diagnostic Laboratory (Urbana, IL) for susceptibility testing and were found to be resistant to metronidazole but susceptible to clindamycin. Once these results were received, metronidazole therapy was

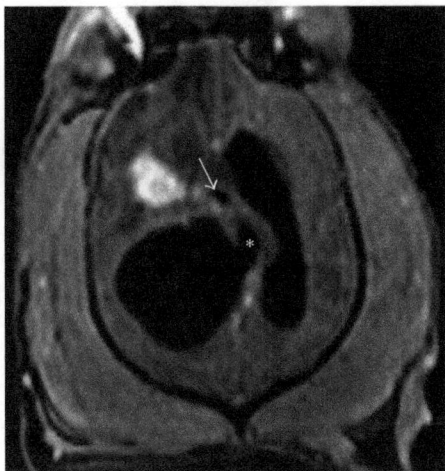

FIGURE 2: Preoperative postcontrast T1-weighted dorsal MR image of the head. There is subfalcine herniation of the right lateral ventricle (asterisk) with subsequent suspected isolation of the lateral ventricle from the third ventricle (arrow).

discontinued, and the patient was continued on clindamycin alone in addition to phenobarbital.

The patient returned approximately 14 weeks after surgery. She had had no known seizures since surgery, and mentation and activity level were normal. She was still receiving phenobarbital, but clindamycin had been discontinued without instruction about two weeks earlier (the intended course was at least 16 weeks long). She continued to circle occasionally to the right, though the owners felt this had improved. Left-sided menace and postural reaction deficits persisted.

The patient was anesthetized for a brain MRI, and there was marked T2W hyperintensity in the rostral right cerebral hemisphere with loss of normal tissue architecture. The right lateral ventricle was no longer dilated, but its shape was abnormal and came to a point dorsally in the area of the previous abscess (presumably where it was penetrated during surgery) (Figure 5(a)). A midline shift was present, but it was toward the right due to parenchymal loss on that side (Figure 5(b)). Within the right cerebral cortex and white matter, there were pockets of T2W hyperintensity suppressed on T2W FLAIR images but did not correspond with the lateral ventricle, suggestive of hydrocephalus ex vacuo (Figure 5(b)). The cervical spinal cord appeared normal.

There was a peripheral rim of heterogeneously T2-hyperintense, T1-hypointense material conforming to the surface of the right cerebral hemisphere that extended ventrally over the piriform lobe and caudally over the surface of the occipital lobe (Figure 5(c)); in areas this rim had layers of mixed signal on T2-weighted images (Figure 5(d)). Areas of the rim showed susceptibility artifact on T2*-weighed sequences, consistent with hemorrhage (Figure 5(e)). The majority of this plaque-like rim, especially its outer border, was strongly and homogenously enhanced following contrast administration. The enhancement extended along the entire convexity of the hemisphere (Figures 5(f) and 5(g)) with

sharp margins along the plane of the falx cerebri and tentorium cerebelli; it did not extend into the parenchyma.

A sample of cerebrospinal fluid obtained from the cerebellomedullary cistern contained two nucleated cells (mononuclear monocytoid cells and small lymphocytes) and 2 red blood cells per microliter; protein content was mildly elevated at 42.2 mg/dL. Aerobic and anaerobic bacterial cultures were negative.

At the time of writing (44 months after surgery), the patient is reportedly doing well at home. Blindness in the left visual field and occasional circling to the right persist, but activity level is normal, and personality is normal to slightly more reserved than prior to presentation. She is maintained on 8.2 mg phenobarbital twice daily and has a seizure approximately once every four months.

3. Discussion

CT and MRI characteristics of brain abscesses have been described in humans and domestic animals [1–8]. The MR appearance of the abscess in this case is typical of a mature brain abscess, including pockets of T2-hyperintense material surrounded by a T2-hypointense rim, large amounts of vasogenic edema, and strong peripheral contrast enhancement [7–9]. One apparently distinct and as yet unexplained MRI feature of brain abscesses that was present in this case is the appearance of multiple rims on T2-weighted sequences (Figure 1(a) and inset). When this feature is present, the central hyperintense cavity of the abscess is bordered by concentric rings that are hypo-, then hyper-, and then hypointense; hyperintense edema then surrounds the lesion, giving it a target appearance. There is no known histopathologic correlate to these rings, though they may represent different layers of necrotic debris and inflammation or may be caused by an unknown artifact [7, 10].

The imaging appearance of the abscess in this case was consistent with a multiloculated abscess. In human case series, up to 20% of brain abscesses are multiloculated [11–15]. This is thought to result from poor abscess encapsulation. In general, abscesses tend to grow toward white matter and away from well-vascularized gray matter, and the medial wall of the capsule tends to be thinner, which allows "daughter abscesses" to bleb off. While not known to be prognostically significant in people, multiloculated abscesses more often require surgical excision rather than CT-guided aspiration to achieve resolution [13, 16].

The mortality rate in humans with brain abscesses has declined significantly since the advent of CT and is currently between 8 and 25% [15, 17]. Abscesses are treated surgically (by excision or drainage) whenever possible; indications to delay or avoid surgical excision include multiple distantly located abscesses, abscesses in deep or vital brain structures, and concurrent meningitis or ependymitis [16, 18, 19]. An additional indication to promptly perform surgery in the case reported here was the presence of obstructive hydrocephalus of the right lateral ventricle, as evidenced by severe ventricular dilation with periventricular T2 hyperintensity (consistent with interstitial edema) on the MRI. This is an unusual manifestation of focal hydrocephalus known as

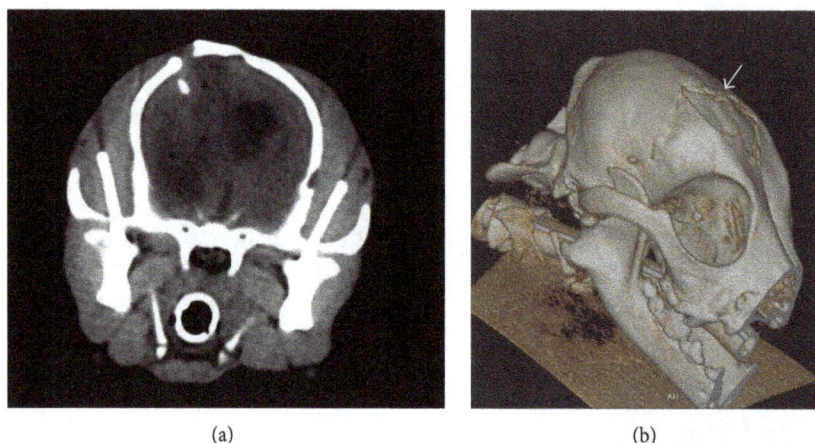

FIGURE 3: Preoperative, precontrast computed tomography (CT) images of the head. (a) Image in a soft tissue window at the level of mandibular rami. There is midline shift toward the left caused by a large hypodensity in the right cerebrum (asterisks), a calvarial defect, and a mineral fragment within the brain parenchyma. (b) Three-dimensional CT reconstruction of the skull in a bone window. Note the smoothly scalloped edges of the elevated bone flap (arrow) and calvarial defect as well as the size discrepancy between the two.

a "trapped ventricle" [20, 21]. In this dog's case the temporal horn of the lateral ventricle was "trapped"; this can occur when the interventricular foramen on one side is occluded and to the authors' knowledge has not been previously reported in a dog. When the interventricular foramen is occluded, the cerebrospinal fluid that is continually produced by the choroid plexus of the lateral ventricle accumulates. Hypertensive hydrocephalus develops, and the ventricle itself can behave as a space-occupying mass. In people, trapped temporal horn has been reported secondary to multiple causes including extraventricular compression by a tumor, intraventricular masses, ventricular trauma, and intraventricular hemorrhage [22–24]. A trapped ventricle requires expedient surgical intervention to either remove the cause of obstruction or shunt CSF away from the ventricle [21, 25, 26]. The apparent cause of obstruction in the case presented here was the extraventricular mass effect created by the abscess and surrounding edema in the area of the right interventricular foramen (Figures 1(d) and 2). We did not measure intraventricular pressure to document hypertension, but eventual occlusion of the interventricular foramen by a slowly growing abscess may explain this patient's relatively rapid neurologic deterioration following the otherwise insidious clinical course for the first 18 to 24 months of her life.

Another interesting feature of this case that, to our knowledge, has not previously been reported as a natural finding in a dog is the presence of what is termed a "growing skull fracture." This is a well-described but incompletely understood injury seen in children who suffer head trauma while both the skull and brain are rapidly growing (usually at less than one year and rarely more than three years of age) [27]. Four requisite features of a growing skull fracture have been described: (1) skull fracture at a young age, (2) dural tear, (3) brain injury underlying the fracture, and (4) subsequent enlargement of the fracture to form a cranial defect [27]. Children with this condition often present several weeks to years following the initial injury; the most common complaint is

a pulsatile scalp mass, although neurologic deficits can also be present. The bone edges are usually scalloped and thickened and are occasionally elevated away from the brain surface as they were in the case presented here [28].

The pathogenesis of growing skull fractures remains unclear, but current theories are based on abnormal lines of force in the area of the dural and bony defect caused by the physiologic pulsations of the brain and ventricular cerebrospinal fluid. The resultant pressure cone may promote brain herniation through the defect; this combined with normal growth of the brain and skull contributes to continued enlargement of the fracture [29]. In the majority of cases, fracture resolution relies on exposing the edges of the dura and creating a water-tight dural closure to normalize lines of intracranial pressure [29]. In the case presented here, we did not attempt to create a water-tight dural seal or repair the calvarial defect, rather relying on SIS as a dural substitute and polypropylene mesh and the temporalis musculature to provide a protective scaffold over the defect. We elected not to perform cranioplasty (e.g., with polymethylmethacrylate or titanium mesh) to minimize possible substrates for bacterial colonization. Use of polypropylene mesh also increases the risk of bacterial colonization; the use of a temporalis fascial graft instead would potentially have reduced this risk. However, the functional and cosmetic outcomes with the technique used in this patient were excellent; in the absence of direct focal trauma to that area we do not anticipate any drawbacks to this approach.

There was no evidence of residual abscess on the postoperative MRI. There was loss of brain parenchyma from the right cerebral hemisphere as well as hydrocephalus ex vacuo and T2 hyperintensity in the cortical gray matter suggestive of gliosis. The extra-axial heterogeneously contrast-enhancing material is most consistent with a chronic subdural hematoma (CSDH), which refers to a fluid collection within the layers of the dura mater with preservation of the underlying arachnoid space [30]. Subdural hematomas tend

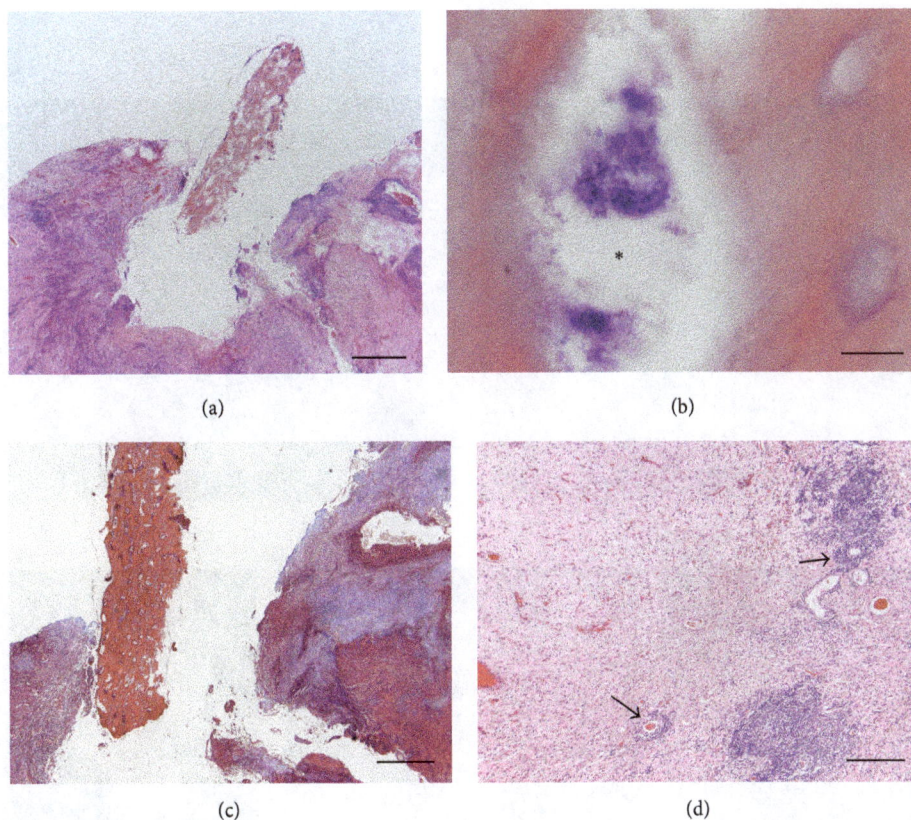

FIGURE 4: (a) Necrotic bone fragment surrounded by cavitated and inflamed neuropil. Hematoxylin and eosin ×2, scale bar = 650 μm. (b) Gram-positive cocci within the marrow space (asterisk) of the necrotic bone fragment. Gram stain ×100, scale bar = 8 μm. (c) Fibrosis (blue) of the neuropil surrounding the necrotic bone fragment (red). Masson's trichrome stain ×4, scale bar = 400 μm. (d) Lymphoplasmacytic perivascular cuffs (arrows) and diffuse gliosis throughout the neuropil at the periphery of the sample. Hematoxylin and eosin ×10, scale bar = 175 μm.

to have a crescent shape and conform to dural attachments such as the falx cerebri (in contrast to epidural hematomas, which are biconvex in shape and can cross dural attachments but not calvarial sutures) [31]. The MR imaging characteristics of the different stages of SDH have been described [32]. CSDH are often hyperintense on T2W images and commonly have a layered appearance, as was appreciated in this case (Figure 5(d)) due to the development of internal septations and membranes joining the inner and outer membranes of the hematoma [33]. Rebleeding within the hematoma occurs frequently in people and also contributes to their heterogeneous appearance on MRI as well as to their potential for continued expansion [31]. It is common for both the membrane and the subdural collection to be enhanced following contrast administration, because the capsule surrounding the hematoma is a capillary-rich membrane that allows active exchange of contrast material [31, 34]. It is therefore important to consider other causes of extra-axial contrast enhancement such as meningitis, subdural empyema, or en plaque meningioma in these cases.

CSDH is a potential complication of therapeutic procedures that significantly decrease the volume of the intracranial contents and thereby lead to intracranial hypotension; for example, CSF shunting is a well-recognized risk factor for CSDH in people [30, 35]. This patient likely developed a postoperative subdural hematoma as a result of the rapid decrease in both tissue and CSF intracranial contents that occurred at the time of surgery. If not removed, subdural hematomas typically persist for months to over a year as they undergo compaction and fibrosis to eventually form a dense fibrous connective tissue layer much like the dura [31]. Surgical removal is recommended if the hematoma continues to increase in size on serial imaging or if the patient clinically deteriorates [30]. However, noncompressive mixtures of blood, CSF, and air are expected MRI findings in human patients after craniotomy; epidural collections are more common than subdural, but both are possible and typically do not require intervention [36]. Based on this, the lack of significant mass effect on the postoperative MRI, and the patient's continued clinical improvement, we did not perform further imaging to monitor the suspected SDH.

This case presents several interesting and novel findings: the potential for a brain abscess to have a chronic and insidious course prior to causing rapid neurologic deterioration, the importance of performing anaerobic bacterial culture and sensitivity in cases of suspected brain abscess, and the possibility of ventricular entrapment by an intracranial mass leading to partial hydrocephalus and intracranial

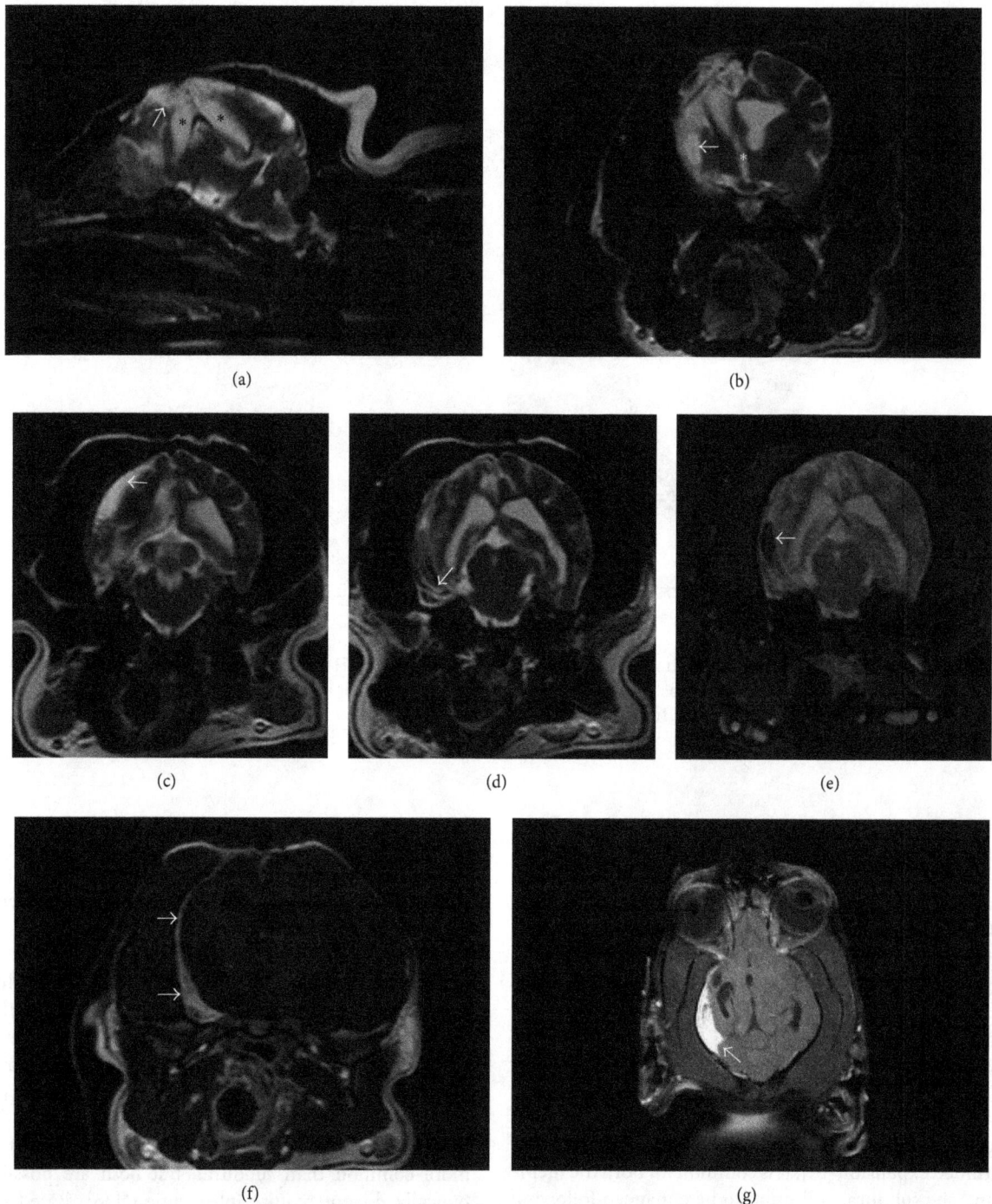

FIGURE 5: Postoperative MR images of the head. (a) T2-weighted right parasagittal image. The shape of the right lateral ventricle is abnormal (asterisks), and there is T2-hyperintense tissue in the area previously occupied by the abscess (arrow). (b) T2-weighted transverse image at the level of the rostral third ventricle (asterisk). There is parenchymal loss on the right side, with resulting midline shift toward the right. There are extraventricular fluid pockets within the parenchyma suppressed on T2-weighted FLAIR imaging (arrow). (c) T2-weighted transverse image at the level of the caudal colliculi. There is a peripheral rim of predominantly T2-hyperintense material along the right side of the cerebrum (arrow). (d) T2-weighted transverse image at the level of the midbrain. The peripheral rim is seen ventrally and has mixed T2 signal and a layered appearance (arrow). (e) T2*-weighted transverse image at the level of the midbrain. Signal voids within the rim (arrow) are consistent with hemorrhage. (f) Postcontrast T1-weighted transverse image at the level of the thalamus. The peripheral rim strongly and, in most areas, uniformly contrast enhanced (arrows). (g) Postcontrast T1-weighted dorsal image at the level of the mesencephalic aqueduct. Note the sharply defined margin of the peripheral contrast-enhancing material along the tentorium cerebelli (arrow).

hypertension. This case also documents for the first time a naturally occurring growing skull fracture in a dog. Finally, this case provides imaging findings consistent with a subdural hematoma that can be seen following removal of a large intracranial mass.

Disclosure

Preliminary results were presented at the 2nd Annual Southeastern Veterinary Neurology Group Conference, Athens, GA, October 2011.

Conflict of Interests

The authors declare that there is no conflict of interests regarding the publication of this paper.

Acknowledgment

The authors would like to thank Dr. Andy Shores for sharing his knowledge of growing skull fractures.

References

[1] A. L. Bilderback and D. Faissler, "Surgical management of a canine intracranial abscess due to a bite wound: Case Report," *Journal of Veterinary Emergency and Critical Care*, vol. 19, no. 5, pp. 507–512, 2009.

[2] E. G. H. Wouters, M. Beukers, and L. F. H. Theyse, "Surgical treatment of a cerebral brain abscess in a cat," *Veterinary and Comparative Orthopaedics and Traumatology*, vol. 24, no. 1, pp. 72–75, 2011.

[3] C. Costanzo, L. S. Garosi, E. N. Glass, C. Rusbridge, C. E. Stalin, and H. A. Volk, "Brain abscess in seven cats due to a bite wound: MRI findings, surgical management and outcome," *Journal of Feline Medicine and Surgery*, vol. 13, no. 9, pp. 672–680, 2011.

[4] I. Mateo, V. Lorenzo, A. Muñoz, and M. Pumarola, "Brainstem abscess due to plant foreign body in a dog," *Journal of Veterinary Internal Medicine*, vol. 21, no. 3, pp. 535–538, 2007.

[5] D. R. Enzmann, R. H. Britt, and R. Placone, "Staging of human brain abscess by computed tomography," *Radiology*, vol. 146, no. 3, pp. 703–708, 1983.

[6] R. H. Britt, D. R. Enzmann, and A. S. Yeager, "Neuropathological and computerized tomographic findings in experimental brain abscess," *Journal of Neurosurgery*, vol. 55, no. 4, pp. 590–603, 1981.

[7] A. B. Haimes, R. D. Zimmerman, S. Morgello et al., "MR imaging of brain abscesses," *American Journal of Roentgenology*, vol. 152, no. 5, pp. 1073–1085, 1989.

[8] L. S. Klopp, J. T. Hathcock, and D. C. Sorjonen, "Magnetic resonance imaging features of brain stem abscessation in two cats," *Veterinary Radiology and Ultrasound*, vol. 41, no. 4, pp. 300–307, 2000.

[9] R. D. Zimmerman and A. B. Haimes, "The role of MR imaging in the diagnosis of infections of the central nervous system," *Current Clinical Topics in Infectious Diseases*, vol. 10, pp. 82–108, 1989.

[10] J. Pyhtinen, E. Pääkö, and P. Jartti, "Cerebral abscess with multiple rims on MRI," *Neuroradiology*, vol. 39, no. 12, pp. 857–859, 1997.

[11] S.-Y. Yang and C.-S. Zhao, "Review of 140 patients with brain abscess," *Surgical Neurology*, vol. 39, no. 4, pp. 290–296, 1993.

[12] S. Stephanov, "Experience with multiloculated brain abscesses," *Journal of Neurosurgery*, vol. 49, no. 2, pp. 199–203, 1978.

[13] T.-M. Su, C.-M. Lan, Y.-D. Tsai et al., "Multiloculated pyogenic brain abscess: experience in 25 patients," *Neurosurgery*, vol. 52, no. 5, pp. 1075–1080, 2003.

[14] A. Danziger, H. Price, and M. M. Schechter, "An analysis of 113 intracranial infections," *Neuroradiology*, vol. 19, no. 1, pp. 31–34, 1980.

[15] N. Nathoo, S. S. Nadvi, P. K. Narotam, and J. R. van Dellen, "Brain abscess: management and outcome analysis of a computed tomography era experience with 973 patients," *World Neurosurgery*, vol. 75, no. 5-6, pp. 716–726, 2011.

[16] C.-H. Lu, W.-N. Chang, and C.-C. Lui, "Strategies for the management of bacterial brain abscess," *Journal of Clinical Neuroscience*, vol. 13, no. 10, pp. 979–985, 2006.

[17] S.-Y. Yang, "Brain abscess: a review of 400 cases," *Journal of Neurosurgery*, vol. 55, no. 5, pp. 794–799, 1981.

[18] H. Çavuşoglu, R. A. Kaya, O. N. Türkmenoglu, I. Çolak, and Y. Aydin, "Brain abscess: analysis of results in a series of 51 patients with a combined surgical and medical approach during an 11-year period," *Neurosurgical Focus*, vol. 24, no. 6, p. E9, 2008.

[19] D. P. Calfee and B. Wispelwey, "Brain abscess," *Seminars in Neurology*, vol. 20, no. 3, pp. 353–360, 2000.

[20] S. Bhagwati, "A case of unilateral hydrocephalus secondary to occlusion of one Foramen of Monro," *Journal of Neurosurgery*, vol. 21, no. 3, pp. 226–229, 1964.

[21] H. L. Rekate, "A contemporary definition and classification of hydrocephalus," *Seminars in Pediatric Neurology*, vol. 16, no. 1, pp. 9–15, 2009.

[22] R. S. Maurice-Williams and M. Choksey, "Entrapment of the temporal horn: a form of focal obstructive hydrocephalus," *Journal of Neurology Neurosurgery and Psychiatry*, vol. 49, no. 3, pp. 238–242, 1986.

[23] P. Bret, S. Gharbi, F. Cohadon, and J. Remond, "Meningioma of the lateral ventricle: 3 recent cases," *Neurochirurgie*, vol. 35, no. 1, pp. 5–12, 1989.

[24] T. W. Eller and J. F. Pasternak, "Isolated ventricles following intraventricular hemorrhage," *Journal of Neurosurgery*, vol. 62, no. 3, pp. 357–362, 1985.

[25] A. P. Amar, S. Ghosh, and M. L. J. Apuzzo, "Ventricular tumors," in *Youmans Neurological Surgery*, R. H. Winn, Ed., vol. 1, pp. 1237–1263, Saunders, Philadelphia, Pa, USA, 5th edition, 2004.

[26] H. L. Rekate, "Hydrocephalus in children," in *Youmans Neurological Surgery*, R. H. Winn, Ed., vol. 3, pp. 3387–3404, Saunders, Philadelphia, Pa, USA, 5th edition, 2004.

[27] R. A. Lende and T. C. Erickson, "Growing skull fractures of childhood," *Journal of Neurosurgery*, vol. 18, no. 4, pp. 479–489, 1961.

[28] F. Goldstein, T. Sakoda, J. J. Kepes, K. Kavidson, and C. E. Brackett, "Enlarging skull fractures: an experimental study," *Journal of Neurosurgery*, vol. 27, no. 6, pp. 541–550, 1967.

[29] M. G. Muhonen, J. G. Piper, and A. H. Menezes, "Pathogenesis and treatment of growing skull fractures," *Surgical Neurology*, vol. 43, no. 4, pp. 367–373, 1995.

[30] J. K. Krauss, L. F. Marshall, and R. Weigel, "Medical and surgical management of chronic subdural hematomas," in *Youmans Neurological Surgery*, R. H. Winn, Ed., pp. 535–543, Saunders, St. Louis, Mo, USA, 6th edition, 2011.

[31] V. L. Williams and J. P. Hogg, "Magnetic resonance imaging of chronic subdural hematoma," *Neurosurgery Clinics of North America*, vol. 11, no. 3, pp. 491–498, 2000.

[32] E. S. Fobben, R. I. Grossman, S. W. Atlas et al., "MR characteristics of subdural hematomas and hygromas at 1.5 T," *American Journal of Roentgenology*, vol. 153, no. 3, pp. 589–595, 1989.

[33] M. Kitagawa, M. Okada, H. Koie, K. Kanayama, and T. Sakai, "Magnetic resonance imaging and computed tomography appearance of chronic subdural haematoma in a dog," *Australian Veterinary Journal*, vol. 86, no. 3, pp. 100–101, 2008.

[34] S. Blitshteyn, L. L. Mechtler, and R. Bakshi, "Diffuse dural gadolinium MRI enhancement associated with bilateral chronic subdural hematomas," *Clinical Imaging*, vol. 28, no. 2, pp. 90–92, 2004.

[35] B. O'Neill, J. Wilberger, and A. Wilberger, "Pathophysiology of subdural hematomas," in *Youmans Neurological Surgery*, R. H. Winn, Ed., pp. 532–534, Saunders, St. Louis, Mo, USA, 6th edition, 2011.

[36] A. G. Sinclair and D. J. Scoffings, "Imaging of the post-operative cranium," *Radiographics*, vol. 30, no. 2, pp. 461–482, 2010.

6

Maple Syrup Urine Disease in a Central Indiana Hereford Herd

Mark E. Robarge,[1] Jonathan E. Beever,[2] Stephen D. Lenz,[1] Christopher J. Lynch,[3] and William L. Wigle[1]

[1]*Department of Comparative Pathobiology and Indiana Animal Disease Diagnostic Laboratory, Purdue University, 406 S. University Street, West Lafayette, IN 47907, USA*
[2]*Department of Animal Sciences, University of Illinois, 1207 West Gregory Drive, Urbana, IL 61801, USA*
[3]*Department of Cellular and Molecular Physiology, Penn State University College of Medicine, 500 University Drive, Hershey, PA 17033, USA*

Correspondence should be addressed to William L. Wigle; wwigle@purdue.edu

Academic Editor: Renato L. Santos

Maple syrup urine disease (MSUD) and further cases were identified in herd mates of a small Hereford herd in Indiana based on history, clinical signs, microscopic lesions, and biochemical and genetic testing. This aminoacidopathy has been diagnosed in polled Shorthorn, polled Hereford, and Hereford cattle in Australia, Uruguay, Argentina, and Canada and is the result of a mutation of the branched-chain alpha-ketoacid dehydrogenase complex. The Indiana index calf case was confirmed by showing the classic accumulation of ketoacids in liver that results from a defect in the E1-alpha subunit (248 C/T haplotype) in the mitochondrial branched-chain α-ketoacid dehydrogenase complex. The presence of the mutation was confirmed in the index case, the dam, and four related herd mates that represent the first confirmed cases of bovine MSUD mutation in United States cattle.

1. Introduction

Maple syrup urine disease (MSUD) is an inherited, autosomal recessive, aminoacidopathy resulting from branched-chain α-ketoacid dehydrogenase complex (BCKDH) dysfunction (Skvorak [1]). The BCKDH complex is a mitochondrial multisubunit enzyme composed of three catalytic components including E1, E2, and E3 [1–3]. MSUD naturally occurs in humans and polled Shorthorn, polled Hereford, and Hereford calves resulting in central nervous system dysfunction approximately 2–4 days after birth in calves [1, 4]. In polled Herefords, disease is caused by premature termination of translation, of the E1-alpha subunit, that is induced by a cytidine to thymidine transition at nucleotide 248 (248C-->T) that converts the glutamine codon −6 to a stop codon (Zhang et al. [5]). Since MSUD is an autosomal recessive condition, consanguineous breeding in cattle, as has been shown in humans, would presumably lead to a greater incidence of disease (Skvorak [1]). A deficiency in BCKDH results in an inability to oxidize the branched-chain ketoacids of

the branched-chain amino acids leucine, isoleucine, and valine (Maxie and Youssef [4]). Loss of this activity results in the accumulation of the branched-chain amino acids along with their respective ketoacids: ketoisocaproic, keto-β-methylvaleric, and ketoisovaleric acids in cerebrospinal fluid, blood, and tissues. The mechanism by which these metabolites cause central nervous system dysfunction is not fully understood (Maxie and Youssef [4]).

MSUD could represent a subset of the hereditary neuraxial edema disease complex described in Hereford calves in the United States but these cases were never confirmed to have the currently known genetic mutations or biochemical changes consistent with MSUD and spongy vacuolation was described in the spinal cord which is not consistent with MSUD (Cordy et al. [6]). A syndrome similar to MSUD was also reported in Gelbvieh-cross calves in Nebraska but genetic analysis failed to show a mutation in the E1-α subunit (O'Toole et al. [7]). To the authors' knowledge, no case report of naturally occurring MSUD in cattle has been published in the United States. In the current report, MSUD in an Indiana

Hereford herd is described to inform veterinarians and owners of the presence of this disease mutation in the Hereford cattle population and the possibility of this mutation resulting in clinical disease.

2. Case Presentation

The affected male Hereford calf came from a small herd (7 cow/calf pairs) in Indiana. This was the owners' first year raising cattle and they obtained the herd from the previous owner without any known pedigree information. The cattle were kept on a small pasture with a small calf barn for shelter. No other calves from this farm were affected and all calves had the same sire. At three days of age, the owner noted that the calf was "not acting normally." The following day the calf was recumbent and depressed. The calf was given oxytetracycline and milk replacer with no clinical improvement. On the subsequent morning, the animal was presented to the Purdue University Veterinary Teaching Hospital for evaluation.

Upon presentation to the Purdue University Veterinary Teaching Hospital, the animal was depressed, was laterally recumbent, and had bilateral nystagmus. Temperature, pulse, and respiration were within normal limits. Based on the age of the calf and limited diagnostic work-up, the suspected diagnosis at that time was bacterial meningitis. Due to financial restrictions associated with diagnostics and treatment, euthanasia was elected and the calf was submitted to the Animal Disease Diagnostic Laboratory for necropsy. Neither a chemistry panel nor a complete blood count was performed prior to euthanasia.

Gross necropsy examination was unremarkable. No gross abnormalities were observed in the brain. No obvious urine odor was noted. Specimens of major organs and tissues were collected, fixed in neutral buffered 10% formalin, routinely processed, embedded in paraffin, sectioned, stained with H&E, luxol fast blue, oligodendrocyte transcription factor (Olig-2), and glial fibrillary acidic protein (GFAP), and examined by light microscopy. Histologic abnormalities on H and E staining were confined to the white matter of the cerebrum, cerebellum, and brain stem and consisted of severe spongy vacuolation of myelin with the long axis of vacuoles parallel to axons (status spongiosus) (see Figure 1). Lesions were not observed in sections of peripheral nerve. Virchow Robin's space in the white matter was also variably expanded by increased clear space (edema). Astrocytes in the white matter had an increased amount of eosinophilic cytoplasm (reactive). No abnormalities in myelination were observed with luxol fast blue staining compared to routinely used control brain sections. The relative number of oligodendrocytes and astrocytes were compared using Olig-2 and GFAP, respectively, between the calf with MSUD and an age-matched control calf. No appreciable difference was observed between the calf with MSUD and the age-matched control calf by two observers (William L. Wigle and Mark E. Robarge). The author's acknowledge that a difference may have been present since edema in the calf with MSUD made observations on numbers of oligodendrocytes and astrocytes in these areas difficult to compare to the age-matched control.

Each of the nine amplicons corresponding to the exons of bovine BCKDHA were successfully amplified using the

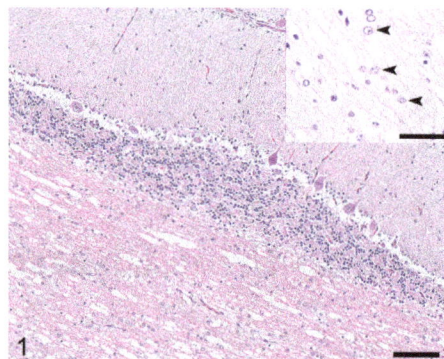

FIGURE 1: Brain from index case: note marked vacuolation of cerebellar white matter (status spongiosus) with sparing of gray matter. Vacuoles (edema) are empty with the long axis parallel to axons. Bar = 100 μm. Inset: cerebellum at 100x magnification: many astrocytes in the white matter are reactive with an increased amount of eosinophilic cytoplasm (arrowheads). Bar = 35 μm. Hematoxylin and Eosin stain.

genomic DNA isolated from the original calf, and herd mates, submitted for analysis. Direct sequencing of the PCR products revealed that the affected calf was homozygous for the previously identified mutation in polled Herefords caused by premature termination of translation, of the E1-alpha subunit, that is induced by a cytidine to thymidine transition in exon 2 (248C-->T) that converts the glutamine codon −6 to a stop codon (Zhang et al. [5]). In polled Shorthorns, the mutation results in a substitution of leucine in place of a highly conserved proline at codon 372 due to a cytidine to thymidine transition at nucleotide 1380 (1380C-->T) resulting in dysfunction of the E1-alpha subunit (Dennis and Healy [8]). The dam of the affected calf was shown to be heterozygous for the 248 C/T haplotype, which is consistent with the reported recessive inheritance of the disease. Of the eight additional individual samples collected from the subject herd, four were found to be heterozygous for the mutation (corresponding to one carrier cow and three carrier calves) with the remainder being homozygous for the normal allele. The sire of the affected calf had been sold and was unavailable for testing.

Sections of frozen liver from the calf affected with MSUD and three "healthy" age-matched but not breed-matched control calf frozen livers were evaluated for branched-chain ketoacid levels (Olson et al. [9]) of ketoisovaleric (KIV), ketoisocaproic (KIC), and keto-β-methylvaleric (KMV) acids which are the ketoacids of valine, leucine, and isoleucine, respectively, and showed marked elevations consistent with MSUD. "Healthy" control calves of a comparable age but different breed were diagnosed with pneumonia, ventricular septal defect, and coccidiosis, respectively, which presumably should minimally affect the branched-chain ketoacid levels in the liver. Results are summarized in Table 1.

3. Discussion

The history, histologic findings, homozygous mutation in the E1-α subunit, and increased branched-chain ketoacid detection in liver of submitted Hereford calf are consistent with MSUD. Multiple animals (one cow and three calves)

TABLE 1: Branched-chain ketoacid concentrations.

Animals	KIV (nmol/g)	KIC (nmol/g)	KMV (nmol/g)
MSUD Suspect calf	24.92	>362	24.25
3 "Healthy Calves"	1.97	10.92	0.63
Increase in MSUD calf from healthy calves	12.6X	>33X	38.4X

Ketoacid concentrations in the liver of the Hereford calf with maple syrup urine disease versus the average of three "healthy" age-matched but not breed-matched control calves are summarized. KIV: ketoisovaleric, KIC: ketoisocaproic, and KMV: keto-β-methylvaleric acids, respectively.

in the herd were heterozygous for the mutation in the E1-α subunit as well.

Status spongiosus, the histologic hallmark of MSUD, is a term that describes neural tissue that has a microvacuolar, sieve-like change by light microscopy [2, 10, 11]. This appearance may be from swelling of astrocyte/oligodendrocyte cytoplasm, processes in neuropil, or myelin sheaths [4, 11, 12]. Although the presence of this lesion in myelin is distinctive on light microscopic evaluation, electron microscopy is needed to definitively define the change (Maxie and Youssef [4]). In MSUD, myelin vacuolation is due to splitting of myelin lamellae at the intraperiod line which produces vacuoles within the myelin sheath mostly involving the outer myelin lamellae [13]. Status spongiosus has many causes in animals including idiopathic, toxic, metabolic, and infectious conditions [4, 5, 7, 11, 14, 15].

Many different categories of disease, as mentioned above, in calves can cause status spongiosis of white matter and were considered in this index case before ancillary testing confirmed this calf to have MSUD. One such cause is idiopathic spongiform myelinopathy that has been documented in horned Hereford calves in New Zealand and in polled Hereford calves in Britain (Maxie and Youssef [4]). Idiopathic myelinopathies were ruled out after positive ancillary testing confirmed MSUD. Hepatic and to a lesser extent renal encephalopathy are possible etiologies; however, the kidney and liver were normal in this case, and Alzheimer type II cells, reactive astrocytes in the gray matter with a clear nucleus, and increased amount of cytoplasm found singly or in groups were not observed [4, 11]. Hexachlorophene, a polychlorinated phenolic compound used as a topical antiseptic, and halogenated salicylanilide, an anthelmintic, cause status spongiosus of white matter in both the central and peripheral nervous system (Maxie and Youssef [4]). Toxic compounds like these can be ruled out based on lack of exposure to the compound and no lesions seen in peripheral nervous tissue. Ingestion of corn towards the end of growing season infected with *Stenocarpella maydis* can cause status spongiosus as a result of mycotoxicosis but was ruled out since this fungus is found in southern Africa and Argentina (Maxie and Youssef [4]). Many toxic plants should be considered including *Stypandra* sp., *Hemerocallis* sp., *Tylecodon wallichii*, *Ornithogalum toxicarum*, and *Helichrysum* sp.; however, these plants grow in various countries around the world and are not reported in Indiana (Maxie and Youssef [4]).

To the authors' knowledge, this represents the first documented naturally occurring case of MSUD in cattle in the United States. This finding indicates the presence of the genetic mutation for MSUD within the US cattle population and suggests the possible need for genetic screening to eliminate the trait.

Conflict of Interests

The authors declare that there is no conflict of interests regarding the publication of this paper.

Acknowledgment

The authors would like to thank Dr. Margaret Miller for help in histological interpretation and IHC selection.

References

[1] K. J. Skvorak, "Animal models of maple syrup urine disease," *Journal of Inherited Metabolic Disease*, vol. 32, no. 2, pp. 229–246, 2009.

[2] R. A. Harris, M. Joshi, and N. H. Jeoung, "Mechanisms responsible for regulation of branched-chain amino acid catabolism," *Biochemical and Biophysical Research Communications*, vol. 313, no. 2, pp. 391–396, 2004.

[3] S. J. Yeaman, "The 2-oxo acid dehydrogenase complexes: recent advances," *Biochemical Journal*, vol. 257, no. 3, pp. 625–632, 1989.

[4] M. Maxie and S. Youssef, "Nervous System," in *Jubb, Kennedy & Palmer's Pathology of Domestic Animals*, M. G. Maxie, Ed., pp. 292–389, Elsevier, Edinburgh, UK, 2007.

[5] B. Zhang, J. Healy, Y. Zhao et al., "Premature translation termination of the pre-E1alpha subunit of the branched chain alpha-ketoacid dehydrogenase as a cause of maple syrup urine disease in polled Hereford calves," *The Journal of Biologic Chemistry*, vol. 265, no. 5, pp. 2425–2427, 1990.

[6] D. R. Cordy, W. P. Richards, and C. Stormont, "Hereditary neuraxial edema in Hereford calves," *Pathologia Veterinaria*, vol. 6, no. 6, pp. 487–501, 1969.

[7] D. O'Toole, D. L. Montgomery, L. Steadman, B. O'Rourke, W. Russell, and J. Dennis, "Status spongiosus of white matter in newborn Gelbvieh-cross calves," *Journal of Veterinary Diagnostic Investigation*, vol. 17, no. 6, pp. 546–553, 2005.

[8] J. A. Dennis and P. J. Healy, "Definition of the mutation responsible for maple syrup urine disease in poll shorthorns and genotyping poll shorthorns and poll herefords for maple syrup urine disease alleles," *Research in Veterinary Science*, vol. 67, no. 1, pp. 1–6, 1999.

[9] K. C. Olson, G. Chen, and C. J. Lynch, "Quantification of branched-chain keto acids in tissue by ultra fast liquid chromatography-mass spectrometry," *Analytical Biochemistry*, vol. 439, no. 2, pp. 116–122, 2013.

[10] P. A. Harper, P. J. Healy, and J. A. Dennis, "Maple syrup urine disease as a cause of spongiform encephalopathy in calves," *Veterinary Record*, vol. 119, no. 3, pp. 62–65, 1986.

[11] B. A. Summers, J. F. Cummings, and A. de Lahunta, "Degenerative disease of the central nervous system," in *Veterinary Neuropathology*, B. A. Summers, J. F. Cummings, and A. de Lahunta, Eds., pp. 3–298, Mosby, St. Louis, Mo, USA, 1995.

[12] M. B. Graeber, W. F. Blakemore, and G. W. Kreutzberg, "Cellular pathology of the central nervous system," in *Greenfield's Neuropathology*, D. I. Graham and P. L. Lantos, Eds., Arnold, London, UK, 2002.

[13] P. A. W. Harper, P. J. Healy, and J. A. Dennis, "Ultrastructural findings in maple syrup urine disease in Poll Hereford calves," *Acta Neuropathologica*, vol. 71, no. 3-4, pp. 316–320, 1986.

[14] G. Hagen and I. Bjerkås, "Spongy degeneration of white matter in the central nervous system of silver foxes (*Vulpes vulpes*)," *Veterinary Pathology*, vol. 27, no. 3, pp. 187–193, 1990.

[15] S. L. Wood and J. S. Patterson, "Shetland sheepdog leukodystrophy," *Journal of Veterinary Internal Medicine*, vol. 15, no. 5, pp. 486–493, 2001.

7

Ultrasonographic, Surgical, and Histopathological Findings of a Uterine Leiomyoma in a Cow

Arvind Sharma,[1] Adarsh Kumar,[1] Sheikh Imran,[1] Pankaj Sood,[2] and Rajesh Kumar Asrani[3]

[1] Department of Veterinary Surgery and Radiology, College of Veterinary and Animal Sciences, CSK HP Agriculture University, Himachal Pradesh, Palampur 176062, India
[2] Department of Veterinary Gynaecology and Obstetrics, College of Veterinary and Animal Sciences, CSK HP Agriculture University, Himachal Pradesh, Palampur 176062, India
[3] Department of Veterinary Pathology, College of Veterinary and Animal Sciences, CSK HP Agriculture University, Himachal Pradesh, Palampur 176062, India

Correspondence should be addressed to Sheikh Imran, sheikhimran_08@rediffmail.com

Academic Editor: L. Espino López

The objective of this case report was to describe the ultrasonographic, surgical, and histopathological findings of a rare clinical case of uterine leiomyoma in a 5-year-old Holstein crossbred cow presented for diagnosis and treatment of infertility. Transrectal palpation revealed a large nonpainful mass suspected to be an abscess or a tumor in the caudal abdomen on the right side. Transabdominal ultrasonography revealed a round mass with irregular hypoechogenic/echogenic foci and a thin echogenic capsule around it. Ultrasonographic-guided centesis of the lesion under local analgesia did not yield any foul smelling aspirate leading to a tentative diagnosis of an intra-abdominal tumor. The lesion was later confirmed by exploratory laparotomy and histopathology as a case of uterine leiomyoma. The cow gave birth to a live normal calf 12 months following the surgery. Rectal examination after parturition revealed no evidence of the tumor at the surgical site. Ultrasonography enabled prompt, noninvasive diagnosis of uterine leiomyoma and proved to be a useful decision-making tool in the abdominal surgery of the cow. This is an interesting case which broadens the spectrum of the causes of infertility in cattle.

1. Introduction

A leiomyoma, histopathologically classified as mesenchymal tumor, is a benign neoplasia of smooth muscle. Leiomyomas of the genitalia occur far more frequently in females than males, and they are among the most commonly encountered tumors of the female reproductive system in almost all domestic species. In an abattoir study, leiomyomas were found to have a low frequency of occurrence as they represented only 1% to 2% of all neoplasia in sheep, cattle, and pigs [1]. Few case reports of vaginal and cervical leiomyomas in cows have been previously reported [2, 3]; however, reports on ultrasonographic and surgical findings of uterine leiomyomas in cows have not been published in peer-reviewed journals until now. The purpose of this paper was to document a rare case of leiomyoma of the uterus in an infertile cow and her return to production following excision of the neoplasm.

2. Case Presentation

A 5-year-old Holstein crossbred cow was admitted to the Teaching Veterinary Clinic Complex, College of Veterinary and Animal Sciences in October 2009 with a history of repeat breeding for last 5 months. The cow had been vaccinated regularly and dewormed appropriately and had no other relevant medical history. The physical examination was normal, and results from a complete blood count (CBC) and biochemical profile were within normal limits. On transrectal palpation, the cervix, uterus, and both the ovaries were normal in size, consistency, and texture; however, detailed examination revealed a large nonpainful mass (~10 cm

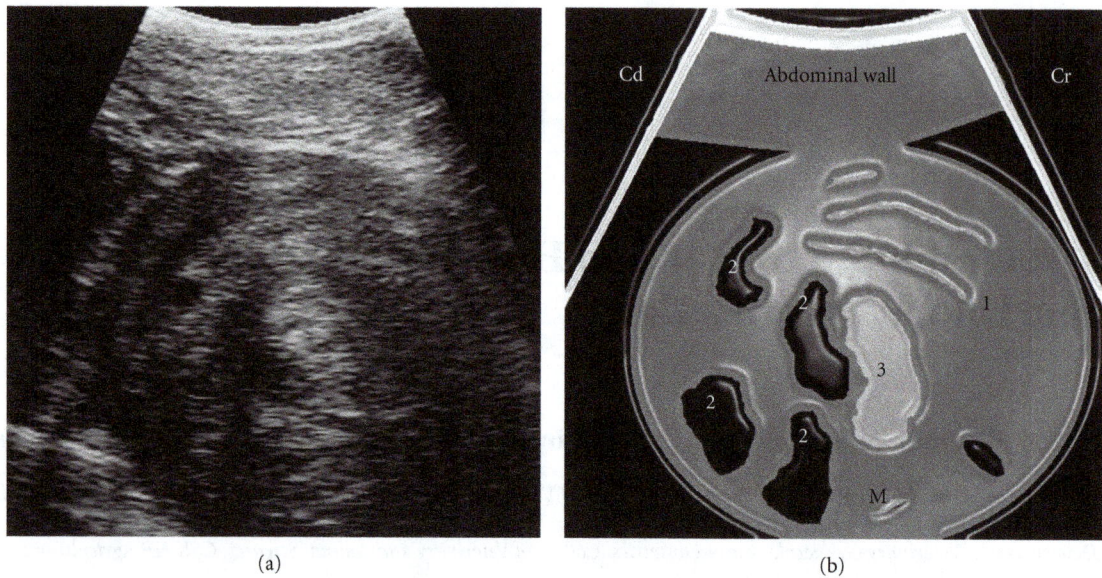

(a)   (b)

Figure 1: Ultrasonogram of the uterine tumour, imaged from the right paralumbar fossa, after bringing it closer to the abdominal wall by transrectal manipulation and placing the transducer parallel to the longitudinal axis of the cow. 1: uterine tumour, 2: hypoechogenic areas, 3: echogenic areas, Cd: caudal, Cr: cranial, and M: medial.

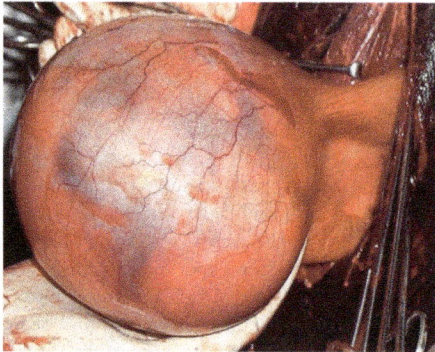

Figure 2: Uterine mass exteriorized after performing the right flank exploratory laparotomy.

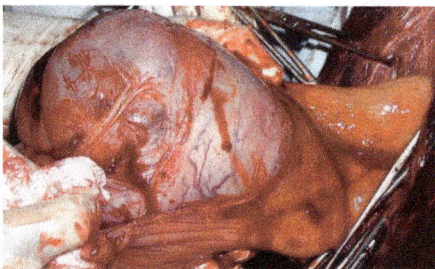

Figure 3: Hysterotomy depicting the intraluminal location of the mass in the right uterine horn.

diameter) suspected to be an abscess or a tumor in the caudal abdomen on the right side.

Transabdominal ultrasonography was done from right paralumbar fossa using a 3.5 MHz curvilinear transducer with an assistant holding the mass transrectally towards abdominal wall. The lesion with a diameter of 7.8 cm appeared as a round mass with irregular hypoechogenic/echogenic foci and a thin echogenic capsule around it (Figure 1). Ultrasonographic-guided centesis of the lesion under local analgesia did not yield any foul smelling aspirate, which precluded the presence of an abscess, thereby hinting towards a possibility of an intra-abdominal tumor.

Standing caudal right flank celiotomy was recommended which would also allow the histological assessment. As expected, the pendulous mass was found attached to the uterine wall (Figure 2). A hysterotomy was made outside the abdomen to avoid contamination of the peritoneal cavity. Superficial incision revealed the intraluminal location of the mass (Figure 3). The uterine mass was excised from the right uterine horn and sent for the histological evaluation. Representative pieces of tissues from the tumor mass were collected in 10% neutral buffered formalin for histopathologic studies. Fixed tissues were trimmed, embedded in paraffin, sectioned at 3–5 μm, and stained with routine haematoxylin and eosin (H&E) stain.

The uterine serosa and muscular layers were reapposed using a double inverting pattern with number 2 plain catgut. Sutures were placed only partial thickness incorporating the serosa and muscular layer of the uterus. The abdominal wound was lavaged and the incision closed routinely. The cow received general medical support including analgesics (Meloxicam (Melonex, Intas Pharmaceuticals Limited, India) at 0.5 mg/kg BW, IM, q24h for 3 days), antibiotics (Streptopenicillin (Dicrysticin-S LD, Zydus Animal Health Limited, India) at 2.5 gm, IM, q12h for 5 days), exercise with fresh water and electrolytes available at all times. The recovery of the cow was uneventful and was discharged 5 days postoperatively with no further medication but with instructions for no artificial insemination up to 2 months.

35

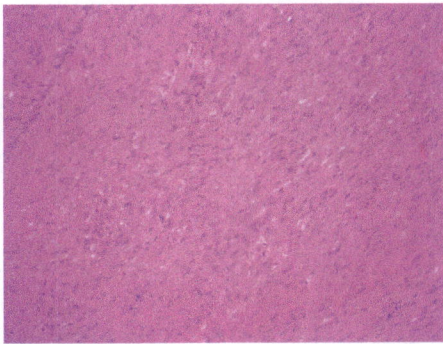

FIGURE 4: Photomicrograph depicting well-differentiated multiple layers of hypercellular and hyperchromatic interwoven bundles of smooth muscle cells. H&E ×66.

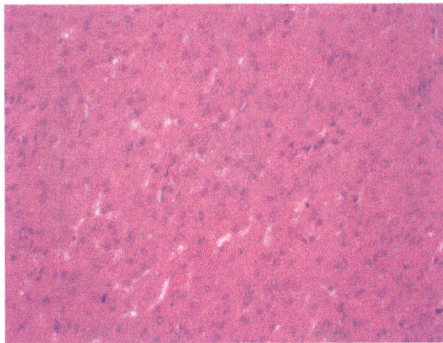

FIGURE 5: Photomicrograph from an area of tumor showing marked increase in its cellularity and occasional mitotic elements. H&E ×132.

Histopathological report of the excised uterine mass showed that it was a leiomyoma with hypercellular and hyperchromatic interlacing bundles of smooth muscle cells running in different layers (Figures 4 and 5). Mitotic figures were not uncommon. The tumor cells were uniform in size. In a few places, there were small areas of necrosis.

The past estrous activity of the cow was regular and periodic (interestrus interval of 19 to 22 days). However, the first estrus postsurgery was manifested after 40 days, with a regain in normal rhythm *per se* thereafter. During all overt estrous periods after surgery, the physical properties of genital discharge were normal.

3. Discussion

The etiology of the uterine leiomyoma is not known [3]. It consists of neoplastic cells of smooth muscle differentiation accompanied by varying quantities of connective tissue and lacks a glandular component [4, 5]. Macroscopically, leiomyoma can reach up to 10–12 cm in diameter without being invasive. Initially, when the tumor is small, it has a fleshy consistency which becomes firm or even hard as it develops due to stromal connective tissue. In most cases, the leiomyoma projects like a nodular tumor into the uterine, vaginal, or cervical lumen [6].

The reason behind the cow's infertility in this case was uncommon in being associated with a progressive uterine growth. A logical explanation for this has been provided in case of a uterine leiomyoma in a mare [7]. A low-grade endometritis associated with uterine tumor, impairing of the implantation of the embryo due to mucosal damage caused by the tumor, and lastly an impediment to the transuterine migration of the embryo caused by the uterine mass itself could contribute to infertility.

Ultrasonographic-guided centesis was useful to reach at a tentative diagnosis; however, it could not ascertain the origin of the mass. Since the identification and histological typing of gastrointestinal tumours on the basis of the ultrasonographic appearance is not reliable, fine-needle aspiration or biopsy is almost always indicated when trying to establish a diagnosis [8]. The reason for not being able to pinpoint the origin of the mass ultrasonographically was the greater depth of the abdomen in the cow as the ultrasonographic waves gradually attenuated due to acoustic impedance of the tissues during the travel.

The future fertility of the cow was in question due to two possibilities—the recurrence of the tumor and the postoperative intra-abdominal adhesions around the uterus and ovaries. Adhesions affecting a section of or the entire reproductive tract are probably the most frequent sequelae of an ovariectomy, and they can have serious consequences on the future reproductive performance of the animal [9]. There are very few studies that have followed a large number of cows after surgery to determine postoperative fertility. In this case, the cow gave birth to a live normal calf 12 months following the surgery. Rectal examination after parturition revealed no evidence of the tumor at the surgical site.

In conclusion, ultrasonography enabled prompt, noninvasive diagnosis of the uterine leiomyoma and proved to be a useful decision-making tool in the abdominal surgery of the cow. This is an interesting case which broadens the spectrum of the causes of infertility in cattle.

References

[1] T. J. Hulland, "Tumors of muscle," in *Tumors in Domestic Animals*, J. E. Moulton, Ed., University of California Press, 2nd edition, 1978.

[2] R. O. Ramadan, W. S. Abu-El Fadle, A. M. El Hassan, M. Bindary, and A. Gomaa, "Vaginal leiomyoma in a cow," *Reproduction in Domestic Animals*, vol. 28, pp. 39–43, 1993.

[3] S. Sendag, Y. Cetina, M. Alana, F. Ilhana, F. Eskia, and A. Wehrendb, "Cervical leiomyoma in a dairy cattle," *Animal Reproduction Science*, vol. 103, pp. 355–350, 2008.

[4] R. S. Brodey and J. F. Roszel, "Neoplasms of the canine uterus, vagina, and vulva: a clinicopathologic survey of 90 cases," *Journal of the American Veterinary Medical Association*, vol. 151, no. 10, pp. 1294–1307, 1967.

[5] N. J. MacLachlan and P. C. Kennedy, "Tumors of the genital systems," in *Tumors in Domestic Animals*, D. J. Meuten, Ed., pp. 547–573, Iowa State Press, Ames, Iowa, USA, 4th edition, 2002.

[6] P. C. Kennedy and R. B. Miller, "The female genital system," in *Pathology of Domestic Animals*, K. V. F. Jubb, P. C. Kennedy, and N. Palmer, Eds., pp. 349–470, Academic Press, New York, NY, USA, 1993.

[7] C. Berezowski, "Diagnosis of a uterine leiomyoma using hysteroscopy and a partial ovariohysterectomy in a mare," *Canadian Veterinary Journal*, vol. 43, no. 12, pp. 968–969, 2002.

[8] M. Frame, "Gastro-intestinal tract including pancreas," in *Diagnostic Ultrasound in Small Animal Practice*, P. Mannion, Ed., pp. 90–92, Blackwell, 2006.

[9] A. S. Turner and C. W. McIlwraith, *Techniques in Large Animal Surgery*, Lea and Febiger, Philadelphia, Pa, USA, 2nd edition, 1989.

8

Addisonian Crisis due to Metastatic Adenocarcinoma in a Pygmy Goat

Nora Nogradi,[1] Amanda L. Koehne,[1] F. Charles Mohr,[2]
Sean D. Owens,[2] and Meera C. Heller[3,4]

[1] William R. Pritchard Veterinary Medical Teaching Hospital, University of California, Davis, One Shield Avenue, Davis,
   CA 95616, USA
[2] Department of Pathology, Microbiology and Immunology, School of Veterinary Medicine, University of California Davis,
   Davis, One Shield Avenue, Davis, CA 95616, USA
[3] Department of Medicine and Epidemiology, School of Veterinary Medicine, University of California Davis, Davis,
   One Shield Avenue, Davis, CA 95616, USA
[4] Department of Veterinary Medicine and Surgery, University of Missouri, 900 East Campus Drive, Columbia, MO 65211, USA

Correspondence should be addressed to Meera C. Heller; hellerme@missouri.edu

Academic Editors: N. D. Giadinis, C. Hyun, L. G. Papazoglou, and M. Pizarro

A 15-year-old Pygmy doe was evaluated for acute onset of lethargy, anorexia, and weakness. Adrenal insufficiency was diagnosed based on physical exam findings, blood work abnormalities (hyponatremia, hyperkalemia, azotemia, and hypoglycemia), and lack of cortisol response to the ACTH stimulation test. Abdominal ultrasound exam revealed an intact urinary tract and multiple bilateral peri-renal masses. The doe was treated with intravenous fluid therapy aimed at correcting the electrolyte abnormalities and intravenous corticosteroids. She responded favorably to medical therapy in 24 hours, with dramatic improvement in attitude and appetite. Fluid therapy was discontinued, and the doe was discharged from the hospital on steroid supplementation. She deteriorated rapidly and died at home 36 hours after discharge. Necropsy results revealed metastatic adenocarcinoma originating from the uterus that infiltrated the urinary bladder, the region of the adrenal glands, the left and right renal lymph nodes, the left kidney, the caudal vena cava, the submandibular lymph nodes, the diaphragm, the lungs, and the omentum. Addison's syndrome in ruminants should be considered as an uncommon sequel of intra-abdominal neoplastic processes.

1. Introduction

To the authors' knowledge, this is the first clinical report of Addison's syndrome in a goat. Addison's syndrome describes a clinical phenomenon when the adrenal cortex is unable to produce steroid hormones, in particular the corticosteroid cortisol and the mineralocorticoid aldosterone. Cortisol is produced by the zona fasciculata of the adrenal cortex, and its primary functions are in the maintenance of blood pressure, cardiovascular function, and physiologic glucose levels as well as the regulation of protein, carbohydrate, and fat metabolism. Aldosterone is produced by the zona glomerulosa of the adrenal cortex and acts on the collecting ducts and the distal convoluted tubules in the kidneys. It is responsible for conservation of sodium, water retention, maintenance of blood pressure, and secretion of potassium [1].

Addison's disease is a well-described clinical syndrome in dogs, characterized by diarrhea, vomiting, lethargy, anorexia, muscle weakness, hyperkalemia, hyponatremia, hypoglycemia, and lack of corticosteroid-induced stress leukogram despite illness [2]. The doe in this case report presented with similar, nonspecific clinical signs and, along with the characteristic serum electrolyte and biochemical abnormalities, raised the clinician's suspicion for primary hypoadrenocorticism.

2. Case Presentation

A 15-year-old Pygmy doe was presented to the Veterinary Medical Teaching Hospital of the University of California, Davis, for an acute onset of anorexia, lethargy, and weakness of 2-day duration that progressed into recumbency on the evening of evaluation. The doe was individually housed in a barn, had access to a grass pasture, and was supplemented with wheat hay. At the time of presentation, she was not current on routine vaccinations, had not recently been treated for endo- or ectoparasites, and had not received any medical treatment, including pharmacologic agents, prior to presentation. At presentation, she weighed 19 kg and had a body condition score of 2 out of 5. She was obtunded and exhibited profound weakness. On physical examination, a normal rectal temperature and respiratory rate were noted, and mild tachycardia (100 bpm) was observed. Mucous membranes were pale and tacky with a capillary refill time of 3 seconds. Skin turgor was delayed, and peripheral pulse quality was weak. Eyes, ears, and nose were clean; lice infestation of the skin was evident. No murmurs or arrhythmias were evident on cardiac auscultation; normal bronchovesicular sounds were auscultated in all lung fields bilaterally. No ruminal contractions could be auscultated; however, the doe was observed to pass feces at the time of presentation, and a fecal occult blood test was negative. A brief neurologic exam revealed obtundation, intact cranial nerves and spinal reflexes, and profound muscle weakness, and the doe was unable to stand with assistance. Abnormalities on blood work available after hours included anemia (17%, ref.: 23–36%) with normal total protein concentration (7 g/dL; ref.: 6.8–8.3 g/dL), hyponatremia (132 mmol/L; ref.: 140–150 mmol/L), hyperkalemia (6.8 mmol/L; ref.: 3.4–5.7 mmol/L), hypoglycemia (<20 mg/dL; ref.: 45–80 mg/dL), and azotemia (creatinine: 2.4 mg/dL; ref.: 0.7–1 mg/dL). A urinalysis was not performed as urine could not be obtained at the time of presentation. Abdominal ultrasound was performed, and free abdominal fluid was not observed. The urinary bladder was found to be intact, and bilateral renomegaly with abnormal renal echogenicity and thickened renal cortices (1 cm) was noted. Multiple diffusely hyperechoic masses were observed in the inguinal and perirenal regions (Figure 1). The uterus, containing hypoechoic fluid, was identified in the right inguinal region, and a wall thickness of 5 mm was observed. Small intestinal bowel loops were visualized in the ventral abdomen. Decreased peristaltic activity and increased wall thickness (4 mm) were noted.

The doe was started on replacement fluid therapy with isotonic sodium-chloride solution at a dose of 20 mL/kg in order to treat the electrolyte abnormalities, with 5% dextrose added to the fluids to treat the severe hypoglycemia. Attitude and vital parameters improved after the fluid bolus, blood glucose levels normalized, and the doe was maintained on isotonic sodium-chloride supplemented with 2% dextrose at a rate of 4 mL/kg/hr overnight to promote diuresis and ameliorate the azotemia. The doe's attitude slightly improved on day 2: she stood on her own and was picking at food; she was passing feces and urinating normally. Complete blood count revealed normocytic, normochromic anemia with increased reticulocyte count suggestive of a regenerative process. The leukogram was unremarkable, and total protein and fibrinogen concentrations were within normal limits. Serum biochemistry panel on day 2 revealed improvement in

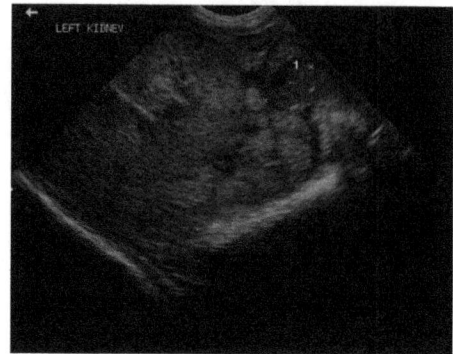

FIGURE 1: Ultrasonographic image of the left kidney obtained from the right paralumbar fossa. Note the increased thickness of the renal cortex and the multiple masses in the perirenal region. Obtained with a 5 MHz microconvex transducer. Left is dorsal; right is ventral.

the hyponatremia (139 mmol/L; ref.: 140–150 mmol/L), normal glucose concentration (75 mg/dL; ref.: 45–80 mg/dL) but no significant change in the azotemia (creatinine: 2.4 mg/dL; ref.: 0.7–1 mg/dL, BUN: 104 mg/dL; ref.: 19–31 mg/dL) and hyperkalemia (6.7 mmol/L; ref.: 3.4–5.7 mmol/L). The doe was also hypercalcemic (11.6 mg/dL; ref.: 8.9–11.2 mg/dL) and had a decreased albumin concentration (2.7 g/dL; ref.: 3.8–4.5 g/dL). Urinalysis revealed isosthenuria (USG: 1.010) and no other abnormal findings. An abdominal ultrasound exam was repeated which was found to be consistent with the findings from the previous day. The problem list in this doe included low body condition score, fatigue, obtundation, anemia, azotemia, hyperkalemia, hyponatremia, hypercalcemia, hypoalbuminemia, and perirenal masses detected on the abdominal ultrasound examination.

This doe had no history of prolonged anorexia, and her daily feed determined to be of good quality. As such, a systemic disease process or endoparasitism was considered the most likely differentials for her decreased body condition score. Her acute onset of fatigue and obtundation was thought to be due to the severe hypoglycemia, as her mentation and strength improved after dextrose supplementation. Hypoglycemia in an adult animal may result from excessive glucose utilization, neoplasia (insulinoma), impaired hepatic gluconeogenesis and glycogenolysis (hepatic insufficiency), diabetogenic hormone (cortisol) deficiency, sepsis, or a combination of these mechanisms [3]. This doe had normal liver enzymes and no evidence of sepsis based on the physical exam and the leukogram, so increased glucose uptake by the cells, hyperinsulinemia due to insulin producing tumor, and cortisol deficiency were considered likely causes of her severe hypoglycemia. This patient's azotemia and severe electrolyte disturbances in light of normal or adequate urine production were suggestive of polyuric renal failure or hypoadrenocorticism. Unfortunately, a urine specific gravity was not obtained prior to initiation of fluid therapy. However, the persistently elevated creatinine in the face of fluid therapy and diuresis was suggestive of impaired renal function. Although hyperkalemia is often observed with oliguric renal failure, the magnitude of the hyperkalemia in this patient and the lack of response to intravenous fluid therapy and glucose supplementation in addition to the severe hypoglycemia and fatigue were suggestive of adrenal insufficiency. Further, the presence of regenerative anemia, in concert with the low serum albumin concentration, and the absence of evidence to support hemolysis suggested blood loss. As the doe had no history of external hemorrhage and fecal occult blood test was negative, the ectoparasitism detected on the physical exam was considered the most likely cause of the anemia and hypoalbuminemia. The observed hypercalcemia in this patient is an uncommon finding in ruminants and is usually associated with hypervitaminosis D due to iatrogenic or toxic causes [4]. Additionally, elevated total calcium levels in ruminants can also be associated with pseudohyperparathyroidism due to a neoplastic process, and hypercalcemia can also be associated with hypoadrenocorticism in other species [5].

Following the initial diagnostic tests, additional diagnostic tests performed included fecal egg count determination (which was negative) and performance of an ACTH (adrenocorticotropic hormone) stimulation test to evaluate the function of the adrenal cortex. Baseline cortisol concentrations were undetectable, and thus a follow-up ACTH stimulation test was performed using a dosage of synthetic ACTH of $10 \mu g/kg$. This dose was extrapolated from the results of a previous report [6]. Serum cortisol concentrations 1 hour after ACTH administration remained below detection range levels, and the diagnosis of adrenal insufficiency was made. An intra-abdominal neoplastic process was considered most likely with direct involvement of the adrenal glands. A biopsy of the peri-renal masses and the kidneys was not performed due to lack of owner consent. As the owner elected for supportive care only, the doe was treated with a single dose of prednisolone sodium succinate intravenously (2 mg/kg) to address the glucocorticoid deficiency and then maintained on once daily intravenous dexamethasone (0.2 mg/kg). The severe hyperkalemia was a concern, but unfortunately, mineralocorticoid administration was not an option in this doe due to financial constraints. She was given low dose furosemide intravenously (0.25 mg/kg) once to increase urinary excretion of potassium, while maintenance fluid therapy with dextrose supplementation was continued. The doe was significantly brighter and stronger on day 3; she had normal vital parameters and rumen contractions, maintained a good appetite, and was passing manure and urine normally. Blood work revealed resolution of the electrolyte abnormalities and persistent azotemia, therefore fluid therapy was continued with Normosol-R. She was able to maintain physiologic glucose levels with voluntary feeding and the steroid therapy, and she was subsequently weaned off dextrose supplementation. Glucose and electrolyte concentrations were normal on day 4, while the azotemia was unchanged (creatinine: 2.3 mg/dL; ref.: 0.7–1 mg/dL; BUN: 123 mg/dL; ref.: 19–31 mg/dL), and the diagnosis of chronic renal insufficiency was made. She was tapered off the intravenous fluid therapy and given a dose of long acting methylprednisolone acetate (1 mg/kg intramuscular) in order to prepare her for discharge on day 5. The owner reported signs of abdominal discomfort and restlessness the day following discharge and brought the doe

back to the hospital 36 hours after discharge, but she was deceased on arrival. A full necropsy revealed widespread neoplasia, which was histologically confirmed as adenocarcinoma. The largest and presumably primary mass was in the uterus with infiltration into the lungs, diaphragm, left kidney, urinary bladder, omentum, sublumbar, and left and right renal lymph nodes and to the region of the adrenal glands where adrenal tissue could not be identified grossly or histologically. Adjacent to the right kidney, the neoplasm extended into the caudal vena cava and occluded the lumen. In addition, a thrombus was attached to the intravascular tumor (Figure 2). Effacement of the adrenal glands by the neoplasm presumably led to the doe's clinical presentation consistent with hypoadrenocorticism. The acute onset of abdominal pain and rapid deterioration of the doe may have been due to the occluding tumor metastasis and thrombus in the caudal vena cava.

3. Discussion

Primary hypoadrenocorticism has been previously reported in South African angora goats, resulting in increased sensitivity of these animals to weather changes [6], which appears to be genetic in this breed [7]. Diagnosis of Addison's syndrome is based on results of the ACTH stimulation test [3]. As this test is not routinely performed in goats, the ACTH dose used in this doe was selected based on a previous study, where it was successfully used to evaluate adrenal function in healthy Angora and Boer goats [6]. Another experimental model successfully used both the low dose (0.4 IU/kg = 4 μg/kg) and high dose (2.5 IU/kg = 25 μg/kg) ACTH stimulation tests in Angora and Spanish wethers [7]. Physiologic resting cortisol concentrations have been reported to be between 1 and 15 ng/mL in healthy, adult goats [6–8], and a normal response was considered to be a minimum of 3-4-fold elevation of plasma cortisol after ACTH administration [6, 7]. In dogs, a standard dose of synthetic ACTH (250 μg/dog) is used for evaluation of adrenocortical function, regardless of the size of the dog, and a normal response is considered to be an 8-10-fold elevation in the cortisol concentration when compared to resting levels [9]. However, a validated testing protocol has not been described in goats with primary hypoadrenocorticism. Based on previous research [6, 7] and our findings in this case, we conclude that the ACTH stimulation protocol used in this goat proved to be a reliable way to diagnose Addison's syndrome.

Addison's syndrome most commonly occurs in young, female dogs and is due to an immune mediated process destructing the adrenal cortices [10]. There is one case report of a 12-year-old dog diagnosed with Addison's syndrome due to bilateral adrenal neoplasia [11]. That dog presented with clinical signs and laboratory alterations consistent with Addison's disease but had an uncharacteristic signalment and bilaterally enlarged adrenal glands on the abdominal ultrasound exam. The dog was started on standard replacement therapy with dexamethasone and fludrocortisone, and after an initial positive response to therapy, it acutely deteriorated in 5 days showing signs of restlessness and abdominal

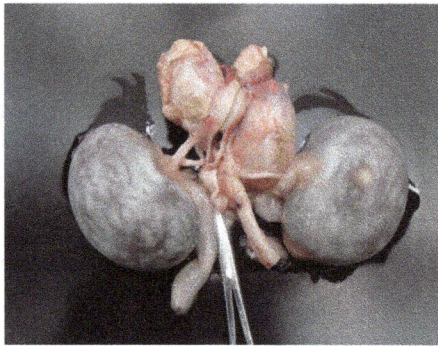

FIGURE 2: Gross image of kidneys and tumor masses. Tumor nodules are present between the kidneys in the region of the adrenal glands and renal lymph nodes and also within the caudal vena cave (asterisk). The left kidney has a small tumor nodule underneath the capsule. Top: cranial, bottom: caudal. The ruler spans 2 cm.

discomfort. Histological examination of the adrenal glands after euthanasia revealed highly anaplastic bilateral adrenal neoplasia. According to a recent retrospective study, the average rate of metastatic involvement of the adrenal glands is 21% in dogs, 26.9% in horses, and 31.3% in cattle [12]. No goat necropsies were involved in that study. Common tumor types that metastasize to the adrenal gland include carcinoma, adenocarcinoma, and lymphoma. Only one dog was reported to have developed Addison's disease secondary to the metastatic neoplasia [12]. Necropsy findings in this doe revealed that the metastatic adenocarcinoma originated from the uterus and infiltrated multiple abdominal organs. There are a couple of single case reports of uterine neoplasia of muscle origin in goats [13, 14] and one report of metastasized adenocarcinoma of the uterus [15], but no case series of uterine neoplasia are described. Based on studies in other species [16], we may assume that they are more common in the geriatric population.

Dogs diagnosed with Addison's syndrome often have azotemia, which is considered to be prerenal in origin and due to the dehydration [10]. The azotemia in this doe was unresponsive to diuresis, suggestive of renal origin. Dogs diagnosed with primary hypoadrenocorticism require lifelong replacement therapy with corticosteroids and mineralocorticoids and are reported to maintain a good quality of life [17]. Treatment of the doe in this case report was aimed at correcting the severe electrolyte abnormalities with intravenous fluid therapy and corticosteroid supplementation. As mineralocorticoid administration was not an option due to financial constraints, she was given a single dose of furosemide to increase urinary excretion of potassium. Such treatment is controversial in animals with hypoadrenocorticism, due to the risk of exacerbating the hypotension, although, a partial, single dose with concurrent administration of intravenous fluids was considered to be a safe alternative to mineralocorticoid supplementation in this case. While dexamethasone has no activity on the mineralocorticoid receptors, methylprednisolone and prednisolone both have significant effects on this receptor type [18]. No previous reports described treatment of Addison's disease with corticosteroids only; it

was attempted in this doe as the sole option to lengthen the animal's life. As the doe deteriorated shortly after discharge, while the long acting corticosteroids were still supposed to have adequate circulating levels, inadequate stress response was not considered to be the primary cause of her death but could have contributed to the pain and discomfort of this animal because of its role in promoting a hypercoagulable state [19] leading to thrombosis of the caudal vena cava.

In conclusion, Addison's syndrome as sequelae to neoplasia can occur in goats, and an ACTH stimulation test using synthetic ACTH intravenously can be used to diagnose the disease. As no other causes of primary hypoadrenocorticism have been previously reported in goats, consideration of an intra-abdominal neoplastic process is recommended. The success of replacement therapy likely depends on the initiating cause and potential involvement of organs other than the adrenal glands.

References

[1] S. R. Bornstein, "Predisposing factors for adrenal insufficiency," *The New England Journal of Medicine*, vol. 360, no. 22, pp. 2328–2339, 2009.

[2] S. C. Klein and M. E. Peterson, "Canine hypoadrenocorticism: part I," *Canadian Veterinary Journal*, vol. 51, no. 1, pp. 63–69, 2010.

[3] R. W. Nelson, G. H. Turnwald, and M. D. Willard, "Endocrine, metabolic, and lipid disorders," in *Small Animal Clinical Diagnosis By Laboratory Methods*, M. D. Willard and T. Harold, Eds., pp. 165–207, Elsevier, St. Louis, Mo, USA, 2004.

[4] G. P. Carlson, "Clinical chemistry tests," in *Large Animal Internal Medicine*, B. P. Smith, Ed., pp. 375–397, Mosby, St. Louis, Mo, USA, 2009.

[5] P. A. Schenck, D. J. Chew, L. A. Nagode, T. J. Rosol et al., "Disorders of calcium: hypercalcemia and hypocalcemia," in *Fluid, Electrolyte, and Acid-Base Disorders in Small Animal Practice*, S. P. DiBartola, Ed., Elsevier, St. Louis, Mo, USA, 3rd edition, 2006.

[6] Y. Engelbrecht, T. Herselman, A. Louw, and P. Swart, "Investigation of the primary cause of hypoadrenocorticism in South African Angora goats (*Capra aegagrus*): a comparison with Boer goats (*Capra hircus*) and Merino sheep (*Ovis aries*)," *Journal of Animal Science*, vol. 78, no. 2, pp. 371–379, 2000.

[7] C. A. Toerien, R. Puchala, J. P. McCann, T. Sahlu, and A. L. Goetsch, "Adrenocortical response to ACTH in Angora and Spanish goat wethers," *Journal of Animal Science*, vol. 77, no. 6, pp. 1558–1564, 1999.

[8] L. Eriksson and T. L. Teravainen, "Circadian rhythm of plasma cortisol and blood glucose in goats," *Australian Journal of Applied Science*, pp. 202–203, 1989.

[9] B. P. Meij and J. A. Mol, "Adrenocortical function," in *Clinical Biochemistry of Domestic Animals*, J. J. Kaneko, J. W. Harvey, and M. Bruss, Eds., pp. 605–622, Elsevier, St. Louis, Mo, USA, 2008.

[10] R. W. Nelson, "Disorders of the adrenal gland," in *Small Animal Internal Medicine*, R. W. Nelson and C. G. Couto, Eds., pp. 778–815, Mosby, St. Louis, Mo, USA, 2003.

[11] P. H. Kook, P. Grest, U. Raute-Kreinsen, C. Leo, and C. E. Reusch, "Addison's disease due to bilateral adrenal malignancy in a dog," *Journal of Small Animal Practice*, vol. 51, no. 6, pp. 333–336, 2010.

[12] P. Labelle and H. E. V. De Cock, "Metastatic tumors to the adrenal glands in domestic animals," *Veterinary Pathology*, vol. 42, no. 1, pp. 52–58, 2005.

[13] F. A. Uzal and B. Puschner, "*Cervical leiomyoma* in an aged goat leading to massive hemorrhage and death," *Canadian Veterinary Journal*, vol. 49, no. 2, pp. 177–179, 2008.

[14] K. M. Whitney, B. A. Valentine, and D. H. Schlafer, "Caprine genital *Leiomyosarcoma*," *Veterinary Pathology*, vol. 37, no. 1, pp. 89–94, 2000.

[15] P. Pfister, U. Geissbuehler, D. Wiener, G. Hirsbrunner, and C. Kaufmann, "Pollakisuria in a dwarf goat due to pathologic enlargement of the uterus," *Veterinary Quarterly*, vol. 29, no. 3, pp. 112–116, 2007.

[16] S. J. Woodhouse and C. S. Hanley, "What is your diagnosis? Uterine adenocarcinoma," *Journal of the American Veterinary Medical Association*, vol. 238, no. 3, pp. 289–290, 2011.

[17] S. C. Klein and M. E. Peterson, "Canine hypoadrenocorticism: part II," *Canadian Veterinary Journal*, vol. 51, no. 2, pp. 179–184, 2010.

[18] M. J. Day, "Glucocorticoids and antihistamines," in *Small Animal Clinical Pharmacology*, J. E. Maddison, S. W. Page, and D. B. Church, Eds., pp. 261–269, Elsevier, 2008.

[19] M. A. Kerachian, D. Cournoyer, E. J. Harvey et al., "Effect of high-dose dexamethasone on endothelial haemostatic gene expression and neutrophil adhesion," *Journal of Steroid Biochemistry and Molecular Biology*, vol. 116, no. 3–5, pp. 127–133, 2009.

9

Diagnosis, Surgical Treatment, Recovery, and Eventual Necropsy of a Leopard (*Panthera pardus*) with Thyroid Carcinoma

Ashley Malmlov,[1] Terry Campbell,[2] Eric Monnet,[2] Craig Miller,[1] Becca Miceli,[3] and Colleen Duncan[1]

[1] *Department of Microbiology, Immunology and Pathology, Colorado State University, Fort Collins, 200 West Lake Street, 1644 Campus Delivery, Fort Collins, CO 80523, USA*
[2] *Veterinary Teaching Hospital, Colorado State University, Fort Collins, CO 80523, USA*
[3] *The Wild Animal Sanctuary, Keenesburg, CO 80643, USA*

Correspondence should be addressed to Ashley Malmlov; ash.malmlov@colostate.edu

Academic Editor: Lysimachos G. Papazoglou

An 18-year-old, male, castrated, captive-born leopard (*Panthera pardus*) presented to Colorado State University's Veterinary Teaching Hospital with a two-week history of regurgitation. Thoracic radiographs and ultrasound revealed a well-differentiated cranioventral mediastinal mass measuring 7.5 × 10 × 5.5 cm, impinging the esophagus. A sternotomy followed by mass excision was performed. The mass was diagnosed as an ectopic thyroid carcinoma. The leopard recovered from surgery with minimal complications and returned to near-normal activity levels for just under 6 months before rapidly declining. He had an acute onset of severe dyspnea and lethargy and was euthanized. On postmortem examination the tumor was found to involve the lung, liver, thyroid, parietal pleura, bronchial lymph nodes, and the internal intercostal muscles. This case report describes the history, diagnosis, surgical treatment, postoperative care, and recovery as well as the eventual decline, euthanasia, and necropsy of a leopard with thyroid carcinoma. When compared to thyroid carcinomas of domestic animals, the leopard's disease process more closely resembles the disease process seen in domestic canines compared to domestic cats.

1. Introduction

While it is difficult to estimate the number of captive big cats within USA, it is thought there may be between 10,000 and 20,000 kept in private facilities [1]. In addition to these numbers, there are approximately 1,000 within American Zoological Association accredited zoos (Denver Zoo, pers. Com.). Considering the population size of big cats in captivity, relatively little is known about the diseases they acquire and even less about the best course for medical intervention when compared to domestic animals. A retrospective study focused on the years 1979–2003, based out of Knoxville Zoological Gardens, determined there was a 51% incidence of neoplasia found at necropsy in their large cat collection, of which 27.7% was identified as the cause of death [2]. This was an increase from an older publication based out of Philadelphia

Zoological Gardens that retrospectively reviewed postmortem records and found a 3.6% neoplastic incidence in their felid population between 1901 and 1934. Between the years 1935 and 1955, an incidence of 24.9% was found [3]. In both publications it was suggested that the increase of neoplastic processes over time may be attributed to a longer lifespan associated with better husbandry. Exposure to environmental carcinogens was also considered as a possible explanation [2, 3]. It may also be due, in part, to advancements in diagnostic technology.

With so many big cats in captivity and the increased incidence in neoplasia, it is critical to make known not only what maladies these animals acquire but also methods of diagnosis and the treatment protocols implemented, to help future animals that may be inflicted with a similar disease. In this case report we describe the patient history, diagnosis, surgical treatment, postoperative care, and necropsy findings of a geriatric, captive-born leopard (*Panthera pardus*) with thyroid carcinoma.

2. Case Presentation

The animal described in this case report was an 18-year-old, male, castrated leopard. In 2001 he became a resident of The Wild Animal Sanctuary (TWAS, 501c3 public nonprofit) in Keenesburg, Colorado, USA, where he remained for the duration of his life. There is no information in regard to the leopard's genealogy. Prior to arrival at TWAS, the leopard lived in two different non-AZA accredited zoological parks. At TWAS, the leopard lived in an approximately 24 × 30 m outdoor habitat with four other leopards. The habitat contained 5 insulated concrete dens as shelter, 2 of which measure 2 × 3 m and 3 of which were round dens, 2 m in diameter. He was fed a commercial carnivore-specific diet manufactured by Triple A Brand Meat Company (Burlington, CO), as well as raw meat supplemented with Fresh + Oasis Feline T vitamins. Visual physical examinations were conducted daily by the animal keepers. At the end of February, 2012, the onset of regurgitation was observed in the leopard—which seemed to correlate with the rapid consumption of a whole chicken wing. Prior to this, the leopard had no major medical history and had always been apparently healthy. His caretakers began dicing raw meat into 1 cm cubes, of which he was able to keep down if fed small amounts, frequently. Episodes of regurgitation persisted for two weeks, and the leopard was brought to Colorado State University's Veterinary Teaching Hospital (CSU-VTH) on March 7, 2012.

Upon presentation at CSU-VTH the leopard was quiet, alert, and responsive, with a body condition score of 4 out of 9, and weighed 40 kg. He was tranquilized using DAN-INJECT ApS (Sellerup Skovvej 116, Børkop, Denmark) in the right gluteal muscle with dexmedetomidine (0.015 mg/kg), ketamine (3 mg/kg), and midazolam (0.1 mg/kg) and maintained on isoflurane.

Initial diagnostics included a complete blood count (CBC) and biochemistry panel, thoracic and abdominal radiographs, and thoracic ultrasound. The CBC and biochemistry panel were within normal limits, using reference ranges for domestic house cats. Thoracic radiographs and ultrasound revealed a well-differentiated, cranioventral, mediastinal mass measuring 7.5 × 10 × 5.5 cm, impinging the esophagus and deduced as the cause of regurgitation. No abnormalities were seen on radiographs in the cervical region that might have suggested the thyroid glands were involved. A fine needle aspirate and cytology of the mass identified it as a carcinoma. Cells were small and cuboidal, with moderately basophilic and vacuolated cytoplasm and round nuclei with coarsely granular chromatin and inconspicuous nucleoli. Anisocytosis and anisokaryosis were moderate.

On the same day diagnostics were conducted, a medial sternotomy was performed. The leopard was not taken off general anesthesia during the interim between diagnostics and surgery. The mass was located between the cranial vena cava and external jugular veins—completely occluding the

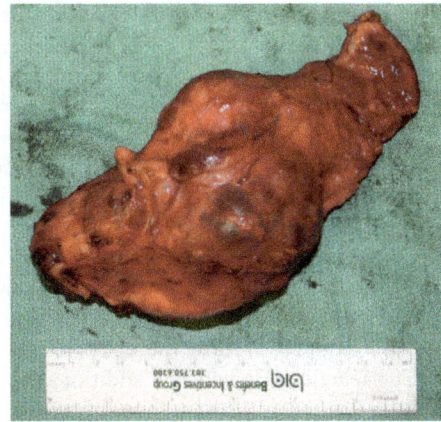

FIGURE 1: Gross image of the highly vascular and well-circumscribed mass excised during sternotomy, measuring 10 × 10 × 13 cm.

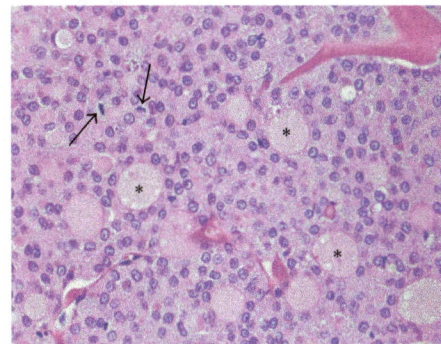

FIGURE 2: Mediastinal mass excised during sternotomy. Ectopic thyroid carcinoma characterized by neoplastic polygonal cells supported by a fine fibrovascular stroma and frequently arranged in follicular structures filled with colloid (asterisk). Numerous mitotic figures (arrows) are present throughout this neoplastic cell population. H&E stain (400x).

veins—and adhered to both the esophagus and trachea. Grossly, the mass appeared well circumscribed and highly vascular. It was dissected away from the surrounding tissue and removed from the chest cavity. The mass measured 10 × 10 × 13 cm (Figure 1). A chest tube was placed in the right ventrolateral thorax to remove fluid accumulation in the dead space formed by excision of the mass and to maintain negative pressure. A 10 mg fentanyl patch was placed between the shoulder blades. The chest tube was removed just prior to extubation. The leopard recovered from anesthesia with no complications and returned to TWAS the same day. Following surgery, the mass was submitted to the Colorado State University Veterinary Diagnostic Laboratories (CSU-VDL) where it was diagnosed as an ectopic thyroid carcinoma (Figure 2) with capsular and vascular invasion. It is believed that this was the tumor of origin and not metastasis from a tumor in the thyroid gland because of the large size of the tumor, coupled with the radiographically normal thyroid glands.

At TWAS, the leopard was kept in a small enclosure measuring 2 × 2 m within the on-site hospital, to closely monitor his postoperative progress. For two days following surgery he was quiet, alert, and responsive. He was given tramadol at 5 mg/kg PO q 24 hours as needed for pain management and ate small quantities of raw meat, frequently. There was mild hemorrhage and edema associated with the incision but no visible drainage or odor that may indicate infection. The fourth day after surgery the leopard had an episode described as a "frantic agonal breathing fit" by his caretakers. He was placed on oxygen and monitored. The tramadol was temporarily discontinued in case the episode was due to an adverse drug reaction. He had one additional episode of frantic breathing that was less severe than the first. The cause of these episodes was never determined, but pain or anxiety was suspected.

Eleven days after surgery the leopard was moved from the TWAS hospital to an outdoor enclosure, separate from the other leopards, measuring 4 × 30 m on the grounds. His caretakers continued to closely monitor his food intake, refrained from giving him any meat with bones, and cut the meat into small cubes. He made a near-full recovery with periodic episodes of regurgitation occurring every 2 to 3 weeks, usually coinciding with either excitement or when the caretakers attempted to increase the size of the meat cubes he received. Famotidine was prescribed, 0.5 mg/kg PO q 24 hours, for an indefinite period of time. Episodes of regurgitation decreased in conjunction with daily administration of famotidine. No additional medical treatment for the thyroid carcinoma was pursued.

On August 18, five and a half months after the initial surgery, the leopard's condition began to decline; his appetite decreased and his caretakers noticed mild respiratory congestion. Clavamox 375 mg tablets PO SID for 11 days were initiated for possible respiratory tract infection. One week later the leopard became acutely anorexic and dyspneic. There was concern that there was metastasis to the lungs and he was humanely euthanized at TWAS on August 28. The carcass was brought to CSU-VDL for necropsy.

On postmortem examination, the left lobe of the thyroid gland was enlarged up to 2 times normal, measuring 4 × 2 × 2 cm. Upon cut section, the thyroid parenchyma was expanded and effaced by a poorly demarcated mass that was pale, homogenous, and slightly firm. The right lobe of the thyroid gland was not identified. Approximately 1L of serosanguinous fluid was present in the thoracic cavity and contained abundant fibrin tags which diffusely adhered to the adjacent visceral and parietal pleura. At the location of the previous surgery site, there was a regionally extensive area in which the left and right cranial lung lobes were adhered together by moderate to marked amounts of fibrous connective tissue, which was accompanied by moderate, segmental dilatation of the esophagus extending caudal to the cardiac sphincter. Throughout the lung lobes, greater than 50% of the pulmonary parenchyma was expanded and effaced by multifocal to coalescing pale, firm nodules ranging from 5 to 15 mm in diameter (Figure 3). Similar nodules were observed multifocally expanding the parietal pleura of the mediastinum, within the skeletal muscle of the internal

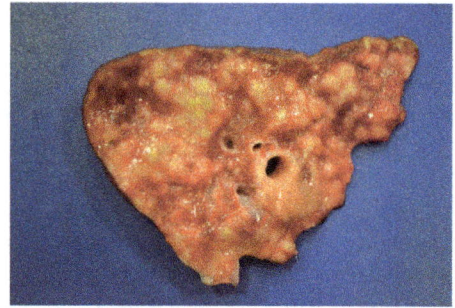

FIGURE 3: Lung. The pulmonary parenchyma is effaced by multifocal to coalescing, pale, firm nodules similar in appearance to those observed in the parietal pleura, thyroid, liver, bronchial lymph nodes, and internal intercostal muscles.

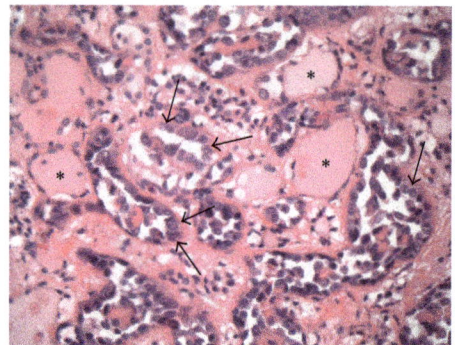

FIGURE 4: Left lobe of the thyroid gland. The normal thyroid follicular architecture (asterisks) is effaced by nests of neoplastic polygonal cells that occasionally form primitive follicles lacking colloid (arrows). H&E stain (400x).

intercostal muscles and throughout the liver. The bronchial lymph node was completely effaced by a mass with characteristics the same as previously described.

Upon histological evaluation, the left lobe of the thyroid gland was expanded and effaced by sheets and nests of neoplastic polygonal cells supported by a fine fibrovascular stroma and arranged in sheets and primitive follicular structures that lacked colloid (Figure 4). Neoplastic cells exhibited marked anisocytosis with varying amounts of eosinophilic cytoplasm. Nuclei were round to ovoid with 0–2 nucleoli and marked anisokaryosis. The mitotic index was approximately 10 per single high-powered field (400x). Large coalescing areas of coagulative necrosis were present throughout the neoplastic cell populations, characterized by areas of hypereosinophilic cellular debris and karyorrhectic nuclei. In addition, the normal tissue architecture of the lung (Figure 5), parietal pleura of the mediastinum, tracheobronchial lymph nodes, and liver were similarly effaced by neoplastic cells as previously described.

Based on gross and histological findings, disseminated thyroid carcinoma of the lung, liver, thyroid, and parietal pleura was diagnosed, with fibrinosuppurative and necrohemorrhagic pleuritis, serosanguinous pleural effusion, and megaesophagus.

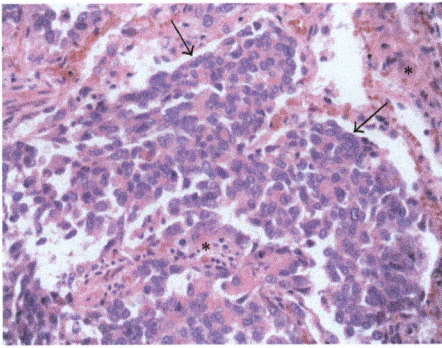

FIGURE 5: Lung. Alveoli are expanded by sheets and nests of neoplastic polygonal cells as observed in the thyroid gland (arrows). Multifocal to coalescing areas of necrosis (asterisk) are present throughout this neoplastic cell population (400x). H&E stain.

3. Discussion

It is generally accepted that nondomestic felids resemble house cats in both their anatomy and physiology, and therefore the better defined disease processes of domestic cats are extrapolated back to nondomestic felids. In domestic cats thyroid adenomas and adenomatous hyperplasia are more common than carcinomas [4–8]. The thyroid is active in these cases and causes hyperthyroidism and heart disease [5]. Feline thyroid carcinomas are less common and account for 2% of hyperthyroid cases but may also be nonfunctioning [8]. They tend to be larger in size than their benign counterparts and may impinge the trachea or esophagus, resulting in dyspnea or dysphagia. Feline thyroid carcinomas are highly metastatic with metastasis most commonly seen in regional lymph nodes [5]. Treatment consists of surgical extraction or radioiodine therapy [5].

In contrast, thyroid carcinomas more commonly afflict domestic dogs, compared to adenomas [4–7]. The incidence of thyroid carcinoma in dogs 8 to 12 years is 1.1% and increases to 4.4% for dogs between 12 and 15 years. The most common presentation is a large, nonpainful mass in the cervical region with clinical signs secondary to the mass: dysphagia, dyspnea, dysphonia, and coughing. Tumors may also be associated with ectopic thyroid tissue and can occur anywhere from the base of the tongue to the base of the heart. The rate of metastasis on necropsy is 80%, with 15% to 38% of dogs already demonstrating metastasis on initial diagnosis. The incidence of metastasis correlates to the size of the primary tumor, with tumors less than $20 \, cm^3$ metastasizing less than 20% of the time and tumors greater than $100 \, cm^3$ metastasizing nearly 100% of the time [9]. The lungs are the most common site for metastasis, followed by the regional lymph nodes. Treatment options include surgery, radioiodine treatment, and medical management [5]. The pattern of disease seen in the leopard's case more closely resembled a thyroid neoplastic process seen in a domestic dog compared to a domestic cat with the type of tumor being a carcinoma with metastasis to lungs and bronchial lymph nodes.

Although the leopard did not have thyroid levels tested, it is assumed that he had a nonfunctioning thyroid carcinoma.

CBC revealed neither erythrocytosis nor excitatory leukogram, and his biochemistry panel lacked an increase in BUN, ALT, or AST—changes which may suggest hyperthyroidism. Furthermore, the leopard had no observed clinical signs of hyperthyroidism prior to surgery, such as polyphagia, weight loss, or polydipsia and polyuria. In addition to this, if the thyroid carcinoma had been functioning, the leopard may have displayed signs of hypothyroidism after excision of which he did not.

After surgical treatment for thyroid carcinoma, the leopard survived for 176 days. At the time of diagnosis he did not have any radiographic evidence of metastasis; however, there was widespread metastasis upon postmortem examination. Due to the rarity of feline thyroid carcinomas, it is not well documented what the life expectancy is for cats that have undergone treatment, but the average age of cats diagnosed with malignant thyroid neoplasms is 15.8 years [7]. The median survival times for dogs with thyroid carcinoma are variable within the literature, but they have been reported to be 2 weeks to 3 months [6]. Comparatively, the leopard lived longer than documented in domestic animals. This may be in part due to the stoic nature of wild-felids, allowing the leopard's disease to be extensive without him demonstrating clinical signs and extending his survival time.

Thyroid carcinomas have been documented in two leopards, a lion (Panthera leo), a puma (Puma concolor), and a jungle cat (Felis chaus) [3, 10]. The cases in the leopards, lion, and puma occurred prior to 1950 and it was speculated that they may have been associated with a lack of dietary supplemental iodine [3]. The jungle cat had concurrent gastric adenocarcinoma, renal adenoma, and a Sertoli cell tumor found on necropsy after the animal was euthanized at the age of 23 for its poor condition and age [10]. The leopard was always given a large carnivore diet. Prior to TWAS the leopard's diet consisted of Zupreem Exotic Feline Diet (Shawnee, Kansas), Nebraska Brand Feline Diet (Central Nebraska Packing, Inc., North Platte, NE), and horse meat. At TWAS his diet was specially formulated for large carnivores and both USDA and CDA regulated, and so it can be concluded that his neoplasia was not secondary to diet.

This leopard's case is unique, not only because of the disease process but also because of the completeness of documentation in the medical progression. We were able to follow the course of disease from initial onset of symptoms to diagnosis, treatment, and eventual outcome of euthanasia and necropsy.

Conflict of Interests

The authors declare that there is no conflict of interests regarding the publication of this paper.

Acknowledgments

The authors would like to thank Pat Craig, staff, and volunteers at The Wild Animal Sanctuary for all they did for the leopard in this case report and what they continue to do for captive-bred large carnivores.

References

[1] *Big Cats and Public Safety Protection*, Welfare IFfA, Yarmouth Port, Mass, USA, 2013.

[2] M. A. Owston, E. C. Ramsay, and D. S. Rotstein, "Neoplasia in felids at the Knoxville zoological gardens, 1979–2003," *Journal of Zoo and Wildlife Medicine*, vol. 39, no. 4, pp. 608–613, 2008.

[3] L. S. Lombard and E. J. Witte, "Frequency and types of tumors in mammals and birds of the Philadelphia zoological garden," *Cancer Research*, vol. 19, no. 2, pp. 127–141, 1959.

[4] D. B. Bailey and R. L. Page, "Tumors of the endocrine system," in *Withrow and MacEwen's Small Animal Clinical Oncology*, S. J. Withrow and D. M. Vail, Eds., vol. 4th, pp. 583–606, Elsevier, St. Louis, Mo, USA, 2007.

[5] L. G. Barber, "Thyroid tumors in dogs and cats," *Veterinary Clinics of North America: Small Animal Practice*, vol. 37, no. 4, pp. 755–773, 2007.

[6] C. C. Capen, "Tumors of the endocrine glands," in *Tumors of Domestic Animals*, D. J. Meuten, Ed., pp. 638–656, Iowa State Press, Ames, Iowa, USA, 4th edition, 2002.

[7] I. Leav, A. L. Schiller, A. Rijnberk, M. A. Legg, and P. J. der Kinderen, "Adenomas and carcinomas of the canine and feline thyroid," *The American Journal of Pathology*, vol. 83, no. 1, pp. 61–122, 1976.

[8] J. C. Scott-Moncrieff, "Thyroid disorders in the geriatric veterinary patient," *Veterinary Clinics of North America: Small Animal Practice*, vol. 42, no. 4, pp. 707–725, 2012.

[9] H. S. Kooistra, "Endocrine disorders," in *Textbook of Veterinary Internal Medicine*, S. J. Ettinger and E. C. Feldman, Eds., vol. 2, pp. 1777–1779, Elsevier, St. Louis, Mo, USA, 7th edition, 2011.

[10] J. W. Sagartz, F. M. Garner, and R. M. Sauer, "Multiple neoplasia in a captive jungle cat (*Felis chaus*)—thyroid adenocarcinoma, gastric adenocarcinoma, renal adenoma, and Sertoli cell tumor," *Journal of Wildlife Diseases*, vol. 8, no. 4, pp. 375–380, 1972.

10

Mesothelioma in Two Nondomestic Felids: North American Cougar (*Felis concolor*) and Cheetah (*Acinonyx jubatus*)

Amanda Whiton,[1] Juergen Schumacher,[1] Erika E. Evans,[1] Janelle M. Novak,[2] Amanda Crews,[2,3] Edward Ramsay,[1] and Robert Donnell[2]

[1] Department of Small Animal Clinical Sciences, College of Veterinary Medicine, University of Tennessee, 2407 River Drive, Knoxville, TN 37996, USA

[2] Department of Biomedical and Diagnostic Sciences, College of Veterinary Medicine, University of Tennessee, Knoxville, TN 37996, USA

[3] Professional Veterinary Pathology Services, Columbia, SC 29203, USA

Correspondence should be addressed to Juergen Schumacher; jschumacher@utk.edu

Academic Editors: L. Espino López, N. D. Giadinis, J. S. Munday, F. Mutinelli, and J. Orós

A 15-year-old male North American cougar (*Felis concolor*) presented with a 2-day history of anorexia, restlessness, and dyspnea. White blood cell count (22.5×10^3 cells/μL) and absolute segmented neutrophil count (21.09×10^3 cells/μL) were increased, and BUN (143 mg/dL), creatinine (6.3 mg/dL), and phosphorus (8.5 mg/dL) concentrations indicated chronic renal disease. Thoracic radiographs showed severe pleural and pericardial effusion. During attempts to remove the fluid, cardiac tamponade developed and the cat died. At necropsy, nodular masses decorated the pericardium at the level of the base of the heart. The final microscopic diagnosis was mesothelioma of the pericardium, tunica adventitia of the main pulmonary artery, left auricle epicardium, and left ventricular epicardium. A 15-year-old female cheetah (*Acinonyx jubatus*) was evaluated for acute respiratory distress. The white blood cell count (25.5×10^3 cells/μL) and absolute segmented neutrophil count (22.19×10^3 cells/μL) were increased. Radiographically pleural effusion and a cranial thoracic mass were seen. The cheetah was euthanized, and a gross diagnosis of disseminated pleural mesothelioma with thoracic effusion was made. Histologically, pleural mesothelioma was confirmed with local invasion of the lung and pulmonary arterial emboli and infarction. In both cases, a diagnosis of mesothelioma was made based on cellular morphology, microscopic architecture, and neoplastic cell coexpression of cytokeratin and vimentin.

1. Introduction

Mesothelioma is a neoplasm involving cells that line the coelomic cavities of the body and can occur as either a widespread nodular mass or multifocal masses. Mesothelial tumors are considered malignant due to their ability to seed throughout a body cavity resulting in numerous tumors and implantation metastasis; however, spread into noncommunicating body cavities is considered rare [1]. In domestic dogs, primary mesothelial tumors have been reported affecting the thoracic cavity, pericardial sac, abdominal cavity, and vaginal tunics of the scrotum [1]. In domestic cats, primary mesotheliomas have been reported in the pericardium, pleura, peritoneum, and the abdomen with pulmonary and nodal metastases [1–6]. While pleural mesotheliomas have been reported in tigers and clouded leopards (*Neofelis nebulosa nebulosa*), pericardial mesotheliomas are rarely reported in both domestic and nondomestic species [7–9].

A common clinical sign of affected animals is pronounced dyspnea caused by pleural effusion or compression from peritoneal effusion. Marked effusions from direct exudation of the tumor or from tumor-obstructed lymphatics can be present. Animals diagnosed with pericardial mesothelioma may present with cardiac tamponade or evidence of right-sided heart failure [1]. A pericardial mesothelioma in a domestic cat with effusion and the clinical presentation and pathologic findings of a pericardial mesothelioma in a Bengal tiger (*Panthera tigris*) have been reported [10, 11]. Histologically, mesotheliomas can appear as either epithelial, mesenchymal, or biphasic.

2. Case Reports

Case 1. A 15-year-old male cougar (*Felis concolor*) from a large felid sanctuary in Tennessee, USA, presented to the University of Tennessee Veterinary Medical Center (UTVMC) with a 2-day history of anorexia, lethargy, and restlessness. Prior to transport to the UTVMC, the cougar received oral midazolam (NovaPlus; Hospira, Lake Forest, IL, USA; 0.12 mg/kg). At presentation, the cougar was mildly sedated but alert. The animal was in good body condition (body weight, 62 kg). Respiratory rate was 28 breaths per minute, and inspiratory phase was prolonged. Mucous membranes were cyanotic. The animal was immobilized via hand injection with a combination of dexmedetomidine (0.01 mg/kg i.m.; DexDomitor; Pfizer Animal Health, Exton, PA, USA) and ketamine hydrochloride (3 mg/kg i.m.; Ketaset; Fort Dodge Animal Health, Fort Dodge, IA, USA). Following endotracheal intubation, anesthesia was maintained with 0.5–2% isoflurane (Aerrane; Baxter Healthcare Corporation, Deerfield, IL) in 100% oxygen. Thoracic auscultation revealed bilaterally decreased lung sounds and muffled heart sounds. The femoral pulse was weak, and heart rate was 98 beats per minute. An intravenous catheter was placed in the left medial saphenous vein, and Normosol-R (Hospira) was administered at 10 mL/kg/hr. Electrocardiography (ECG) leads were attached in a conventional manner, and no abnormalities were recorded. A transmission pulse oximeter probe was placed over a lingual artery, and oxygen saturation (SpO_2) values were <90%, indicating severe hypoxemia. End-tidal carbon dioxide ($EtCO_2$) concentrations were >40 mmHg, indicative of hypercapnia. In order to antagonize the effects of dexmedetomidine and improve cardiopulmonary performance, intramuscular atipamezole (Antisedan; Pfizer Animal Health, New York, NY, USA; 0.05 mg/kg) was administered 10 minutes after endotracheal intubation. A venous blood sample was collected from the jugular vein and submitted for hematology, plasma biochemistry, and feline coronavirus (FCoV) titers.

Right lateral and dorsoventral radiographs of the thorax revealed rounding of the lung lobes and separation of the lung lobes from the body wall by a soft tissue opacity, consistent with pleural effusion. Air bronchograms were seen in the right cranial and right middle lung lobes. Cardiac margins were not seen, and there was a mild right mediastinal shift. Abdominal radiographs showed decreased serosal detail and mottling falciform and omental fat. An approximately 2 cm diameter soft tissue mineral opaque nodule with irregular margins was present over the plane of the liver on lateral radiographs. The radiographic interpretation was bicavitary effusion secondary to a neoplastic process, cardiac disease, or infectious process.

Thoracocentesis revealed a yellow, cloudy, and highly cellular fluid with a total protein of 3.4 g/dL. Small lymphocytes were the predominant cells, but there were also low numbers of foamy macrophages that occasionally exhibited erythrophagocytosis and contained small amounts of hemosiderin-like material. A cytologic diagnosis of a lymphocyte-rich, probable chylous effusion with the presence of red blood cells indicative of prior hemorrhage and increased

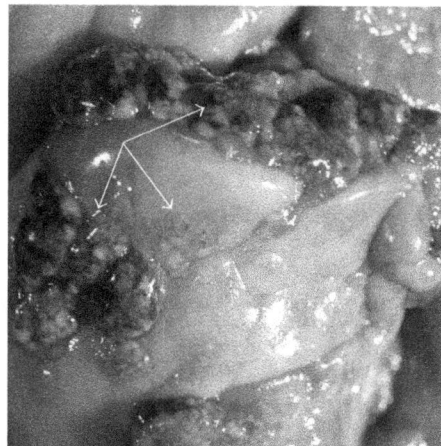

Figure 1: Gross photograph of numerous neoplastic mesothelial, exophytic, and tan to brown masses (arrows) on the epicardial and visceral pericardial surfaces of a 15-year-old cougar (*Felis concolor*).

numbers of mast cells was made. During removal of approximately 2 L fluid from the chest, the cougar developed ventricular premature complexes, became tachycardic, and arrested. Resuscitation efforts were unsuccessful.

Blood work abnormalities included an elevated white blood cell count (22.5×10^3 cells/μL; reference intervals, 3.10–16.90×10^3 cells/μL) and an elevated absolute segmented neutrophil count (21.09×10^3 cells/μL; reference interval, 0.056–11.60×10^3 cells/μL). BUN (143 mg/dL; reference interval, 12–65 mg/dL), creatinine (6.3 mg/dL; reference interval, 0.8–5.3 mg/dL), and phosphorus (8.5 mg/dL) levels were also markedly increased, indicating chronic renal disease. Serum was negative for antibodies to FCoV. Aerobic and anaerobic cultures of the thoracic fluid yielded no bacterial growth. Samples from the thoracic and abdominal effusion were PCR negative for FCoV.

At necropsy, the thoracic cavity contained 3 L of mildly gelatinous serosanguineous fluid. There was diffuse pulmonary atelectasis. Multifocal to coalescing petechial luminal hemorrhages were located throughout the length of the trachea. Fibrinous adhesions were present between the parietal pleura, pericardial/mediastinal pleura, and pulmonary pleura. The wall of the pericardial sac was opaque, thickened, and edematous. The pericardial sac contained 600 mL thick red to purple fluid. Numerous, brown exophytic proliferations, ranging in size from $0.5 \times 0.2 \times 0.3$ to $5.0 \times 2.0 \times 1.5$ cm, covered the epicardial surface of both atria, encircled the main pulmonary artery and aorta, extended to the cardiac apex, and were continuous with masses present on the visceral surface of the pericardium (Figure 1). A $1.0 \times 1.0 \times 0.5$ cm gray to white focal mass expanded the mediastinum. One liter of red-orange-yellow gelatinous fluid was found within the abdominal cavity. The spleen was enlarged, and the gallbladder was distended with a torturous cystic duct.

Histopathologic evaluation of the main pulmonary artery (with exophytic proliferations) revealed an unencapsulated population of polygonal to columnar cells arranged in undulating folds, papillary projections, and dense sheets on a fibrovascular stroma. Along the main pulmonary artery, the neoplastic cells proliferated along the tunica adventitia and blended with adipose tissue (Figure 3(a)). These neoplastic cells incorporated the epicardium and blended with the surrounding epicardial adipose tissue. There was histopathologic evidence of pleural and visceral pericardial involvement. Neoplastic cells had oval euchromatic nuclei, eosinophilic cytoplasm, and indistinct borders. There was moderate anisocytosis (2-3x) and anisokaryosis (2-3x). Mitotic figures averaged 1/10 high-power fields (400x). There was multifocal necrosis with amorphous eosinophilic material and karyorrhectic debris with scattered dystrophic mineralization. Mixed with neoplastic cells were neutrophils, lymphocytes, plasma cells, epitheloid macrophages, siderophages, and hemorrhage. Immunohistochemical staining revealed the presence of both cytokeratin (clones AE1/AE3, DAKO) and vimentin (clone V9, DAKO) intermediate filaments in the neoplastic cells (Figures 3(b) and 3(c)). Other relevant histopathologic findings in the lungs included alveolar histiocytosis with "heart failure cells," alveolar smooth muscle hypertrophy, and hyperplasia with type II pneumocyte hypertrophy, all related to cardiac insufficiency.

The diagnosis was chronic active pericarditis and mesothelioma involving the pericardium, tunica adventitia of the main pulmonary artery, left auricle epicardium, and left ventricular epicardium.

Case 2. A 15-year-old female cheetah (*Acinonyx jubatus*) (body weight, 41.5 kg) from a zoological institution in Tennessee, USA, presented with acute onset of abdominal breathing and a 1-day history of lethargy and anorexia. The cheetah was immobilized with an intramuscular combination of ketamine (3.5 mg/kg; Ketaset; Fort Dodge Animal Health), dexmedetomidine (0.012 mg/kg, DexDomitor; Pfizer Animal Health), and midazolam (0.06 mg/kg, NovaPlus, Hospira) via a remote drug delivery system. Following endotracheal intubation, anesthesia was maintained with 2% isoflurane in 100% oxygen. An intravenous catheter was placed in the cephalic vein, and Normosol-R was administered at 10 mL/kg/hr. A venous blood sample was collected from the jugular vein and submitted for hematology, plasma biochemistry, and FCoV serology.

Thoracic radiographs revealed a cranial thoracic mass and separation of the lung lobes from the body wall, consistent with pleural effusion. Differential diagnoses included lymphoma, thymoma, lymphadenopathy, and thyroid carcinoma. Fluid was also noted in the abdominal cavity. The animal was euthanized due to quality of life concerns and poor prognosis for recovery.

Cytology of the thoracic effusion detected round cells and unidentifiable clusters, which most likely represented mesotheliocytes; however, some features of malignancy, for example, carcinoma, could not be ruled out. Aerobic and anaerobic cultures of the thoracic nodules revealed one colony of a gram-negative, nonfermentative rod, resembling *Acinetobacter* sp. Bacterial culture of a venous blood sample revealed no organisms on a gram stain, no anaerobes, and few colonies of *Klebsiella pneumoniae* and actinomyces-like organisms.

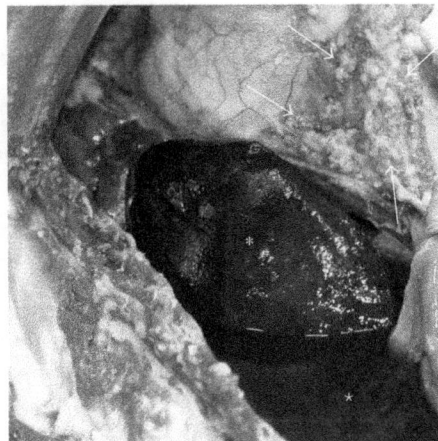

FIGURE 2: Gross photograph of the right thoracic cavity of a 15-year-old cheetah (*Acinonyx jubatus*). There is engorgement of the torsed right middle lung lobe (asterisk), and serosanguineous fluid partially fills the chest cavity (star). Multifocal coalescing tan nodules (mesothelioma) are present on the pleural and mediastinal surface (arrows).

Hematologic abnormalities included an elevated white blood cell count (25.5×10^3 cells/μL; reference range, 3.70–25.20×10^3 cells/μL) and an elevated absolute segmented neutrophil count (22.19×10^3 cells/μL; reference range, 1.34–20.90×10^3 cells/μL). Plasma chemistry and electrolytes values were within normal limits, and serum was negative for antibodies to FCoV.

At necropsy, 2 L of dark red, serosanguineous, and turbid fluid was present within the thoracic cavity (Figure 2). Throughout the chest cavity, small (0.1–0.5 cm), and multifocal, coalescing white to light tan nodules were firmly attached to the pleura. The pericardial sac contained 4.5 mL of clear, light yellow fluid. The right middle lobe was turgid, enlarged, dark red, firm, and torsed 360 degrees. The remaining lung lobes were atelectatic. The left cranial lung lobe, toward the apex, contained multifocal irregular areas that were depressed, firm, and dark red with measurements ranging from $0.5 \times 0.2 \times 0.2$ cm to $3.0 \times 1.0 \times 1.8$ cm. The right adrenal gland had decreased corticomedullary distinction, was irregular and diffusely enlarged, and measured $3.9 \times 2.5 \times 1.3$ cm. The adrenal cortex was enlarged, with a corticomedullary ratio of $1.5 : 1 : 1.4$. The left adrenal gland measured $3 \times 1.5 \times 1$ cm.

The gross diagnosis was disseminated pleural mesothelioma with severe thoracic effusion, diffuse pulmonary atelectasis, and acute right middle lung lobe torsion. Additional diagnoses included hepatic congestion, mild multifocal hepatic telangiectasia, multifocal pancreatic ductular cysts, multifocal pancreatic exocrine nodular hyperplasia, adrenal cortical adenoma, multifocal splenic myelolipomas, moderate subacute multifocal gastric congestion, and focal ovarian bursal cyst.

Microscopically, the thoracic mass was lined by raised to exophytic aggregates of moderately pleomorphic mesothelial cells. The mass was composed of clusters, cords, and islands of

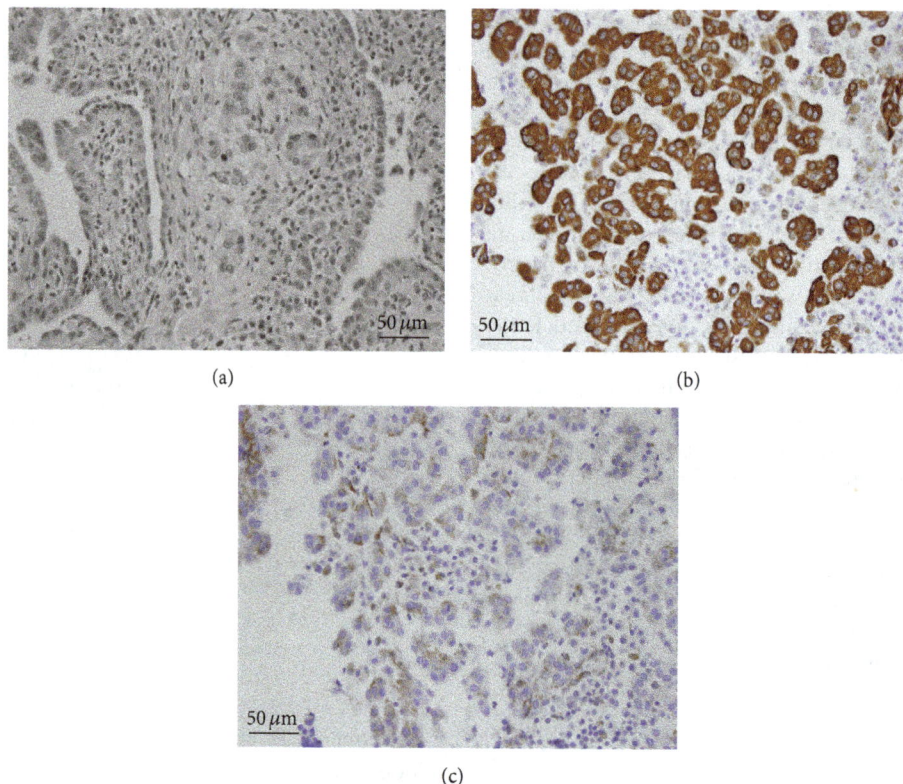

(a)

(b)

(c)

FIGURE 3: Photomicrographs of a mass overlying the epicardium and main pulmonary artery from a 15-year-old cougar. (a) Multiple papillary structures of fibrovascular stroma and nests of anisocytotic pleomorphic polygonal cells are covered by pleomorphic anisocytotic cuboidal to columnar cells (hematoxylin and eosin stain). (b) Clustered and individual cells strongly stain brown for the presence of cytokeratin intermediate filaments (immunohistochemistry, cytokeratin [AE1/AE3] antibody, DAB chromagen, hematoxylin counterstain). (c) The same clustered and individual cells stain brown for the presence of vimentin intermediate filaments (immunohistochemistry, vimentin [V9] antibody, DAB chromagen, hematoxylin counterstain). All figures are at 40x objective. Bar = 50 μM.

polygonal cells confluent with the surface cells. The neoplastic cells had variably distinct cell borders, moderate amphophilic cytoplasm, round euchromatic nuclei with finely stippled chromatin, and prominent nucleoli. Anisocytosis was moderate (2-3x), and anisokaryosis was marked (4-5x). Mitotic figures averaged 3/10 high-power fields (400x). Scattered throughout the tissue were areas of necrosis with neutrophils, lymphocytes, hemorrhage, and amphophilic-fibrillar material. Neoplastic cells exhibited staining for antibody binding to both cytokeratin and vimentin intermediate filaments.

The pulmonary pleura had multiple focal to extensive, superficial to infiltrative aggregates of moderately pleomorphic polygonal cells. Within the left cranial lung lobe, two vessels (arteries, presumptive) contained the same neoplastic cells as previously noted, proximal to a large area of hemorrhage admixed with cellular debris and fibrin extending to the apex (infarction) with diffuse pleural fibrosis.

Sections of the diaphragm had serosal proliferation and diaphragmatic infiltration by the neoplastic cells described above. Subjacent myocytes were shrunken and hypereosinophilic.

The right adrenal gland was effaced by a large area of necrosis surrounded by highly infiltrative cells as described for the pleural lesion. These extended through the cortical parenchyma with a reactive fibrous connective tissue

proliferation on the outer surface. The zona reticularis was thickened in the left adrenal gland. The histopathologic diagnosis was disseminated pleural mesothelioma with local invasion of the lung; pulmonary arterial emboli; and adrenal, diaphragmatic, and hepatic metastases.

A final diagnosis of mesothelioma with marked thoracic effusion and adrenal metastasis was made based on cellular morphology and coexpression of cytokeratin and vimentin.

3. Discussion

In both the cougar and cheetah, a diagnosis of mesothelioma was made based on cytologic, histologic, and immunohistochemical findings. The cougar was diagnosed with pericardial mesothelioma, which is considered rare in all species, and to the authors' knowledge, this is only the second report of a primary pericardial mesothelioma in a large cat [12]. A diagnosis of disseminated pleural mesothelioma was made in the cheetah. Pleural mesotheliomas in large cats have been reported in both tigers and clouded leopards [8, 12].

While mesothelioma in humans and rats is often associated with asbestos exposure [1], this has yet to be definitively associated with the formation of mesothelioma in domestic and nondomestic animals. A study in dogs found increased levels of asbestos in lung tissues of affected animals versus control dogs; however, this has not been documented in domestic cats [13]. In animals, exposure to asbestos may be only a contributing factor for the development of mesothelioma. Golden retrievers developed pericardial mesothelioma after a long history of idiopathic hemorrhagic pericardial effusion, suggesting that chronic inflammation may also lead to neoplastic transformation [14]. Mesothelial tumors are most often associated with older animals, but reports of dogs as young as 7 weeks of age suggest that a congenital form may also be present [1]. While there is a report of pleural mesothelioma in a female lion housed within an enclosure in which asbestos fibers were found, no fibers were identified in either the lung or neoplastic tissues [7]. Although not definitive, that report suggests that asbestos exposure may lead to mesothelioma formation in animals as well. Additionally, asbestos fibers are small and can be easily cleared, making them difficult to detect within sections of the lung. There was no known exposure to asbestos in either the cougar or cheetah in the present cases.

Both the cheetah and cougar were diagnosed with tricavitary effusion. Possible causes of tri-cavitary effusion include congestive heart failure, hypoproteinemia (renal and liver disease, glomerulonephritis, malabsorption, and parasitism), neoplasia, bacterial peritonitis, feline infectious peritonitis (FIP), pansteatitis, toxoplasmosis, tuberculosis, pregnancy, and trauma. An important diagnostic ruleout in feline species is FIP caused by mutation of FCoV, which affects both wild and domestic cats. Serum that is positive for FCoV is highly suggestive, but not a definitive diagnosis, of FIP [15]. Cheetahs in particular are known to be susceptible to FCoV. Both felids in this report were negative for FCoV.

Intrathoracic masses, such as mesotheliomas, can cause chylothorax due to thoracic duct obstruction, which prevents lymph draining into the vena cava. Chylothorax is an accumulation of lymph in the pleural space; it appears milky and has a high triglyceride and lymphocyte content. This accumulation of fluid in the thorax can in turn cause pulmonary atelectasis, as seen in the cougar in this report. Histologically, within the lung of the cougar were increased numbers of macrophages containing hemosiderin consistent with "heart failure cells," likely a result of restriction due to pericardial fluid accumulation.

The diagnosis of mesothelioma in the cheetah was based on the extensive involvement of the pleura with no evidence of a primary carcinoma elsewhere. While the adrenal involvement raised the possibility of an adrenal carcinoma metastasizing to the pleural cavity with carcinomatosis, at the time of gross examination, the histologic findings supported a diagnosis of mesothelioma rather than carcinoma.

A clinical diagnosis of mesothelioma can be difficult and challenging, as it is mainly a diagnosis of exclusion. Clinical presentation of the cougar and cheetah reported here differed when comparing respiratory status. The cheetah presented in respiratory distress, while the cougar's clinical signs were mild and associated with an increased inspiratory phase only. Both animals had radiographic evidence of bicavitary effusion, which was confirmed at necropsy.

Based on the findings of the cases reported here, mesothelioma should be suspected in patients presenting with chronic, nonspecific disease and fluid accumulation in either the thoracic and/or abdominal cavity. Radiography and ultrasonography are not considered the diagnostic imaging modalities of choice due to the presence of effusion, which will make detection of masses difficult. Thoracic/abdominal computed tomography is more sensitive for identifying nodular lesions in the presence of effusion.

Cytologic evaluation of fluid is of diagnostic value for identification of thoracic disease processes. Although mesothelial cells are commonly identified in fluid, these cells will proliferate in multiple pathologic conditions associated with fluid accumulation in a body cavity. This feature makes it difficult to determine whether the mesothelial cell proliferation is reactive or neoplastic. Cytologic evaluation of thoracic effusion obtained via thoracocentesis in the cougar did not demonstrate mesothelial cells but a lymphocyte-rich effusion and increased numbers of mast cells. In the cheetah, round cells and clusters of cells most likely representing reactive mesotheliocytes with some features of malignancy were identified upon cytologic evaluation of the thoracic fluid. Pericardiocentesis in a Bengal tiger with pericardial mesothelioma yielded an extremely cellular hemorrhagic effusion (specific gravity of 1.033), containing reactive mesothelial cells and erythrocytes [11].

Gross evidence of disease differed between the two cases as well. On necropsy, the cougar's final diagnosis was pericardial mesothelioma, whereas pleural mesothelioma with adrenal metastasis was evident in the cheetah. For the cheetah, adrenal carcinoma metastasizing to the pleural cavity with associated carcinomatosis could not be completely ruled out; however, this is considered unlikely.

Histologically, it is important to differentiate mesothelioma from carcinomas, adenocarcinomas, or sarcomas, based on the morphologic type of mesothelioma. Immunohistochemistry to determine biphasic intermediate filament expression is diagnostically useful in that cytokeratin expression is often positive in mesotheliomas and therefore is helpful in differentiating sarcomatous mesotheliomas from sarcomas [1]. Vimentin expression is of diagnostic value in differentiating epithelial mesothelioma from adenocarcinomas, which are typically vimentin-negative [7]. In both animals of this report, sections of the masses were positive for both cytokeratin and vimentin, which further supports a diagnosis of mesothelioma. Although not performed in these cases, the use of calretinin antibody may be beneficial in differentiating between mesotheliomas and adenocarcinomas. Immunohistochemistry demonstrating the concurrent presence of cytokeratin and vimentin played an important role in the final diagnosis of mesothelioma in both cases. A diagnosis of mesothelioma is based on a tumor associated with the lining of the coelomic cavity, presence/absence of effusion, histopathologic differentiation of cell types, and immunohistochemical staining [1]. In most cases, the etiology of the tumor is unidentified, with affected animals having no known exposure to potential causative agents.

Acknowledgments

The authors thank the carnivore staff at the Knoxville Zoo-logical Gardens and Tiger Haven, Kingston, TN, USA, in particular M. L. Haven and D. Chaffins for their care and assistance with the animals presented in this report.

References

[1] L. Garrett, "Mesothelioma," in *Small Animal Clinical Oncology*, S. Withrow and D. Vail, Eds., pp. 804–808, Elsevier, St. Louis, Mo, USA, 2007.

[2] C. P. Raflo and S. P. Nuernberger, "Abdominal mesothelioma in a cat," *Veterinary Pathology*, vol. 15, no. 6, pp. 781–783, 1978.

[3] A. N. Al-Dissi and H. Philibert, "A case of biphasic mesothe-lioma with osseous and chondromatous differentiation in a cat," *Canadian Veterinary Journal*, vol. 52, no. 5, pp. 534–536, 2011.

[4] B. Bacci, F. Morandi, M. de Meo, and P. S. Marcato, "Ten cases of feline mesothelioma: an immunohistochemical and ultrastructural study," *Journal of Comparative Pathology*, vol. 134, no. 4, pp. 347–354, 2006.

[5] T. M. J. Heerkens, J. D. Smith, L. Fox, and J. M. Hostetter, "Peri-toneal fibrosarcomatous mesothelioma in a cat," *Journal of Vet-erinary Diagnostic Investigation*, vol. 23, no. 3, pp. 593–597, 2011.

[6] Y. Kobayashi, H. Usuda, K. Ochiai, and C. Itakura, "Malignant mesothelioma with metastases and mast cell leukaemia in a cat," *Journal of Comparative Pathology*, vol. 111, no. 4, pp. 453–458, 1994.

[7] E. Bollo, F. E. Scaglione, M. Tursi et al., "Malignant pleural mesothelioma in a female Lion (*Panthera leo*)," *Research in Veterinary Science*, vol. 91, no. 1, pp. 116–118, 2011.

[8] A. A. Cunningham and A. P. Dhillon, "Pleural malignant mesothelioma in a captive clouded leopard: (*Neofelis nebulosa nebulosa*)," *Veterinary Record*, vol. 143, no. 1, pp. 22–24, 1998.

[9] N. S. Shin, S. W. Kwon, D. Y. Kim, O. K. Kweon, I. B. Seo, and J. H. Kim, "Metastatic malignant mesothelioma in a tiger (*Panthera tigris*)," *Journal of Zoo and Wildlife Medicine*, vol. 29, no. 1, pp. 81–83, 1998.

[10] L. P. Tilley, J. M. Owens, R. J. Wilkins, and A. K. Patnaik, "Peri-cardial mesothelioma with effusion in a cat," *Journal of the American Animal Hospital Association*, vol. 11, no. 1, pp. 60–65, 1975.

[11] E. B. Wiedner, R. Isaza, W. A. Lindsay, A. L. Case, J. Decker, and J. Roberts, "Pericardial mesothelioma in a Bengal tiger (*Panthera tigris*)," *Journal of Zoo and Wildlife Medicine*, vol. 39, no. 1, pp. 121–123, 2008.

[12] A. Th. Weiss, A. B. da Costa, and R. Klopfleisch, "Predominantly fibrous malignant mesothelioma in a cat," *Veterinary Medicine International*, vol. 2010, Article ID 396794, 4 pages, 2010.

[13] L. T. Glickman, L. M. Domanski, T. G. Maguire, R. R. Dubielzig, and A. Churg, "Mesothelioma in pet dogs associated with expo-sure of their owners to asbestos," *Environmental Research*, vol. 32, no. 2, pp. 305–313, 1983.

[14] N. Machida, R. Tanaka, N. Takemura, Y. Fujii, A. Ueno, and K. Mitsumori, "Development of pericardial mesothelioma in golden retrievers with a long-term history of idiopathic haem-orrhagic pericardial effusion," *Journal of Comparative Pathol-ogy*, vol. 131, no. 2-3, pp. 166–175, 2004.

[15] L. W. Myrrha, F. M. F. Silva, E. F. Peternelli, A. S. Junior, M. Resende, and M. R. Almeida, "The paradox of feline coronavirus pathogenesis: a review," *Advances in Virology*, vol. 2011, Article ID 109849, 8 pages, 2011.

11

Scleral Rupture Secondary to Idiopathic Non-Necrotizing Scleritis in a Dog

Lori J. Best, Shelley J. Newman, Daniel A. Ward, and Diane V. H. Hendrix

University of Tennessee, 2407 River Drive, Knoxville, TN 37919, USA

Correspondence should be addressed to Daniel A. Ward; dward@utk.edu

Academic Editors: C. Hyun, J. Lakritz, F. Mutinelli, and J. Orós

Background. Canine granulomatous scleritis is an uncommon disease that can be classified as necrotizing or non-necrotizing. Clinical signs associated with scleritis are typically severe, resulting in pain and loss of vision, and response to treatment is often poor. Necrotizing scleritis has been previously associated with scleral rupture. *Case Presentation.* A 10-year-old male castrated Chihuahua was presented for periocular pain, tissue swelling adjacent to the limbus superiorly, chemosis, mild corneal edema and neovascularization adjacent to the superotemporal limbus in the right eye. The left eye was within clinically normal limits. Surgical exploration of the right eye revealed a scleral rupture at the inferonasal aspect of the globe. Histopathology revealed a non-necrotizing granulomatous scleritis with no infectious organisms visualized. Infectious disease testing and special histopathologic staining did not reveal an underlying infectious etiology. *Conclusion.* Granulomatous scleritis is a painful and vision-threatening disease that needs to be treated early and aggressively in order to avoid loss of vision or loss of the eye. Globe rupture secondary to severe non-necrotizing scleritis is an uncommon, but detrimental, clinical manifestation of this disease. This is the first case report of scleral rupture secondary to severe non-necrotizing scleritis and therefore represents a unique and interesting disease manifestation.

1. Background

Scleritis is an uncommon and poorly understood disease process in dogs [1]. The sclera comprises approximately 80% of the fibrous outer portion of the eye and is the posterior continuation of the transparent cornea. The sclera is closely associated with several ocular tissues and for this reason secondary keratitis, conjunctivitis, chorioretinitis, orbital cellulitis, and blepharitis may be seen in cases of primary scleritis [2]. The etiology of canine scleritis is often presumed to be immune-mediated due to the characteristic presence of granulomatous inflammatory infiltrates, response to immunosuppressive therapy, and inability to identify microorganisms by histopathology [3]. Other potential underlying causes of scleritis include *Ehrlichia canis, Onchocerca spp., Toxoplasma gondii,* trauma (including surgical trauma), and extension of panophthalmitis or orbital cellulitis [1, 3, 4]. In humans, granulomatous scleritis is often associated with systemic vascular or autoimmune collagen disorders including rheumatoid arthritis [5], Wegener's granulomatosis [6], and systemic

lupus erythematosus [7]. Some reported cases of scleritis in dogs have tested negative for canine rheumatoid factor, anti-DNA antibody, and LE cell identification, and there has not been a clearly established link between scleritis and systemic autoimmune disease in dogs [8].

Clinical signs associated with canine scleritis include ocular hyperemia, ocular pain, and exophthalmos, as well as clinical signs associated with secondary anterior uveitis, posterior uveitis, conjunctivitis, or keratitis. Clinical signs are frequently unilateral upon initial admission but the disease will often progress to affect the other eye [9]. A definitive diagnosis of scleritis can be achieved histologically with a partial thickness biopsy or after enucleation [10]. Canine scleritis is not well described in the peer-reviewed literature, so it is difficult to accurately determine prognosis. In one series canine scleritis cases showed little improvement with local and systemic immunosuppressive treatment and the prognosis for affected eyes was considered guarded to poor [1].

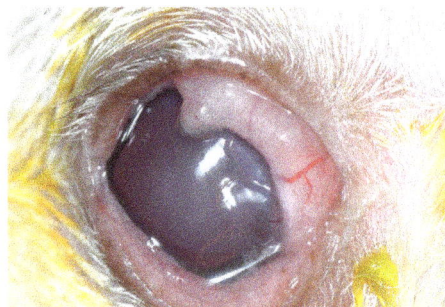

FIGURE 1: Appearance of right eye on initial presentation. Notice fluctuant swelling of the conjunctiva. There is also mild corneal edema and neovascularization.

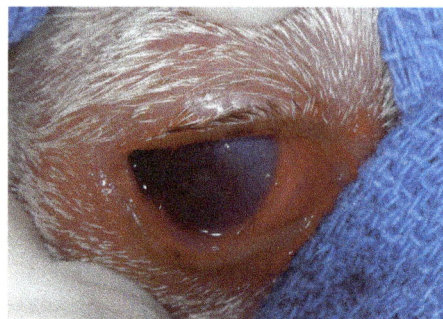

FIGURE 2: Appearance of right eye 2 weeks after initial presentation. Notice severe periorbital swelling, conjunctival hyperemia, and corneal edema and neovascularization.

Histologically, canine scleritis is characterized by a diffuse granulomatous cell infiltrate composed predominantly of tissue macrophages, lymphocytes and plasma cells. In severe cases, the inflammatory cells may completely efface normal scleral tissue [1]. Granulomatous scleritis is further categorized as necrotizing or non-necrotizing based on whether or not there is lysis or merely separation of scleral collagen [9]. In cases of chronic scleritis, thinning of the scleral collagen with subsequent severe staphyloma formation can occur [9]. One review suggests that the scleral degeneration seen with necrotizing scleritis can result in scleral malacia and perforation [11]. Necrotizing scleritis and scleral rupture have been associated with *Ehrlichia canis* [12].

The purpose of this report is to highlight the clinical and histopathological features of a case of presumed immune-mediated non-necrotizing granulomatous scleritis in a dog. This is a unique presentation of the disease because of the associated scleral rupture, and has not been previously reported to the authors' knowledge.

2. Case Presentation

A 10-year-old male castrated Chihuahua was presented to the University of Tennessee College of Veterinary Medicine ophthalmology service for evaluation of blepharospasm, mucoid ocular discharge, and progressive swelling of the superior conjunctiva of the right eye (OD) (Figure 1). There was an approximately 1 week history of blepharospasm, epiphora, chemosis, corneal edema, and a pale yellow nodule on the superonasal conjunctiva that was being treated three times daily with bacitracin/neomycin/polymyxin B/dexamethasone ophthalmic ointment (BNP-Dex) OD. The corneal edema and conjunctival nodule appeared to resolve with BNP-Dex treatment. Diarrhea was noticed by the owners at approximately the same time as the development of blepharospasm. The dog was exposed to a lemur that had been diagnosed with *Yersinia pseudotuberculosis*, had no previous history of ophthalmic or systemic disease, and had no significant travel history.

There were no abnormalities on general physical examination aside from a mild fever of 39.4°C. On ophthalmic examination, pupillary light reflexes and menace responses were normal in both eyes (OU). Schirmer tear tests and intraocular pressures were within normal limits OU and both eyes were negative for fluorescein stain uptake. The left eye (OS) was normal on slit lamp biomicroscopy and indirect ophthalmoscopy. The following abnormalities were observed in the OD: moderate blepharospasm, mucoid ocular discharge, pain on palpation of the periorbital tissues, conjunctival swelling and chemosis, mild corneal edema and neovascularization adjacent to the superotemporal limbus, and mild aqueous flare. The lens, vitreous and fundus were within normal limits OD. Based on the ocular exam findings, an ocular ultrasound was recommended.

Ultrasonographic images were obtained using a 15 MHz linear array probe. An area of hypoechogencity, possibly representing fluid accumulation or a cyst, was identified adjacent to the ventral limbus OD. Potential differential diagnoses for this structure were staphyloma, occult scleral rupture, or conjunctival foreign body with surrounding seroma formation. Based on these findings, periocular exploratory surgery was recommended. The owner declined surgical intervention and opted to continue therapy with BNP-Dex.

The patient was presented 2 weeks later for a recheck examination. At that time a fever of 40.4°C was present and the OD was markedly more uncomfortable compared to the initial visit. The left eye was normal. Severe periorbital swelling and pain were identified OD (Figure 2). Midstromal neovascularization and severe diffuse corneal edema were present in the right cornea, and moderate aqueous flare was present within the anterior chamber OD.

Based on the worsening clinical course, lack of response to treatment, and with differentials that included surgically treatable lesions, the owner consented to surgical exploration of the right periorbital region.

A complete blood cell count, serum biochemistry panel with electrolytes, and urinalysis were submitted prior to anesthesia. The complete blood cell count revealed a neutrophilia of 15.29×10^3/uL (RR: $2.65-9.8 \times 10^3$/uL) and increased band neutrophils of 550/uL (RR: 0–300/uL) consistent with an inflammatory leukogram. A mild hypochromic microcytic anemia was present with a hematocrit of 39.9% (RR: 41%–60%), MCHC of 30.3 g/dL (RR: 34.5–36.3 g/dL), and MCV of 59.2 fL (RR: 62–74 fL). The serum biochemistry panel revealed an increased total protein of 9.5 g/dL (RR: 5.4–6.8 g/dL) with a decreased albumin of 2.0 g/dL (RR:

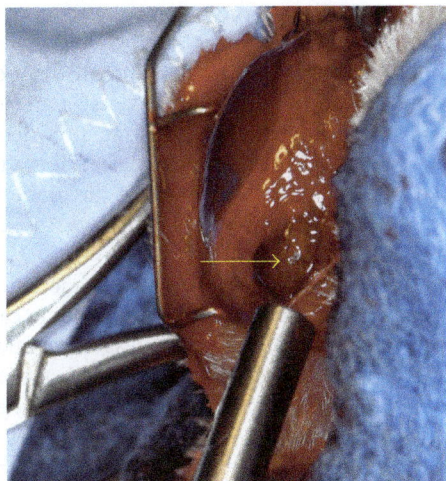

FIGURE 3: Intraoperative appearance. The conjunctiva has been dissected away and uveal tissue can be seen prolapsing through the region of scleral rupture (yellow arrow).

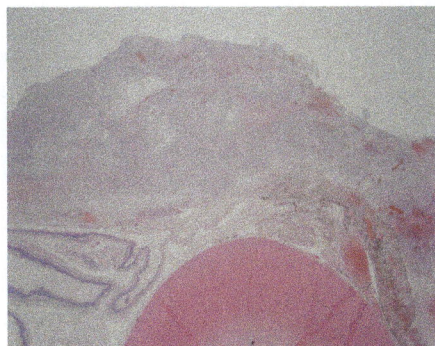

FIGURE 5: At the limbus, a markedly severe multinodular inflammatory infiltrate is present within and expanding from the limbus.

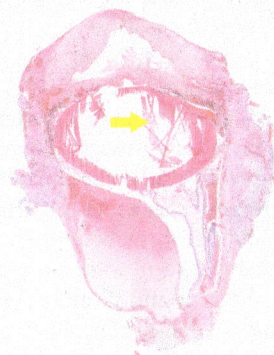

FIGURE 4: Low power view of the globe. The lens is artifactually fragmented (arrow). There is a marked inflammatory response centered at the limbus. In addition, there is retinal detachment and accumulation of fluid in the subretinal space. The cornea is markedly thickened and there is early keratitis.

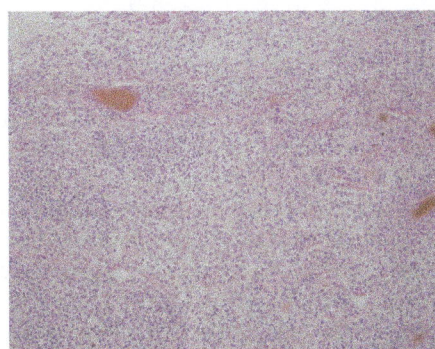

FIGURE 6: The inflammatory infiltrate is distinctive in that it is composed of recurring clusters of neutrophils surrounded by reactive foamy macrophages (pyogranulomas) which coalesce to create the limboscleral inflammation.

3.2–4.1 g/dL) and an increased globulin of 7.5 g/dL (RR: 2–3.2 g/dL). Protein electrophoresis indicated polyclonal gammopathy, indicative of chronic antigenic stimulation.

The patient was placed in sternal recumbency and the right eye was sterilely prepped and draped. A 1 cm lateral canthotomy was made with tenotomy scissors and a 6–0 silk stay suture was placed at the superior limbus. The superior bulbar conjunctiva was then incised approximately 2 mm posterior to the limbus with curved tenotomy scissors and the conjunctiva bluntly dissected with tenotomy scissors while the bulb was rotated inferiorly. Hemorrhagic chemosis, sclerosis, and pockets of fibrinonecrotic material

were encountered throughout the conjunctiva. The periorbital musculature was also noted to be sclerotic. No cystic structures or foreign bodies were encountered superiorly, so exploration was continued nasally and inferonasally. Upon examination of the inferonasal aspect of the globe, a scleral rupture was found at the 4 o'clock position, approximately 3 mm posterior to the limbus (Figure 3). Uveal tissue was herniated through the rupture, and vitreous humor and aqueous humor were leaking from the site. The sclera surrounding the rupture appeared malacic. An attempt to close the scleral rupture was made with 8-0 polyglactin 910 but there was not sufficient normal scleral tissue present to allow suturing. The surgery was then converted to a standard subconjunctival enucleation. The globe was placed in Davidson's solution for fixation and submitted for histopathologic evaluation.

A histologic section of the enucleated globe was made via sagittal section through the entire eye. The tissue sample was stained with hematoxylin and eosin (H&E) and with Masson's trichrome. There was a severe diffuse granulomatous scleritis present, more concentrated at the level of the limbus (Figures 4 and 5). The inflammation was characterized primarily by macrophages that were arranged in aggregates and sheets and accompanied by lymphocytes and fewer neutrophils (Figure 6). In perilimbal regions, the granulomatous infiltrate was more marked and the sclera had an

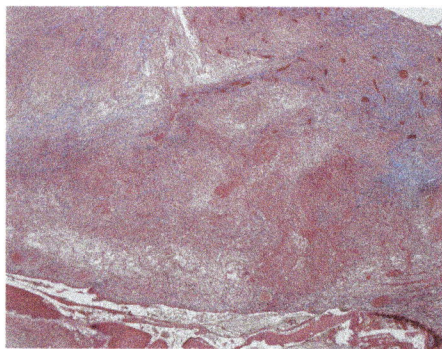

FIGURE 7: Sclera at the limbus. In this Masson trichrome stained section, there is marked separation of collagenous stroma (blue) by the eosinophilic cellular infiltrate. The collagen is not necrotic.

increased thickness, as a result of separation of intact collagen bundles by cellular infiltrate (Figure 7). The corneal stroma was diffusely expanded by edema and there were multifocal small caliber vessels (neovascularization) and scattered neutrophils. The anterior chamber contained red blood cells, neutrophils, epithelioid macrophages, multinucleated giant cells, and fibrin. There was regionally extensive separation of the choroid from the sclera and the cleft was filled with red blood cells and fibrin. The retina was diffusely detached and there was hypertrophy of the retinal pigment epithelium (RPE). Hemorrhage, fibrin, and karyorrhectic debris filled the space separating the retina and RPE. The vitreous chamber contained fibrin and karyorrhectic debris.

Periodic acid-Schiff (PAS) and GMS stains failed to reveal fungi or yeasts and Ziehl-Neelsen (Zn) and Fite's failed to reveal mycobacteria or atypical mycobacteria. A 16sRNA test performed to further rule out infectious causes of scleritis was positive. The cloned PCR products were sequenced, but the sequences did not correlate with any specific microbial species. A conjunctival swab of the right eye was negative for aerobic, anaerobic, and fungal organisms. Urine was negative for blastomyces and histoplasma antigen, and serologies were negative for *E. canis*, *R. rickettsia*, *B. burgdorferi*, and *B. henselae*. Blastomyces and histoplasma agar gel immunodiffusion were both negative and fecal culture for *Yersinia pseudotuberculosis* was also negative. Based on these findings, an infectious cause of granulomatous scleritis was considered highly unlikely.

The patient was discharged the day after surgery on amoxicillin/clavulanic acid oral suspension, carprofen, and omeprazole. The temperature had returned to normal at 39°C. At suture removal 10 days later, the surgical site had healed without complication. On subsequent recheck appointments, the patient's left eye exhibited focal scleral thickening and anterior uveitis that was responsive to an immunosuppressive dose of prednisolone (2 mg/kg/day). The patient also developed ecchymoses on his ventral abdomen. The patient had a normal platelet count, no history of trauma, and normal clotting times when these lesions developed. For this reason, the patient was treated with pentoxifylline for presumptive immune-mediated vasculitis.

3. Conclusions

Canine idiopathic scleritis is an uncommon diagnosis and has been rarely reported [12, 13]. This case represents the first case of scleral rupture secondary to non-necrotizing scleritis to be reported in the peer reviewed literature. The possibility of resultant scleral rupture of the globe in these cases makes early diagnosis and aggressive treatment of utmost importance.

A diagnosis of primary scleritis was made as opposed to scleritis secondary to uveal inflammation because the sclera was affected first clinically and was more affected by granulomatous inflammation than the uvea. Histopathologic findings similar to those reported here have been described in other cases of granulomatous scleritis [13]. A designation of idiopathic granulomatous scleritis was made after special stains failed to reveal the presence of microorganisms and systemic infectious disease tests were negative. This case was further categorized as non-necrotizing scleritis because the characteristic hypereosinophilic staining of collagen seen in necrotizing scleritis was absent [14] and because Masson trichrome staining demonstrated separation of collagen by the inflammatory infiltrate. Although it is not common for canine cases of immune-mediated scleritis to be associated with systemic immune-mediated disease, our case appeared to have evidence of systemic disease.

Scleral thinning has been previously associated with necrotic scleritis and scleritis secondary to *Ehrlichia canis* [12] but antemortem serology in our patient was negative for this agent. Blunt scleral trauma is another cause of scleral rupture. Dogs with scleral rupture secondary to blunt trauma generally present with acute hyphema, subconjunctival hemorrhage, and eyelid or conjunctival swelling [15]. The histological changes seen with blunt trauma include hemorrhage in the anterior and posterior chambers, retinal detachment, choroidal edema, choroidal hemorrhage, and subchoroidal hemorrhage [15]. Our case does not fit with the clinical presentation or histopathologic changes seen with blunt trauma.

Scleral rupture in this case was most likely secondary to scleral thinning and staphyloma formation. The sclera is composed of irregularly arranged collagen and elastic fibers. In scleritis, these fibers are dissected by granulomatous inflammation and in this case the connective tissue fibers were almost completely effaced multifocally. The lack of normal collagen structure creates a weakened focus of sclera where normal intraocular pressure can result in scleral thinning and protrusion of uveal tissue. With severe staphyloma formation, scleral rupture can occur.

Scleral rupture usually results in irreversible vision loss. Cases of scleral rupture secondary to scleritis in dogs have not been well described in the peer-reviewed literature. Surgical repair of these cases is difficult due to the inability of the abnormal sclera to hold suture. Further investigation is warranted to determine the most appropriate treatment and diagnostic recommendation in new cases of scleritis. At this time, it seems most prudent to perform diagnostic tests to rule out infectious causes of scleritis and then institute aggressive immunosuppressive therapy.

Abbreviations

OD: Right eye
OS: Left eye
OU: Both eyes.

Authors' Contribution

Lori J. Best drafted the paper and participated in clinical decision making and case diagnostics. Shelley J. Newman provided interpretation of histopathology and revised paper for appropriate intellectual content. Daniel A. Ward participated in case management and diagnostics and revised paper for appropriate intellectual content. Diane V. H. Hendrix participated in case management, diagnostics, and paper revision.

References

[1] A. R. Deykin, A. Guandalini, and A. Ratto, "A retrospective histopathologic study of primary episcleral and scleral inflammatory disease in dogs," *Veterinary and Comparative Ophthalmology*, vol. 7, pp. 245–248, 1997.

[2] D. J. Maggs, "Cornea and sclera," in *Slatter's Fundamentals of Veterinary Ophthalmology*, D. J. Maggs, P. A. Miller, and R. Ofri, Eds., pp. 175–202, Elsevier Saunders, St. Louis, Mo, USA, 4th edition, 2008.

[3] B. H. Grahn and L. S. Sandmeyer, "Canine episcleritis, nodular episclerokeratitis, sclertitis, and necrotic scleritis," *Veterinary Clinics of North America*, vol. 38, no. 2, pp. 291–308, 2008.

[4] C. L. Martin, "Cornea and sclera," in *Ophthalmic Disease in Veterinary Medicine*, C. L. Martin, Ed., pp. 241–297, Manson, London, UK, 2005.

[5] S. C. Reddy and U. R. K. Rao, "Ocular complications of adult rheumatoid arthritis," *Rheumatology International*, vol. 16, no. 2, pp. 49–52, 1996.

[6] S. L. Harper, E. Letko, C. M. Samson et al., "Wegener's granulomatosis: the relationship between ocular and systemic disease," *Journal of Rheumatology*, vol. 28, no. 5, pp. 1025–1032, 2001.

[7] A. Heiligenhaus, J. E. Dutt, and C. Stephen Foster, "Histology and immunopathology of systemic lupus erythematosus affecting the conjunctiva," *Eye*, vol. 10, no. 4, pp. 425–432, 1996.

[8] B. C. Gilger, O. J. Franck, and E. Bentley, "Diseases and surgery of the canine cornea and sclera," in *Veterinary Ophthalmology*, K. N. Gelatt, Ed., pp. 743–745, Blackwell, Oxford, UK, 2007.

[9] R. R. Dubielzig, K. Ketring, G. J. McLellan, and D. A. Albert, "Granulomatous scleritis, necrotizing scleritis," in *Veterinary Ocular Pathology*, pp. 232–234, Elsevier, 2010.

[10] R. D. Whitley and B. C. Gilger, "Diseases of the canine cornea and sclera," in *Veterinary Ophthalmology*, K. N. Gelatt, Ed., pp. 635–671, Lippincott, Wiliams and Wilkins, Philadelphia, Pa, USA, 3rd edition, 1999.

[11] B. H. Grahn and R. L. Peiffer, "Fundamentals of veterinary ophthalmic pathology," in *Veterinary Ophthalmology*, K. N. Gelatt, Ed., pp. 393–394, Blackwell, Oxford, UK, 2007.

[12] A. A. Komnenou, M. E. Mylonakis, V. Kouti et al., "Ocular manifestations of natural canine monocytic ehrlichiosis (*Ehrlichia canis*): a retrospective study of 90 cases," *Veterinary Ophthalmology*, vol. 10, no. 3, pp. 137–142, 2007.

[13] M. J. Day, J. R. B. Mould, and W. J. Carter, "An immunohistochemical investigation of canine idiopathic granulomatous scleritis," *Veterinary Ophthalmology*, vol. 11, no. 1, pp. 11–17, 2008.

[14] N. Denk, L. S. Sandmeyer, C. C. Lim, B. S. Bauer, and B. H. Grahn, "A retrospective study of the clinical, histological, and immunohistochemical manisfestations of 5 dogs originally diagnosed histologically as necrotizing scleritis," *Veterinary Ophthalmology*, vol. 15, pp. 102–109, 2012.

[15] A. Rampazzo, C. Eule, S. Speier, P. Grest, and B. Spiess, "Scleral rupture in dogs, cats, and horses," *Veterinary Ophthalmology*, vol. 9, no. 3, pp. 149–155, 2006.

12

Atypical Presentation of Constrictive Pericarditis in a Holstein Heifer

Mohamed M. Elhanafy and Dennis D. French

Department of Veterinary Clinical Medicine, Rural Animal Health Management, 1008 W. Hazelwood Drive, 223 Large Animal Clinic, Urbana, IL 61802, USA

Correspondence should be addressed to Mohamed M. Elhanafy, elhanafy@illinois.edu

Academic Editors: L. Arroyo and M. Bugno-Poniewierska

The field diagnosis of constrictive pericardial effusion is often established on the pertinent pathognomonic physical examination findings, but the condition cannot be ruled out based on absence of these cardinal signs. Constrictive pericardial effusion is not always manifested by bilateral jugular venous distention and pulsation, brisket edema, and muffled heart sounds, all of which are considered the key points in the field diagnosis of pericardial effusion and hardware disease. This case will also document that the outcomes of hematology, serum biochemistry panels, and blood gas analysis can be totally inconsistent with passive venous congestion and constrictive pericardial effusion in cattle. Chest radiographic findings revealed radio dense, wire-like objects; the findings were suggestive but not conclusive for pericardial or pleural effusions, due to indistinguishable diaphragmatic outline and cardiopulmonary silhouette. Cardiac ultrasonography was found to be an excellent paraclinical diagnostic procedure for cases that potentially have traumatic pericarditis and constrictive pericardial effusion. Ultrasound-guided pericardiocentesis was also a valuable diagnostic aid in establishing a definitive diagnosis.

1. Introduction

The fundamental task of a veterinarian is making a diagnosis and planning the most effective therapeutic approach. Veterinarians face three challenges on a daily basis: establishing a correct diagnosis, selecting appropriate clinical management, and keeping up to date with useful technological advances [1]. In some instances, routine physical examination fails to detect the clinically significant abnormalities of the body system(s) involved even when conducted by highly skilled practitioners. Additionally, hematology and serum biochemistry are not always effective in determining the disease process, and this lack of specificity renders the diagnosis tentative rather than conclusive.

Diagnostic imaging procedures such as thoracic radiographs or cardiac ultrasonography are not frequently applied in large animal practice due to lack of equipment, time, or economic constraints. These factors limit diagnostic capabilities and may lead to incorrect diagnosis, unnecessary treatments, and the potential for a negative impact on the veterinary-client-patient relationship and unneeded animal suffering.

In large animal patients, this scenario could easily happen with diseases such as constrictive pericarditis or cardiac tamponade. Pericarditis is the most commonly encountered consequence of traumatic reticuloperitonitis in cattle [2] and obtaining a definitive diagnosis can be challenging in certain instances.

It may be assumed that the diagnosis of such cases is often straightforward based on the pertinent cardinal signs and the pathognomonic physical examination findings described in text books such as bilateral jugular venous distention/pulsation, brisket edema, pulmonary edema, and muffled heart sounds [2]. However, variability in history, presenting complaints, physical examination findings, and clinical pathology data often makes the diagnosis somewhat elusive.

This paper describes a challenging, uncommon presentation of constrictive pericarditis in a 9-month-old Holstein heifer and highlights the limitations of routine physical exam, hematology, and serum chemistry in the diagnosis of the disease.

2. Case Presentation

A 9-month-old Holstein heifer was presented to the Veterinary Teaching Hospital, University of Illinois with a three-week history of decreased appetite, decreased fecal output, and intermittent fever. The heifer had been evaluated previously and treated for enzootic pneumonia with oxytetracycline followed by ceftiofur and finally enrofloxacin.

Upon presentation, the heifer was bright, alert, and responsive and had normal ambulation. Rectal temperature was 40.3°C [104.5°F] (reference range 37.8–39.2°C; 100–102.5°F). The respiratory rate was 36 breaths/minute (reference range 24–36 breaths/minute) with an abdominal respiratory pattern. Chest auscultation revealed audible moist rales over the middle third of lung fields bilaterally and high-pitched, hissing rhonchi dorsally. It was noted that there was a slight abduction of both elbows. The heart rate was 72 beats/minute (reference range 55–80 beats/minute) with normal rhythm. Cardiac sounds were barely audible and were overwhelmed by the breathing sounds. The withers pinch test appeared to be normal and no jugular distention or pulsation was detected. Furthermore, the brisket was of normal size and consistency. She appeared slightly dehydrated based on her eye recession. The rumen was completely atonic, the intestines were hypomotile, and the rectum was full of firm dry feces upon rectal exam.

Complete blood count revealed leukocytosis (15.3 × 10^3/uL; reference range 4.0–12.0 × 10^3/uL) with neutrophilia (12.3 × 10^3/uL; reference range 0.6–4.0 × 10^3/uL) and monocytosis (963/uL; reference range 25–800/uL).

Serum chemistry profile showed decreased albumin (1.8 gm/dL; reference range 2.1–3.6 gm/dL) and increased globulin (5.0 gm/dL; reference range 3.6–4.5 gm/dL). Hepatic enzymes and renal values were within normal limits. There was moderate hypocalcemia (7.5 mg/dL; reference range 9.7–12.4 mg/dL), hypokalemia (3.6 mmol/L; reference range 3.9–5.8 mmol/L), hypochloremia (91 mmol/L; reference range 95–100 mmol/L), and hyponatremia (130 mmol/L; reference range 132–152 mmol/L).

Based on the arterial blood gas analysis the heifer was neither hypoxic nor hypercapnic, with moderate alkalosis (pH 7.54; reference range 7.35–7.50). The P_aO_2 (103.0 mm Hg; reference range 85–105 mm Hg), P_aCO_2 (29.9 mm Hg; reference range 34–45 mm Hg), oxygen saturation (98.0%; reference range 97–99% at sea level), and the blood l-lactate (0.9 mmol/L; reference range up to 2.9 mmol/L) were within normal limits.

To rule out pulmonary disease, thoracic radiographs were taken. Images revealed a round circumscribed mass measuring approximately 2.4 × 1.8 cm with a fluid line and a large area of gas dorsally. This mass was superimposed over the cardiac region. Multiple small, round to irregular, gas opacities could be seen throughout the ventral aspect of the thorax. A diffuse interstitial to alveolar pattern was observed on the caudal lung lobes as well as one thin metallic

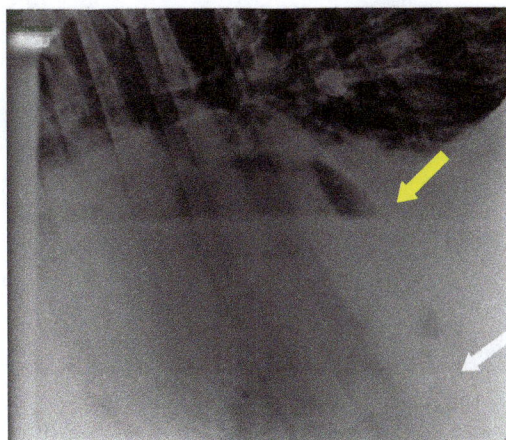

FIGURE 1: Laterolateral radiograph showing circumscribed mass with a fluid line and an area of gas shadows dorsally superimposing in the cardiac region (yellow arrow), thin opaque foreign material in the region of the caudal thorax (white arrow).

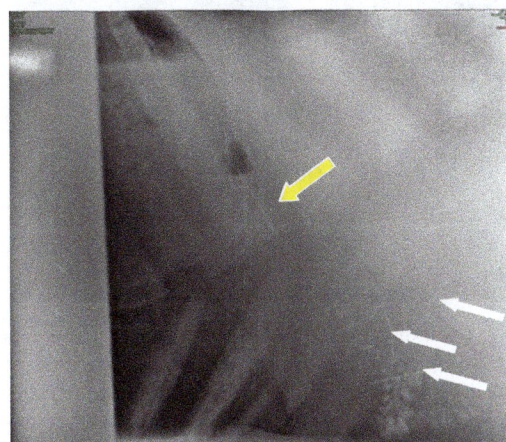

FIGURE 2: Laterolateral radiograph taken at the level of the reticulum and diaphragm. The intrathoracic foreign body and gas shadows could be seen cranial to the reticulum (yellow arrow). The lung and diaphragm could not be differentiated because of the increased soft tissue opacity. Three thin metallic opaque foreign bodies could be seen in the cranial epigastric abdomen in the region of the reticulum (white arrows).

opaque foreign object in the region of the caudal thorax (Figure 1). Three thin metallic opaque foreign bodies were also noted in the cranial abdomen in the region of the reticulum (Figure 2).

Ultrasound was used to better characterize the thoracic mass identified on radiographs. The ultrasonographic evaluation of the left hemithorax revealed moderate-to-large amounts of hypoechoic fluid within the ventral pleural space. Multiple hyperechoic, linear, undulating projections were imaged throughout the pleural cavity indicating chronic fibrinous pleurisy (Figure 3). The surface of pericardium was rugged, with multiple hyperechoic linear pericardial projections imaged throughout, indicative of chronic inflammatory changes with fibrin strand deposition (Figure 4). A large

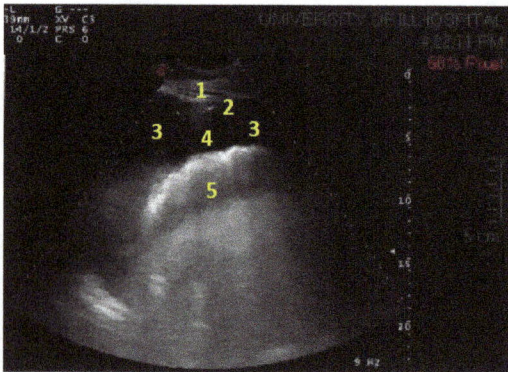

FIGURE 3: Ultrasonogram of the left thorax at the seventh intercostal space using a 3.5 MHz convex transducer showing pleural effusion. 1: thoracic wall; 2: costal pleura; 3: pleural effusion; 4: fibrin strands; 5: lung.

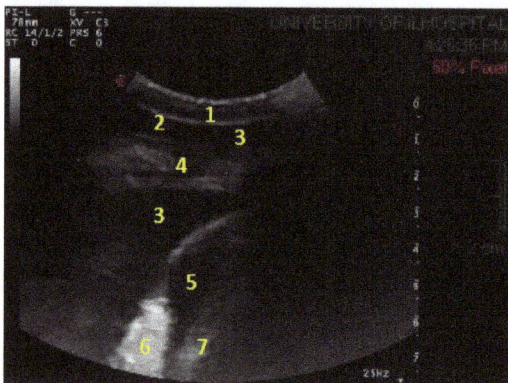

FIGURE 5: Ultrasonogram of pericardial effusion obtained by 3.5 MHz convex transducer placed in the distal fifth intercostal space on the left thorax. 1: thoracic wall; 2: thickened pericardium; 3: massive hypoechogenic pericardial effusion; 4: fibrin strands; 5: ventricular wall.

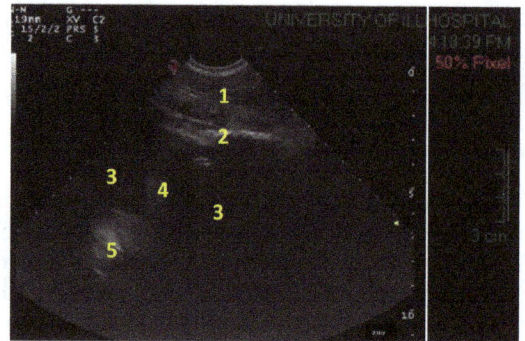

FIGURE 4: Ultrasonogram of pericardial effusion with strands of fibrin on the epicardium obtained by 3.5 MHz convex transducer placed in the fifth intercostal space on the left thorax. 1: thoracic wall; 2: parietal pleura; 3: pleural effusion; 4: lung 5: hypoechogenic pericardial effusion; 6, thickened pericardium with fibrin strands; 7, atrial wall.

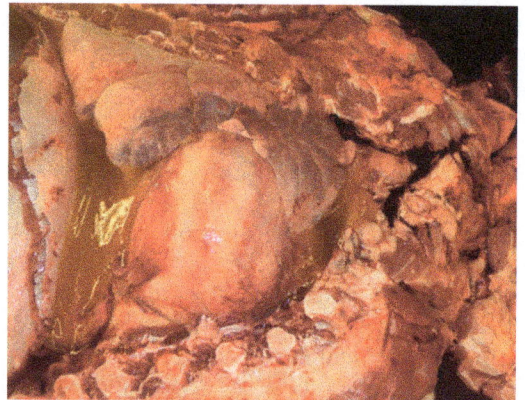

FIGURE 6: Postmortem image of the thoracic cavity showing severely distended pericardium displacing the lung dorsally and yellow gelatinous material within the pleural cavity.

hypoechoic area with irregular margins was also observed in the cranioventral thorax. This was thought to be a massive pericardial effusion that made the evaluation of the cardiac silhouette difficult (Figure 5). Free echogenic fibrin strands were occasionally detected floating within the epicardium.

Ultrasound-guided pericardiocentesis was aseptically performed using a 3-inch 18-gauge needle inserted into the lower third of the 4th intercostal space. It yielded a turbid, gray-colored fluid that contained 4.5 gm/dL (reference range < 2.5 gm/dL) total protein.

Based upon the protracted history of the case, radiographic and ultrasound images and the character of the fluid obtained via pericardiocentesis, a grave prognosis for use and life was made. The owner elected for humane euthanasia and the heifer was submitted for necropsy.

The gross pathology revealed approximately 8 liters of clear yellow fluid in the pleural cavity mixed with yellow gelatinous material (Figure 6). Portions of the ventral aspects of the left and right lungs were adhered to the diaphragm, pericardium, and ventral aspect of the thorax. The intercostal,

sternal, cranial and caudal mediastinal, and tracheobronchial lymph nodes were diffusely enlarged. The pericardium was severely distended, displacing the lung dorsally (Figure 6). Several portions of the pericardium were tightly adhered to the adjacent diaphragm and ventral aspect of the thorax. The pericardial cavity contained approximately 7 liters of clear yellow malodorous fluid admixed with moderate amounts of tan to white friable material. The parietal pericardium was severely thickened measuring approximately 2.5 cm. The pericardial sac and was totally lined by a large mat of thick yellow fibrinous material (Figure 7). Several small to moderately sized abscesses were scattered throughout the abdominal wall, thoracic wall, liver, and reticular serosa. One of the abscesses located on the diaphragmatic surface of the left lobe of the liver contained a thin black 6 cm wire (Figure 8). A similar wire was found free in the reticulum.

3. Discussion

Constrictive pericarditis or cardiac tamponade is the abnormal accumulation of exudate in the pericardial sac. It is the most common sequelae of hardware disease in cattle caused

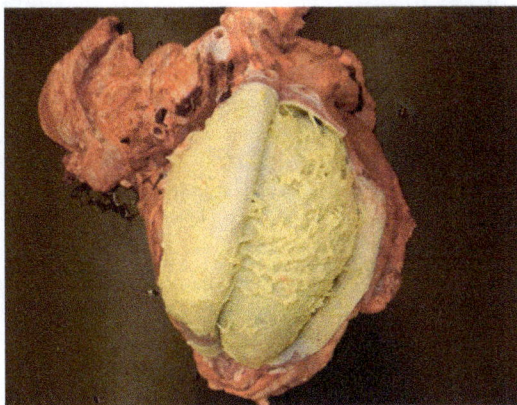

FIGURE 7: Postmortem image of the heart and pericardial sac, which has been opened. Note that the heart is covered with yellow fibrin.

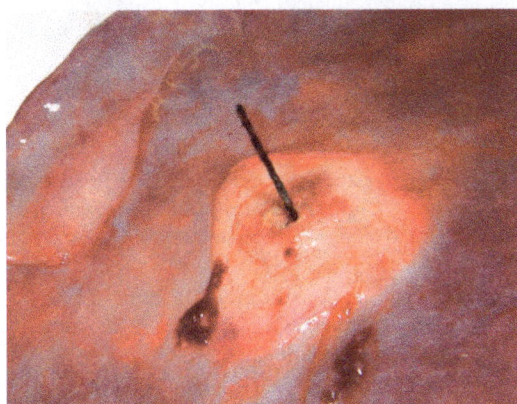

FIGURE 8: Postmortem image revealing a thin black 6 cm wire penetrating the diaphragmatic surface of the left lobe of the liver.

by traumatic perforation of the wall of the reticulum by a sharp foreign body [2]. The classic presentation of constrictive pericarditis has been described in standard text books [2] and some recent case reports [3–5] as muffled heart sounds, bilateral jugular venous distention/pulsation, along with brisket, and pulmonary edema. Brisket edema has been reported to be the most common symptom associated with pericarditis. In 27 out of 40 clinical cases of traumatic pericarditis in water buffaloes, edema of the brisket was recorded as a clinical sign and 37 of the 40 animals had constrictive pericardial effusion on postmortem examination [6]. However, none of these signs were observed in this case despite the presence of voluminous constrictive pericardial effusion recorded by ultrasonography and observed on postmortem examination. The absence of the clinical symptoms considered typical for the disease syndrome made arriving at the final diagnosis challenging.

Constrictive pericardial effusion is expected to lead to the development of generalized venous congestion and edema, as it impairs venous return to the heart. Auricular compression is usually inevitable in the course of the events [2, 4, 7]. Accordingly, some authors [4] related the degree of jugular congestion and brisket edema to the degree of pericardial

effusion. This case presentation illustrates that cardiac tamponade may not always be manifested by venous congestion and brisket edema: the heifer had neither of these signs as part of her physical examination findings. The lack of these signs may have been associated with compensation by cardiac reserve. These compensatory responses comprise the redistribution of the blood flow and increased heart rate [2]. An elevation of heart rate alone is a significant factor in increasing cardiac output and maintaining circulatory equilibrium. It has been documented that cattle can increase their heart rate to four times their resting values [2]. For the case presented here, the heart rate was still normal at presentation suggesting the heart was able to compensate for the pericardial restriction through mechanisms such as increased contractility. Given the severity of the pericarditis, it was surprising that the heart rate was normal. Accumulation of 7 liters of exudate in the pericardial sac would be expected to create sufficient intrapericardial pressure to cause collapse of auricles. However, the fibrinous adhesions between epicardium and the parietal pericardium at the level of the atria may have added extra support to the auricular wall, apparently preventing the collapse.

Muffled heart sounds usually indicate pericardial effusion [8] while heart sound audibility does not rule out pericardial effusion. It has been previously reported that 21 of 28 clinical cases of pericarditis in cows had audible heart sounds on both sides of the chest even though they had pericardial effusion [9]. Fifteen out of 40 reported clinical cases of traumatic pericarditis in water buffaloes had audible heart sounds [6].

In most literature, γ-glutamyltransferase (γ-GT), aspartate aminotransferase (AST) activities, and serum bilirubin concentration were found to be increased with hepatic congestion and right-sided heart failure [10]. Furthermore a strong correlation has been established between liver enzymes activities, especially γ-GT, in cattle and right-sided cardiac insufficiency which indicated that the increased γ-GT is usually a sign of liver congestion and not one of primary liver disease. It has also been reported that some cattle with right-sided cardiac insufficiency were often misdiagnosed with liver disease because of elevated liver enzyme activities, even though they may have had jugular vein distension on clinical examination [10].

For this case, the serum biochemistry liver enzymes were within normal limits. This indicates the animal had not progressed to the point of having significant hepatic venous congestion. The animal's cardiovascular system was still able to compensate for the significant pericardial effusion.

Arterial blood gas analysis was of limited diagnostic value in this case. It revealed the P_aO_2, P_aCO_2, oxygen saturation and the blood l-lactate concentrations to be within normal values. Arterial blood gas is not useful for definitely diagnosing pericarditis but it has some value in being able to rule out a significant loss of functional lung capacity as might occur with diffuse bronchopneumonia, severe pleural effusion, or extensive pulmonary edema.

The anatomical and physiological features of the respiratory system of cattle predispose them to the development of hypoxia faster and more profoundly than other farm animal species [2]. The bovine lung is relatively smaller than other farm animals in relation to the animal size. The ratio of tidal volume to lung volume is much lower in cattle when compared to other large animals such as horses. Cattle also have a small physiological gaseous exchange capacity [11].

Therefore, the 8 liters of pleural fluid effusion in addition to the dorsal displacement of the lung by pericardial distention with 7 liters of fluid would have been expected to build up serious compression atelectasis, ventilation failure, and anoxic anoxia. The respiratory rate on this heifer was assessed to be in the high normal range, but it was difficult to appreciate significant lung disease on physical examination and her P_aO_2 levels were found to be within the normal range.

Radiographs are a helpful diagnostic tool for traumatic reticuloperitonitis with some limitations. The size of the animal makes it challenging to obtain a conclusive radiograph with clear thoracic details. The lack of available equipment in field situations and even in teaching hospitals precludes routine use. In addition, transportation of most bovine patients to a suitable radiology unit may require animal sedation which may further compromise the animal. Furthermore, positioning the animal for imaging requires a team effort and increases risks for handling personnel and potential for excessive radiation exposure.

Definitive diagnosis of this condition by radiography can only be achieved when a foreign body is found perforating the cranial reticular wall and diaphragm (Figure 1), or is located close to the region of the reticulum (Figure 2). A published report [12] suggested that observation of traumatic perforation of the pericardium with radiographs is definitive in only one out of five clinical cases. Chest radiographic findings were suggestive, but not conclusive for pericardial or pleural effusions, due to indistinguishable diaphragmatic outline and cardiopulmonary silhouette.

Cardiac ultrasonography has been suggested as the method of choice for imaging and evaluating the severity of constrictive pericardial effusion [13–15]. Early diagnosis by ultrasonography will prevent unnecessary treatment or animal suffering. In most cases, a large amount of hypoechogenic fluid is seen in the thorax, sometimes containing strands or free clots of fibrin (Figures 4 and 5). In the case presented here, a poor prognosis was concluded based upon the severe disease identified via ultrasonography. The presence of large quantities of fibrin with massive pericardial effusion has been suggested as an important prognostic parameter in cases of pericarditis in human beings [16] and also in cattle [2]. Ultrasound-guided pericardiocentesis was an additional valuable tool that lead to a conclusive diagnosis.

References

[1] O. M. Radostits, I. G. Mayhew, and D. M. Houston, "Making diagnosis," in *Veterinary Clinical Examination and Diagnoses*, pp. 11–52, Elsevier Saunders, Philadelphia, Pa, USA, 1st edition, 2000.

[2] O. M. Radostits, C. C. Gay, K. W. Hinchcliff, and P. D. Constable, "Diseases of the pericardium," in *Veterinary Medicine: A Textbook of the Diseases of Cattle, Horses, Sheep, Pigs, and Goats*, pp. 430–432, Elsevier Saunders, Philadelphia, Pa, USA, 10th edition, 2007.

[3] E. W. Fisher and H. M. Pirie, "Traumatic pericarditis in cattle: a clinical, physiological and pathological study," *British Veterinary Journal*, vol. 121, no. 12, pp. 552–567, 1965.

[4] S. A. Jesty, R. W. Sweeney, B. A. Dolente, and V. B. Reef, "Idiopathic pericarditis and cardiac tamponade in two cows," *Journal of the American Veterinary Medical Association*, vol. 226, no. 9, pp. 1502–1558, 2005.

[5] J. Laureyns, S. de Vliegher, I. Kolkman, L. Vandaele, and A. de Kruif, "Traumatic pericarditis with "steel band-effect" sounds in a young heifer," *Vlaams Diergeneeskundig Tijdschrift*, vol. 74, no. 2, pp. 146–148, 2005.

[6] S. Fubini and T. J. Divers, "Noninfectious diseases of the gastrointestinal tract," in *Rebhun's Diseases of Dairy Cattle*, pp. 130–199, Elsevier Saunders, St. Louis, Mo, USA, 2nd edition, 2007.

[7] T. Mohamed, "Clinicopathological and ultrasonographic findings in 40 water buffaloes (*Bubalus bubalis*) with traumatic pericarditis," *Veterinary Record*, vol. 167, no. 21, pp. 819–824, 2011.

[8] L. Roth and J. M. King, "Traumatic reticulitis in cattle: a review of 60 fatal cases," *Journal of Veterinary Diagnostic Investigation*, vol. 3, no. 1, pp. 52–54, 1991.

[9] U. Braun, B. Lejeune, G. Schweizer, M. Puorger, and F. Ehrensperger, "Clinical findings in 28 cattle with traumatic pericarditis," *Veterinary Record*, vol. 161, no. 16, pp. 558–563, 2007.

[10] U. Braun, "Traumatic pericarditis in cattle: clinical, radiographic and ultrasonographic findings," *Veterinary Journal*, vol. 182, no. 2, pp. 176–186, 2009.

[11] G. J. Gallivan, W. N. McDonell, and J. B. Forrest, "Comparative pulmonary mechanics in the horse and the cow," *Research in Veterinary Science*, vol. 46, no. 3, pp. 322–330, 1989.

[12] S. Imran, S. P. Tyagi, A. Kumar, A. Kumar, and S. Sharma, "Ultrasonographic application in the diagnosis and prognosis of pericarditis in cows," *Veterinary Medicine International*, vol. 2011, Article ID 974785, 10 pages, 2011.

[13] U. Braun, M. Flückiger, and F. Nägeli, "Radiography as an aid in the diagnosis of traumatic reticuloperitonitis in cattle," *Veterinary Record*, vol. 132, no. 5, pp. 103–109, 1993.

[14] T. Moeller, "Clinical and ultrasonographic findings in a cow with pericarditis and ascites -a case report," *Praktische Tierarzt*, vol. 78, no. 5, pp. 403–405, 1997.

[15] S. Buczinski, "Cardiovascular ultrasonography in cattle," *Veterinary Clinics of North America*, vol. 25, no. 3, pp. 611–632, 2009.

[16] M. M. Lewinter, "Pericardial diseases," in *Brunwald's Heart Disease, A Textbook of Cardiovascular Medicine*, P. Libby, R. O. Bonow, D. L. Mann, and D. P. Zipes, Eds., pp. 1829–1854, Saunders, Philadelphia, Pa, USA, 8th edition, 2007.

13

Use of Contrast-Enhanced MR Angiography (CE-MRA) for the Diagnosis of a Vascular Ring Anomaly in a Dog

Silke Hecht, April M. Durant, William H. Adams, and Gordon A. Conklin

Department of Small Animal Clinical Sciences, C247 Veterinary Medical Center,
University of Tennessee College of Veterinary Medicine, 2407 River Dr., Knoxville, TN 37996, USA

Correspondence should be addressed to Silke Hecht, shecht@utk.edu

Academic Editors: C. Hyun and G. Mazzullo

A 4-month-old female mixed breed dog was presented to the University of Tennessee College of Veterinary Medicine with a history of regurgitation and cachexia. Thoracic radiographs revealed focal megaesophagus cranial to the heart base. Magnetic resonance imaging (MRI) was performed. True fast imaging with steady-state precession (TrueFISP), fast low angle shot (FLASH), and short tau inversion recovery (STIR) sequences were acquired prior to contrast medium administration. Contrast-enhanced magnetic resonance angiography (CE-MRA) demonstrated focal megaesophagus and position of the aortic arch to the right of the esophagus. A small ductus diverticulum and an indistinct linear soft tissue band crossing the esophagus were also noted. Surgical exploration confirmed MR diagnosis of a persistent right aortic arch (PRAA) with left ligamentum arteriosum. The dog improved following surgery but was unable to be transitioned to dry food. To our knowledge this is the first report describing the use of CE-MRA for preoperative diagnosis and guided surgical treatment of a vascular ring anomaly in a dog.

1. Introduction

Persistent right aortic arch (PRAA) is the most common vascular ring anomaly in dogs, but other types have been reported and may require a different surgical approach [1]. A definitive diagnosis prior to surgical intervention is desirable to minimize prolonged anesthesia and associated complications. This report describes the successful preoperative diagnosis of a PRAA with left ligamentum arteriosum by means of contrast-enhanced MR angiography (CE-MRA).

2. Case Presentation

A 4-month-old female mixed breed dog, weighing 6.1 kg, was referred to the University of Tennessee College of Veterinary Medicine for evaluation of regurgitation and poor body condition despite a ravenous appetite. A minimum database prior to referral included a complete blood count (CBC) and biochemical profile. There were no significant abnormalities noted on CBC. Biochemical abnormalities included hyperphosphatemia (8.4 mg/dL, reference range 2.9–6.6 mg/dL), hyperglycemia (114 mg/dL, reference range 60–110 mg/dL), hypoproteinemia (5.2 g/dL, reference range 5.4–8.2 g/dL), and hypoglobulinemia (1.5 g/dL, reference range 2.3–5.2 g/dL). On presentation the dog was bright and alert with a body condition score of 2/5. All vital parameters were normal.

Right lateral and ventrodorsal thoracic radiographs were obtained. A dilated mostly gas-filled structure depressing the trachea ventrally consistent with focal megaesophagus was noted cranial to the cardiac silhouette on the right lateral view (Figure 1(a)). On the VD view, there was moderate uniform widening of the cranial mediastinum with the aortic arch located within the right aspect of the cranial mediastinum and the trachea located on midline and deviated to the left at the level of the aortic arch (Figure 1(b)). No additional abnormalities were detected.

MRI was performed using a 1.0 Tesla MR system (Magnetom Harmony; Siemens Medical Solutions, Malvern, PA, USA) to further characterize the suspected vascular ring anomaly. Pre- and postcontrast (Magnevist, Bayer Health-Care Pharmaceuticals Inc., Wayne, NJ, USA; 0.2 mmol/kg

(a)

(b)

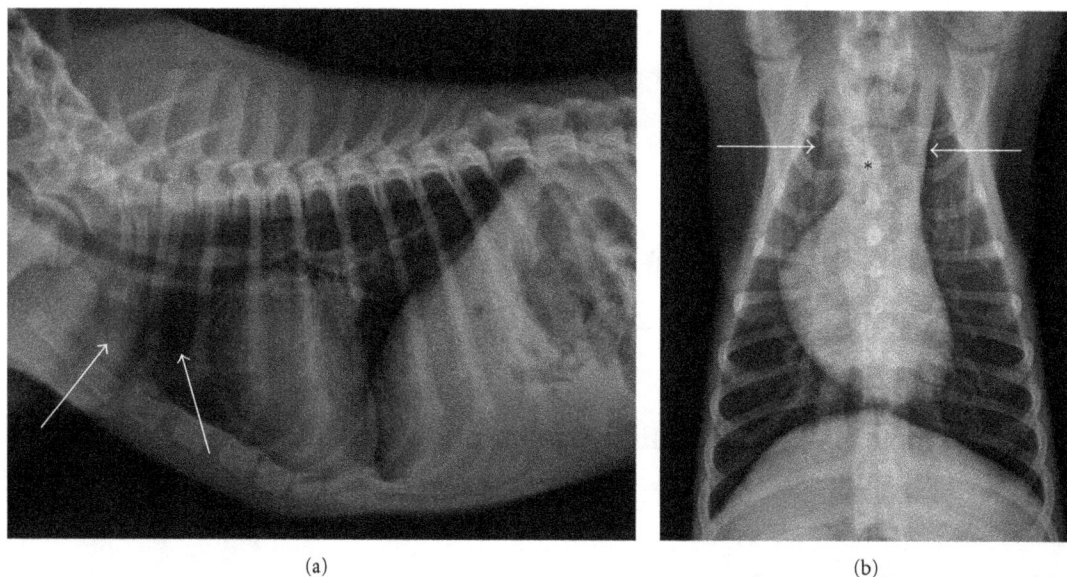

FIGURE 1: Right lateral (a) and ventrodorsal (b) radiographs of the thorax. A dilated mostly gas-filled structure (arrows) consistent with focal megaesophagus is present cranial to the cardiac silhouette on the lateral view (a). On the VD view (b) the aortic arch is located within the right aspect of the cranial mediastinum (∗), the trachea is displaced to the left at the level of the aortic arch, and there is mild widening of the cranial mediastinum (arrows).

TABLE 1: Magnetic resonance imaging parameters.

Pulse sequence	Slice thickness (mm)	Time of repetition (ms)	Time of echo (ms)	Number of averages	Time of inversion (ms)	Flip angle
Transverse TrueFISP	5	6.8	3.4	2		70
Dorsal TrueFISP	3	8.72	4.36	2		70
Sagittal TrueFISP	3	8.72	4.36	2		70
Transverse FLASH 2D	4	433	7.49	1		70
Transverse T2 STIR	5	7070	106	1	145	150
Immediate postcontrast sagittal FLASH 3D (CE-MRA)	1	5.25	2.29	1		30
Delayed postcontrast dorsal FLASH 3D (CE-MRA)	1.5	6.41	3.38	1		10

TrueFISP: true fast imaging with steady-state precession; FLASH: fast low angle shot; STIR: short tau inversion recovery; CE-MRA: contrast enhanced-magnetic resonance angiography.

IV) sequences were obtained, including true fast imaging with steady state precession (TrueFISP), fast low angle shot (FLASH 2D); T2 STIR, and contrast-enhanced angiography (CE-MRA) (immediate and delayed FLASH 3D) (Table 1). The cranial thoracic esophagus was moderately dilated with fluid and gas. The aortic arch and cranial descending aorta were located along the right aspect of the trachea and esophagus (Figure 2(a)), resulting in leftward displacement of these structures. A thin linear band of tissue was present extending from the cranial descending aorta leftward immediately caudal to the level of maximum esophageal dilation (Figure 2(b)). On maximum intensity projection (MIP) of CE-MRA data, there was no evidence of blood flow through the linear structure; however, there was a small focal dilation of the proximal descending aorta consistent with a ductus

diverticulum (Figure 2(c)). 3D reconstructed images of CE-MRA data were less helpful than anticipated due to inability to visualize nonvascular structures such as trachea and esophagus and resultant difficulties in anatomic orientation. An MR diagnosis of persistent right aortic arch with left ligamentum arteriosum and focal megaesophagus was made, and the owners opted for surgical correction.

The patient was placed in right lateral recumbence and prepared for a left thoracotomy. A left fifth thoracotomy was performed and a persistent right aortic arch with left ligamentum arteriosum was confirmed surgically. The mediastinum was bluntly dissected from the left lateral wall of the esophagus in the region of the stricture. The ligamentum arteriosum was bluntly dissected and double ligated. An oroesophageal tube was passed through the strictured region

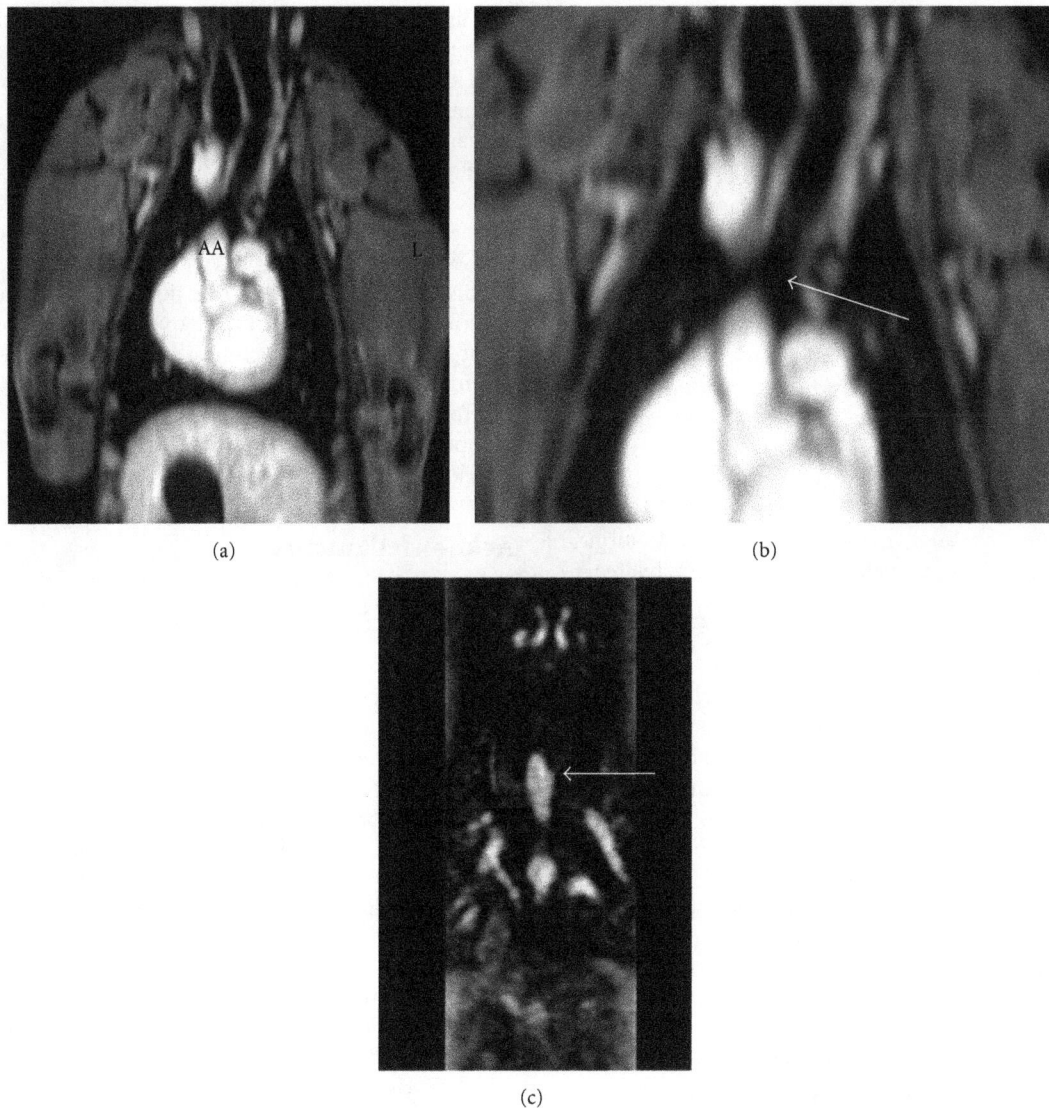

FIGURE 2: CE-MRA images demonstrating persistent right aortic arch with left-sided ligamentum arteriosum and focal megaesophagus. Dorsal plane image (a) shows the location of the aortic arch (AA) on the right and displacing the trachea (T) and dilated esophagus (E) to the left. An indistinct linear soft tissue band extends leftward from the proximal descending aorta immediately caudal to the area of maximum esophageal dilation ((b); arrow) consistent with the left ligamentum arteriosum. Dorsal maximum intensity projection reconstructed image at the level of the cranial descending aorta (c) demonstrates a small focal left-sided dilation of the aorta consistent with the ductus diverticulum (arrow). There is no evidence of blood flow through the ligamentum arteriosum.

to identify any remaining fibrous bands of the ligamentum arteriosum. The thoracotomy was closed routinely. Postsurgical recovery was uneventful. The following day blenderized food was offered in a raised position, and the patient was held in an upright position for 15 minutes after eating. The dog had an excellent appetite and did not exhibit any signs of regurgitation while in the hospital. The owner was instructed to continue elevated feedings with a blenderized diet for 2–4 weeks, with a gradual taper to a dry diet. Instructions to gradually decrease the height of the food bowl were also provided.

A telephone interview with the owner was conducted 8 weeks following surgery. The patient had gained weight,

however, regurgitation resumed during attempts to transition to a dry diet. Follow-up radiographs by the referring veterinarian confirmed continued focal megaesophagus. The patient is currently maintained and asymptomatic on a mash diet that is fed slightly elevated.

3. Discussion

Persistent right aortic arch (PRAA) is a vascular ring anomaly where the right 4th arch, rather than the left 4th, is retained to form the aorta [1]. The presence of a left ligamentum arteriosum, connecting the pulmonary artery to the right aortic arch, results in compression of the esophagus which in turn leads to retention of food and esophageal dilation. The most common clinical signs related to a PRAA are regurgitation, poor body condition, and occasionally coughing, stridor and dyspnea [1]. Clinical signs tend to be noted during the weaning period, and regurgitation occurs shortly after the introduction of solid foods.

PRAA accounts for 95% of all cardiovascular ring anomalies [1–3]. Other vascular ring anomalies include double aortic arch, persistent right ductus arteriosus, aberrant left subclavian artery, aberrant right subclavian artery, and persistent right dorsal aorta. The majority of these anomalies can be identified surgically with a left lateral thoracotomy. However, aberrant right subclavian artery, double aortic arch, or right ductus arteriosus may require an approach via a right lateral thoracotomy [4]. An incorrect surgical approach increases surgical time and morbidity related to postoperative pain and risk of infection. A definitive diagnosis of the type of vascular ring anomaly prior to surgical intervention therefore may decrease morbidity related to prolonged surgical techniques.

A presumptive diagnosis of PRAA is based on historical information and clinical findings. Common radiographic abnormalities that support the diagnosis include enlargement of the cranial mediastinum due to focal megaesophagus, ventral deviation of the trachea cranial to the cardiac silhouette, leftward deviation of the trachea, and absence of the normal left-sided bulge of the ascending aorta [1, 2]. An esophagram may confirm the presence of focal megaesophagus with evidence of esophageal stricture at the level of the heart base but is unable to delineate vascular structures. Angiography may be useful in detection of atypical vascular rings and may aid in the decision of the best surgical approach [1, 3]. However, it is difficult to discern the three-dimensional anatomic relationships of a vascular ring anomaly with two-dimensional images.

Advanced imaging techniques have improved the ability to definitively diagnose vascular ring anomalies. Computed tomography (CT) and magnetic resonance imaging (MRI) are the imaging modalities of choice in human patients with suspected vascular ring anomalies [5]. CT angiography (CTA) has been used successfully in the diagnosis of vascular ring anomalies in dogs [6–8]. While a diagnosis of a persistent right aortic arch is easily made with CTA, identification of a left ligamentum arteriosum is difficult as blood flow through the ligamentum is rarely present [1, 6, 7]. A similar difficulty was encountered when performing contrast-enhanced MR angiography (CE-MRA) in our patient; 3D reconstructed images of CE-MRA data were less helpful than anticipated due to lack of visualization of nonvascular structures such as trachea and esophagus and lack of blood flow through the ligamentum arteriosum, compromising anatomic orientation. We found delayed postcontrast FLASH 3D images most helpful in evaluating thoracic structures. Diagnosis of persistent right aortic arch with left ligamentum arteriosum and focal megaesophagus was based on identification of the relative positions of the aortic arch, trachea, esophagus, and a small ductus diverticulum. A small soft tissue band thought to represent

the ligamentum arteriosum was only indistinctly visible. In contrast, successful identification of a left ligamentum arteriosum with MRI has been documented in a human pediatric case, likely facilitated by larger patient size and a higher magnetic field strength system used [9].

Eight weeks following surgery, the patient was unable to be transitioned to a dry diet. However, the dog was asymptomatic when being fed a mash diet, and the owner was pleased with the outcome. A persistent megaesophagus as in this dog was noted in 13/25 dogs following surgical correction of PRAA [10]. In the same study, 92% of dogs had complete resolution of clinical signs, whereas 8% of dogs improved but had occasional episodes of regurgitation.

To the authors' knowledge this is the first report of preoperative confirmation of a PRAA with left ligamentum arteriosum using magnetic resonance angiography in a dog.

Acknowledgments

This case was presented as a poster at the EVDI Annual Scientific Conference, July 21st–25th 2010, Giessen, Germany.

References

[1] T. VanGundy, "Vascular ring anomalies," *Compendium Small Animal Practice*, vol. 11, pp. 36–45, 1989.

[2] J. W. Buchanan, "Tracheal signs and associated vascular anomalies in dogs with persistent right aortic arch," *Journal of Veterinary Internal Medicine*, vol. 18, no. 4, pp. 510–514, 2004.

[3] M. L. Helphrey, "Vascular ring anomalies in the dog," *Veterinary Clinics of North America—Small Animal Practice*, vol. 9, no. 2, pp. 207–218, 1979.

[4] G. W. Ellison, "Vascular ring anomalies in the dog and cat," *Compendium on Continuing Education for the Veterinary Practitioners*, vol. 2, pp. 693–705, 1980.

[5] L. B. Haramati, J. S. Glicksiein, H. J. Issenberg, N. Haramati, and G. A. Crooke, "MR imaging and CT of vascular anomalies and connections in patients with congenital heart disease: significance in surgical planning," *Radiographics*, vol. 22, no. 2, pp. 337–349, 2002.

[6] S. Pownder and P. V. Scrivani, "Non-selective computed tomography angiography of a vascular ring anomaly in a dog," *Journal of Veterinary Cardiology*, vol. 10, no. 2, pp. 125–128, 2008.

[7] H. Joly, M. A. D'Anjou, and L. Huneault, "Imaging diagnosis—CT angiography of a rare vascular ring anomaly in a dog," *Veterinary Radiology and Ultrasound*, vol. 49, no. 1, pp. 42–46, 2008.

[8] C. R. Henjes, I. Nolte, and P. Wefstaedt, "Multidetector-row computed tomography of thoracic aortic anomalies in dogs and cats: patent ductus arteriosus and vascular rings," *BMC Veterinary Research*, vol. 7, Article ID 57, 2011.

[9] C. H. Zachary, J. L. Myers, and K. D. Eggli, "Vascular ring due to right aortic arch with mirror-image branching and left ligamentum arteriosus: complete preoperative diagnosis by magnetic resonance imaging," *Pediatric Cardiology*, vol. 22, no. 1, pp. 71–73, 2001.

[10] M. M. Muldoon, S. J. Birchard, and G. W. Ellison, "Long-term results of surgical correction of persistent right aortic in dogs: 25 cases (1980–1995)," *Journal of the American Veterinary Medical Association*, vol. 210, no. 12, pp. 1761–1763, 1997.

14

A Case of Contagious Ecthyma (Orf Virus) in a Nonmanipulated Laboratory Dorset Sheep (*Ovis aries*)

Gwynne E. Kinley, Connie W. Schmitt, and Julie Stephens-Devalle

Veterinary Services Program, Walter Reed Army Institute of Research/Naval Medical Research Center, 511 Robert Grant Avenue, Silver Spring, MD 20910, USA

Correspondence should be addressed to Julie Stephens-Devalle; j.stephensdevalle@us.army.mil

Academic Editors: L. G. Papazoglou and M. Pizarro

An approximately 5-month-old laboratory wether, originating from a local vendor with a closed flock and maintained on a preventative medicine plan, presented with a continuum of lesions from hemorrhagic papules, vesicles, and pustules, to multifocal necrotic scabs at the commissure of the lips, medial canthus of the left eye, and distal prepuce. A presumptive diagnosis of Orf virus (ORFV) was made and the sheep was euthanized. A full necropsy was performed, and histopathological evaluation of affected tissues revealed multifocal-to-coalescing necrotizing and proliferative cheilitis and dermatitis with eosinophilic intracytoplasmic inclusion bodies. Electron microscopy findings revealed degenerate keratinocytes containing numerous typical 200–300 nm wide cytoplasmic parapoxvirus virions, confirming the diagnosis of ORFV. We believe that this animal developed a clinical case of ORFV either due to an adverse reaction to an ORFV vaccine, or this animal had a case of preexisting ORFV which manifested after arrival at our facility.

1. Case History and Presentation

On June 13, 2012, an approximately 5-month-old, 24 kg, Dorset wether (*Ovis aries*) was introduced to our facility from a local vendor. Upon arrival, this animal was determined to be healthy based on history, general health, and physical exam. The health certificate that accompanied the animal indicated it had been examined and was clinically free of ORFV, keratoconjunctivitis, contagious foot-rot, and scabies. The WRAIR/NMRC protocol requires all wethers to be sheared, docked, negative for Q fever and ORFV, and dewormed prior to shipment. This animal was acclimated in our vivarium. During the first four days of the acclimation period, the sheep displayed no abnormal behavioral or clinical signs. It demonstrated a healthy appetite and was fed *ad libitum* Rumilab diet 5508 (LabDiet supplier, Quality Lab Products, Elkridge, MD, USA), Timothy Hay (Kaytee Products, Inc., Chilton, WI, USA), and received water *ad libitum*. This Dorset sheep was pair-housed in a standard large animal aluminum run with polyvinyl chloride- (PVC-) coated steel mesh floor racks. The environment was maintained at 68 to 72 degrees F, with a relative humidity range of 30 to 70% and a 12 : 12-hour light : dark cycle. Environmental enrichment was provided in accordance with institute standard operating procedures. All animal handling and husbandry were performed by trained personnel, and the facility was maintained according to accepted animal care and use standards [1]. The sheep was procured for a protocol reviewed and approved by the WRAIR/NMRC Institutional Animal Care and Use Committee (IACUC). WRAIR/NMRC is fully accredited by the Association for the Assessment and Accreditation of Laboratory Animal Care International. Five days after its arrival at our vivarium, the sheep presented with a continuum of lesions from hemorrhagic papules, vesicles, and pustules to multifocal necrotic scabs at the commissure of the lips, medial canthus of the left eye, and distal prepuce. A presumptive diagnosis of ORFV was made, and the sheep was euthanized and submitted to the WRAIR/NMRC Department of Pathology (Silver Spring, MD, USA) to confirm ORFV.

2. Analysis and Findings

A complete necropsy was performed, and sections of the affected haired skin at the mucocutaneous junctions of the

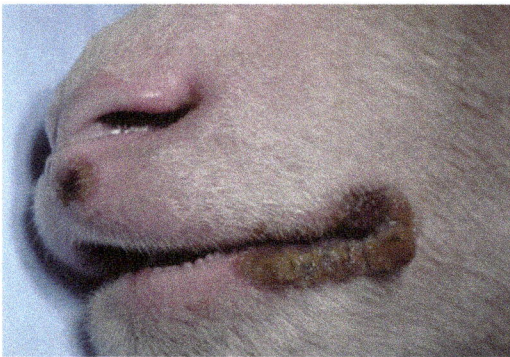

FIGURE 1: Left lips and philtrum. Multifocal-to-coalescing necrotizing and proliferative cheilitis and dermatitis.

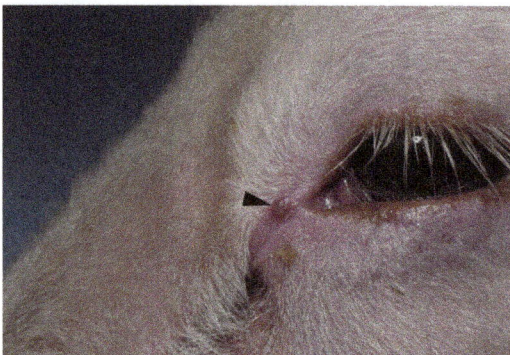

FIGURE 2: Left palpebrae, medial canthus. Focal hemorrhagic pustule (arrowhead).

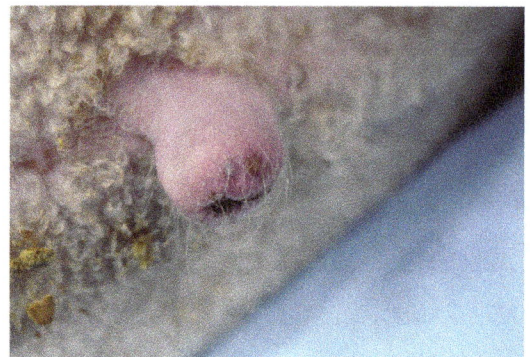

FIGURE 3: Prepuce. Multifocal necrotizing and proliferative posthitis.

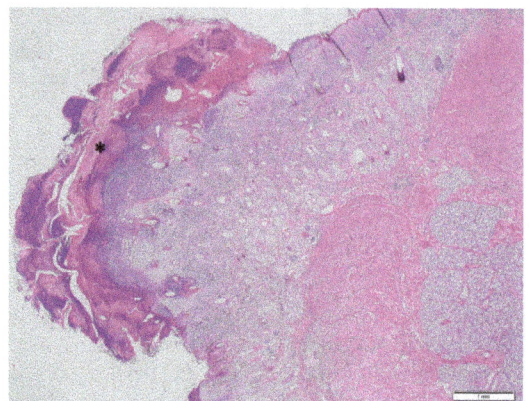

FIGURE 4: Haired skin, lip commissure. Focally extensive, severe, proliferative, and necrotizing dermatitis, with epithelial hyperplasia, necrosis and loss with replacement by a serocellular crust (∗). Hematoxylin and eosin stain, 2x objective.

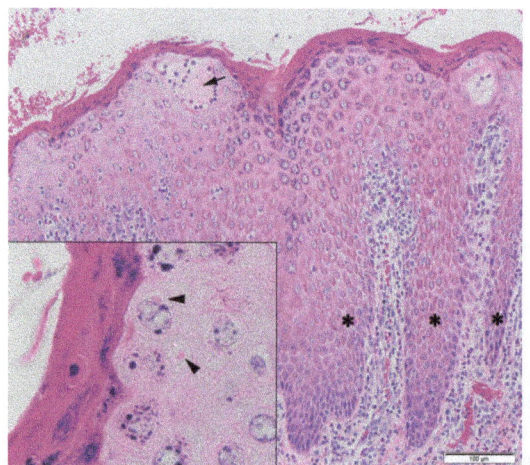

FIGURE 5: Haired skin, lip commissure. Epithelial hyperplasia (∗) with increased thickness up to 10 times normal (acanthosis) with prominent intracellular clear spaces/bridging (spongiosis), anastomosing rete ridges, and a vesicle (arrow). Inset: rarely keratinocytes contain one or more 2–10 μm round, brightly eosinophilic intracytoplasmic inclusion bodies (arrowheads). Hematoxylin and eosin stain, 20x objective.

lips, left eye, and prepuce were submitted for histopathological evaluation. Significant gross necropsy findings included scattered hemorrhagic papules, vesicles, pustules, and numerous multifocal-to-coalescing proliferative and necrotizing scabs affecting haired skin at the mucocutaneous junctions (commissures) of the lips, extending into and affecting the oral papillae, the medial canthus of the left eye, and the distal prepuce (Figures 1, 2, and 3). There were no other significant gross lesions to suggest an underlying immunocompromising condition.

All tissues for histologic assessment were fixed in 10% neutral buffered formalin and routinely processed as 5 μm thick paraffin sections and stained with hematoxylin and eosin stain (H&E). The haired skin at the mucocutaneous junction of the lips (Figures 4, 5, and 6) revealed multifocal epithelial hyperplasia with increased thickness up to 10 times normal (acanthosis) and elongated, anastomosing rete ridges. Multifocally within the epithelium, there was prominent intracellular bridging (spongiosis), neutrophilic inflammation, and multifocal vesicles. Multifocally, the keratinocytes were swollen and often contained clear intracytoplasmic vacuoles (ballooning degeneration) and pyknotic nuclei. Rarely keratinocytes contained one or more 2–10 μm round, brightly eosinophilic intracytoplasmic inclusion bodies. Focally extensive, the epidermis exhibited erosion, loss and

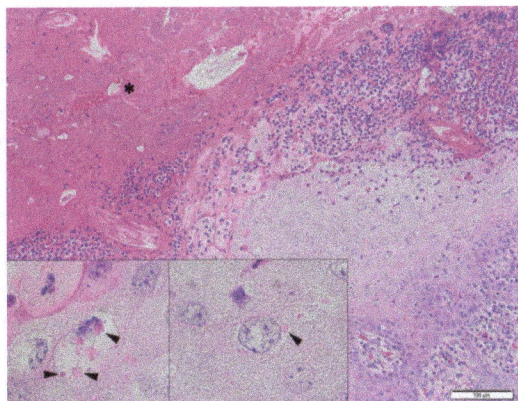

FIGURE 6: Haired skin, lip commissure. Epithelial hyperplasia, necrosis, and loss with overlying serocellular crust (*) composed of keratin, proteinaceous fluid, degenerate neutrophils, and numerous mixed bacteria. Insets: rarely keratinocytes demonstrate large clear cytoplasmic vacuoles (ballooning degeneration) (left) and contain one or more 2–10 μm round, brightly eosinophilic intracytoplasmic inclusion bodies (left and right, arrowheads). Hematoxylin and eosin stain, 20x objective.

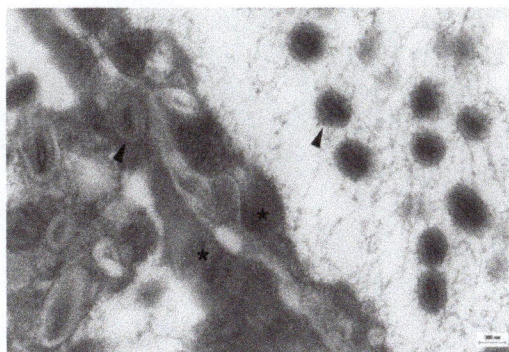

FIGURE 7: Lip. Two keratinocytes with adjacent degenerate cell membranes (*) contain numerous 200–300 nm brick-shaped virions (arrowheads) free within the cytoplasm. Virions show typical parapoxvirus characteristics of an inner core surrounded by an intermediate coat further bounded by an envelope. Transmission electron microscope, lead citrate and uranyl acetate. Bar = 300 nm.

replacement by a thick serocellular crust composed of keratin, proteinaceous fluid, degenerate neutrophils, necrotic cellular debris, and numerous mixed bacteria. Within the subjacent dermis, there were numerous dilated small caliber blood vessels separated by edema, fibrin, and moderate numbers of perivascular and perifollicular neutrophils, histiocytes, and lymphocytes.

All tissues for transmission electron microscopy evaluation were fixed in 4% glutaraldehyde, postfixed in 2% osmium tetroxide, dehydrated ethanol, and embedded in Epon 812 (Electron Microscopy Sciences, Hatfield, PA, USA). Ultrathin sections (70–90 nm) were contrasted with lead citrate and uranyl acetate and examined with a Jeol 100CX II electron microscope. Ultrastructurally, the haired skin at the lip revealed degenerate keratinocytes containing numerous typical 200–300 nm wide cytoplasmic parapoxvirus virions (Figure 7).

3. Discussion

Contagious ecthyma, also called contagious pustular dermatitis, ecthyma contagiosum, and scabby mouth, is a zoonotic disease, called Orf in humans, with worldwide distribution that affects sheep, goats, wild artiodactyls, and man [2–14]. The causative agent is a double-stranded DNA virus that is a member of the family Poxviridae, subfamily Chordopoxvirinae, genus *Parapoxvirus* [2, 4, 6–10, 13, 15]. ORFV gains entry through abraded skin and replicates in epidermal cells [2, 4, 7–10, 13, 14]. Skin lesions progress in an orderly fashion through multiple stages: erythema, macule, papule, vesicle, pustule, scab, and scar [2–7, 9–11, 13, 14]. Infection is confined to the squamous epithelium and may involve the oral cavity, eyelids, teats, and coronary band, subsequently predisposing affected animals to secondary infections [2–7, 9–11, 13, 14]. Rarely, lesions extend to the squamous

epithelium of the esophagus, rumen, and omasum, causing ulcerative gastroenteritis [2, 3, 5, 16]. Residual skin lesions are not infective once the scab falls off, but substantial amounts of infective virus are shed within scabs which can remain infective in the environment for years [2, 4–9, 13]. The disease has high morbidity and low mortality but can cause significant debilitation due to the inability of affected animals to suckle or graze [5, 7–11]. Nursing animals often transfer the virus to adults, typically affecting the teats and udder [2, 4, 5, 7, 8, 10–12, 14]. There are several approved commercial vaccines for ORFV which contain virulent virus [9, 11]. These vaccines are valuable because they limit the severity of disease. The purpose of the vaccine is to produce a lesion at the vaccine site, thus inducing immunity; however, this also causes virus shedding and can contribute to maintenance of infective virus within the environment. Thus, the ORFV vaccine is only recommended for use in endemically infected herds [9, 11].

Gross lesions are characterized by multifocal to coalescing proliferative and ulcerative dermatitis which is localized to the squamous epithelium at mucocutaneous junctions, particularly around the mouth and nares [2, 4–6, 10, 12]. Histologic lesions are characterized by marked epidermal hyperplasia, ballooning degeneration, and eosinophilic intracytoplasmic inclusion bodies within keratinocytes that are only briefly detectable at the vesicular stage [2, 4, 5, 9, 10, 14]. There are frequently superimposed bacterial infections in the affected skin [11]. Ultrastructurally, the cytoplasmic inclusions contain numerous 200–300 nm wide brick-shaped virions typical of parapoxviruses with the characteristic inner core surrounded by an intermediate coat further bounded by an envelope [17].

Sheep previously exposed to ORFV can be repeatedly infected, although the severity of the lesions and time to resolution diminish with each subsequent infection [2, 7, 9, 11]. This indicates that the host immune response can control the severity of disease but cannot prevent reinfection [7]. The reason is partially due to the presence of immunomodulatory proteins expressed by ORFV that suppress elements of the host immune and inflammatory response [3, 6–9, 18]. These immunomodulatory proteins produce a variety of effects, such as protecting the virus from the antiviral effects of interferons, thus allowing viral replication, or inhibiting the biological activity of important immune system cytokines and suppressing inflammation [3, 6–9, 13, 18].

4. Conclusions

According to the limited information from the vendor, this animal originated from a closed flock on site and was subject to the facility's preventive medicine management plan. All sheep receive daily health checks for any abnormalities. Lambs were born on site receive vaccines (BarVac CD/T, Boehringer Ingelheim Vetmedica, St. Joseph, MO, USA, and Scabivax Forte, MSD Animal Health, Summit, NJ, USA) and are dewormed for intestinal parasites. All animals at this vendor remain at the facility their entire life until being sold or used on a protocol.

According to the ORFV vaccine manufacturer's product data sheet, a successful vaccination known as—a "take"—results in vaccine site (axilla or behind the elbow in ewes and lambs) erythema 1–14 days after vaccination, with vesicles and pustules approximately 3–14 days after vaccination. Rupture of the vesicles and pustules, with subsequent scab formation, can be expected from about 7 days after vaccination [19]. The time of exposure to ORFV in the environment and the appearance of clinical signs are about 4 to 14 days, which is similar to that of ORFV vaccine clinical signs [2].

This vaccine is similar to the smallpox vaccine in humans, whereby a live virus (vaccinia virus) is inoculated and a "take" is determined to be a successful correlate of immunity. Generalized vaccinia and progressive vaccinia following vaccination by this live vaccine are among the recognized adverse reactions in immunosuppressed humans [20–23]. They result from blood-borne dissemination of the virus, and lesions emerge 6–9 days after vaccination [20–23]. Although the exact timing of vaccination at the vendor's facility could not be determined in this case, based on this animal's history, clinical signs, histopathological evaluation, and electron microscopy results, we believe that this animal developed a clinical case of ORFV either due to an adverse reaction from the ORFV vaccine, or this animal simply had a case of preexisting ORFV, the severity of which may or may not have been affected by vaccination at the vendor's facility. Contributing factors to either scenario are the stress of transport and new environmental surroundings that likely resulted in immunosuppression of this animal with subsequent ORFV disease manifestations.

Standard procedures taken by a facility after a positive ORFV case is identified should include euthanasia of all animals in direct contact with the positive case, as well as decontamination of the premises. In this case, this animal's penmate was euthanized. Within our facility, all animal rooms are routinely cleaned and disinfected between animal shipments with Sani-Plex 128, a quaternary ammonium chloride (Quip Labs, Wilmington, DE, USA) and Chlordet, a potassium hydroxide mixture (Quip Labs, Wilmington, DE, USA) by

trained personnel wearing proper personal protective equipment (PPE). All removable husbandry and enrichment items are autoclaved. All uneaten food is discarded. All direct contact with animals is conducted by trained personnel wearing disposable PPE consisting of water resistant coveralls, shoe covers, hair bonnet, mask, and gloves.

Research facilities that work with ORFV-susceptible species that will potentially become immunosuppressed, stressed, or undergo significant surgical alteration as part of experimental protocols should consider using animals originating for ORFV-free facilities to prevent potential complications associated with this organism since substantial amounts of infective ORFV are shed within scabs that can remain infective in the environment for years [2, 4–9, 13].

Abbreviations

ORFV: Orf virus
WRAIR/NMRC: Walter Reed Army Institute of Research/Naval Medical Research Center.

Disclaimer

Material has been reviewed by the Walter Reed Army Institute of Research. There is no objection to its presentation and/or publication. The opinions or assertions contained herein are the private views of the author, and are not to be construed as official, or as reflecting true views of the Department of the Army or the Department of Defense. The authors declare no competing interests. Research was conducted in compliance with the Animal Welfare Act and other federal statutes and regulations relating to animals and experiments involving animals and adheres to principles stated in the *Guide for the Care and Use of Laboratory Animals*, 8th edition [1].

Conflict of Interests

The authors declare no potential conflict of interests with respect to the research, authorship, and/or publication of this paper.

Acknowledgments

The authors wish to thank the following individuals from the WRAIR/NMRC Veterinary Services Program: Ms. Marcia Caputo, for animal husbandry and health records; Mr. Michael Proctor, for histologic preparations; Mr. Edward Asafo-Adjei, for electron microscopy; Mr. Bartholomew Taylor and Mr. Matthew Wise, for photography and imaging; and Dr. Jennifer Chapman and Dr. Paul Facemire for technical review.

References

[1] Institute for Laboratory Animal Research, *Guide for the Care and Use of Laboratory Animals*, National Academies Press, Washington, DC, USA, 8th edition, 2011.

[2] D. E. Anderson, D. M. Rings, and D. G. Pugh, "Diseases of the integumentary system," in *Sheep and Goat Medicine*, D. G. Pugh, Ed., pp. 203–204, W.B. Saunders Company, Philadelphia, Pa, USA, 1st edition, 2002.

[3] D. Deane, C. J. Mcinnes, A. Percival et al., "Orf virus encodes a novel secreted protein inhibitor of granulocyte-macrophage colony-stimulating factor and interleukin-2," *Journal of Virology*, vol. 74, no. 3, pp. 1313–1320, 2000.

[4] H. B. Gelberg, "Alimentary system and the peritoneum, omentum, mesentery, and peritoneal cavity," in *Pathologic Basis of Veterinary Disease*, J. F. Zachary and M. D. McGavin, Eds., pp. 326–327, Elsevier, St. Louis, Mo, USA, 5th edition, 2012.

[5] P. E. Ginn, J. E. K. L. Mansell, and P. M. Rakich, "Skin and appendages," in *Jubb, Kennedy, and Palmer's Pathology of Domesic Animals*, M. G. Maxie, Ed., vol. 1, pp. 664–666, Elsevier, Philadelphia, Pa, USA, 5th edition, 2007.

[6] D. M. Haig, "Subversion and piracy: DNA viruses and immune evasion," *Research in Veterinary Science*, vol. 70, no. 3, pp. 205–219, 2001.

[7] D. M. Haig, "Orf virus infection and host immunity," *Current Opinion in Infectious Diseases*, vol. 19, no. 2, pp. 127–131, 2006.

[8] D. M. Haig, C. J. Mcinnes, J. Thomson, A. Wood, K. Bunyan, and A. Mercer, "The orf virus OV20.0L gene product is involved in interferon resistance and inhibits an interferon-inducible, double-stranded RNA-dependent kinase," *Immunology*, vol. 93, no. 3, pp. 335–340, 1998.

[9] D. M. Haig and A. A. Mercer, "Orf," *Veterinary Research*, vol. 29, no. 3-4, pp. 311–326, 1998.

[10] A. M. Hargis and P. E. Ginn, "The integument," in *Pathologic Basis of Veterinary Disease*, J. F. Zachary and M. D. McGavin, Eds., p. 1023, Elsevier, St. Louis, Mo, USA, 5th edition, 2012.

[11] F. A. Murphy, E. P. J. Gibbs, M. C. Horzinek, and M. J. Studdert, "Poxviridae," in *Veterinary Virology*, pp. 289–291, Academic Press, San Diego, Calif, USA, 3rd edition, 1999.

[12] C. B. Navarre, M. Q. Lowder, and D. G. Pugh, "Oral-esophageal diseases," in *Sheep and Goat Medicine*, D. G. Pugh, Ed., pp. 66–67, W.B. Saunders Company, Philadelphia, Pa, USA, 1st edition, 2002.

[13] L. J. Savory, S. A. Stacker, S. B. Fleming, B. E. Niven, and A. A. Mercer, "Viral vascular endothelial growth factor plays a critical role in orf virus infection," *Journal of Virology*, vol. 74, no. 22, pp. 10699–10706, 2000.

[14] I. R. Tizard, "Regulation of adaptive immunity," in *Veterinary Immunology*, p. 217, Elsevier, St. Louis, Mo, USA, 9th edition, 2013.

[15] International Committee on Taxonomy for Viruses, "Virus Taxonomy: 2012 release (current)," http://www.ictvonline.org/virusTaxonomy.asp?version=2012&bhcp=1.

[16] J. F. Zachary, "Mechanisms of microbial infections," in *Pathologic Basis of Veterinary Disease*, J. F. Zachary and M. D. McGavin, Eds., p. 210, Elsevier, St. Louis, Mo, USA, 5th edition, 2012.

[17] N. F. Cheville and H. Lehmkuhl, "Cytopathology of viral diseases," in *Ultrastructural Pathology: The Comparative Cellular Basis of Disease*, pp. 318–327, Wiley-Blackwell, Danvers, Mass, USA, 2nd edition, 2009.

[18] Z. Lateef, S. Fleming, G. Halliday, L. Faulkner, A. Mercer, and M. Baird, "Orf virus-encoded interleukin-10 inhibits maturation, antigen presentation and migration of murine dendritic cells," *Journal of General Virology*, vol. 84, no. 5, pp. 1101–1109, 2003.

[19] MSD Animal Health United Kingdom, "Scabivax Forte Data Sheet," 2012, http://www.msd-animal-health.co.uk/products_public/scabivax_forte/product_data_sheet.aspx.

[20] J. J. Esposito and F. Fenner, "Poxviruses," in *Virology*, pp. 2885–2916, Lippincott Williams and Wilkins, Philadelphia, Pa, USA, 4th edition, 2001.

[21] D. A. Henderson, T. V. Inglesby, J. G. Bartlett et al., "Smallpox as a biological weapon: medical and public health management," *Journal of the American Medical Association*, vol. 281, no. 22, pp. 2127–2137, 1999.

[22] D. J. McClain, "Smallpox," in *Textbook of Military Medicine*, pp. 539–559, Office of the Surgeon General, Borden Institute, Washington, DC, USA, 1997.

[23] J. G. Breman and D. A. Henderson, "Diagnosis and management of smallpox," *New England Journal of Medicine*, vol. 346, no. 17, pp. 1300–1308, 2002.

15

Presumptive Ischemic Brain Infarction in a Dog with Evans' Syndrome

Angelo Pasquale Giannuzzi, Antonio De Simone, Mario Ricciardi, and Floriana Gernone

"Pingry" Veterinary Hospital, Via Medaglie d'Oro 5, 70126 Bari, Italy

Correspondence should be addressed to Mario Ricciardi; ricciardi.mario@alice.it

Academic Editor: Changbaig Hyun

A ten-year-old neutered female mixed breed dog was referred for pale mucous membrane and acute onset of right prosencephalic clinical signs. Brain magnetic resonance imaging was suggestive for right middle cerebral artery ischemic stroke. Based on cell blood count, serum biochemistry and serologic tests and flow cytometric detection of anti-platelets and anti-red blood cells antibodies, a diagnosis of immunomediated haemolytic anemia associated with thrombocytopenia of suspected immunomediated origin was done. Immunosuppresive therapy with prednisone was started and the dog clinically recovered. Two months later complete normalization of CBC and serum biochemistry was documented. The dog remained stable for 7 months without therapy; then she relapsed. CBC revealed mild regenerative anemia with spherocytosis and thrombocytopenia. A conclusive Evans' syndrome diagnosis was done and prednisone and cyclosporine treatment led to normalization of physical and CBC parameters. The dog is still alive at the time the paper submitted. Possible thrombotic etiopathogenetic mechanisms are illustrated in the paper and the authors suggest introducing Evans' syndrome in the differential diagnosis list for brain ischemic stroke in dogs.

1. Case History

A ten-year-old neutered female mixed breed dog, weighing 8,5 Kg (18,7 lbs), was referred to Pingry Veterinary Hospital (Bari, Italy) because of acute onset of disorientation and inability to stand the day before the clinical evaluation. On owner's opinion the clinical signs were improving and at the moment of the evaluation the dog was able to deambulate. General physical examination revealed pale mucous membrane with normal refill time. Systolic arterial blood pressure recorded by Doppler ultrasonography was 140 mm Hg. On neurological exam the dog showed mild depressed mental status, compulsive gait, right circling, decreased postural reactions on the left side, absent menace response on the left eye with normal cotton ball test in both eyes, and absence of conscious nociceptive perception of the left nasal mucosa. Neuroanatomic localization of the lesion was right prosencephalon.

Brain MRI was performed using a 0.25 Tesla permanent magnet (ESAOTE VET-MR GRANDE, Esaote, Genoa, Italy) with the dog in general anaesthesia. MRI sequences protocol included a Fast SE T2-W acquired in sagittal and transverse plane, a fluid attenuate inversion recovery (FLAIR) image, and a SE T1-W acquired in transverse plane before and after intravenous administration of paramagnetic contrast medium (Magnegita, gadopentetate dimeglumine 500 mmol/mL, insight agents; 0.15 mmol/kg BW). T2W ad FLAIR images showed a sharply hyperintense well demarcated lesion at the lateral surface of the right temporal lobe with right caudate nucleus involvement (Figures 1(a), 1(b), and 1(e)). These changes involved both gray and white matter with major involvement of cerebral cortex. The lesion appeared iso-hypointense on T1-W images with mild and irregular enhancement after contrast medium administration (Figures 1(c) and 1(d)). No mass effect was noted. The distribution of the lesion matched the territory of the right middle cerebral artery and its striate branches [1]. Based on MRI features and distribution of the lesions, the acute onset of the neurological abnormalities, and spontaneous improvement a presumptive diagnosis of ischemic territorial infarct was supposed. Inflammatory and neoplastic lesions were considered less likely.

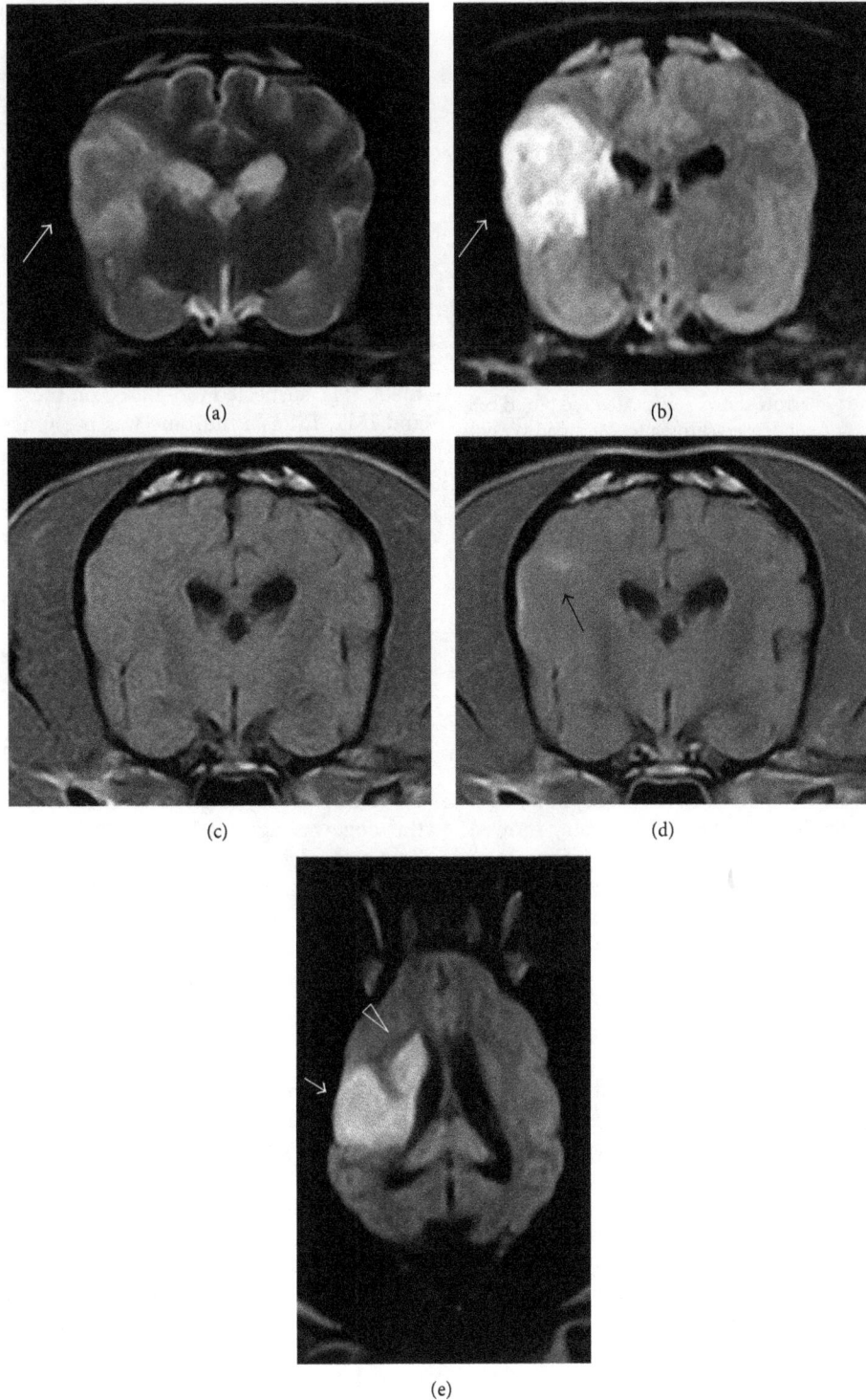

FIGURE 1: Magnetic resonance images of the brain. Transverse T2-weighted (a), FLAIR (b), T1-weighted (c), and T1-weighted, after IV gadolinium administration, (d) images at level of the thalamus; (e) dorsal FLAIR image at level of the dorsal part of the lateral ventricles. There are extensive focal grey and white matter T2 and FLAIR hyperintensity in the right temporal lobe without mass effect (white arrows). The lesion appears isointense to the normal gray matter (c) with mild contrast enhancement (black arrow) (d). The signal changes are most marked within the cortical gray matter (a). On dorsal plane the lesion extends to the right caudate nucleus (arrowhead) (e). Based on MRI features and distribution, the lesion appeared compatible with ischemic infarct in the territory of the right middle cerebral artery and its striate branches.

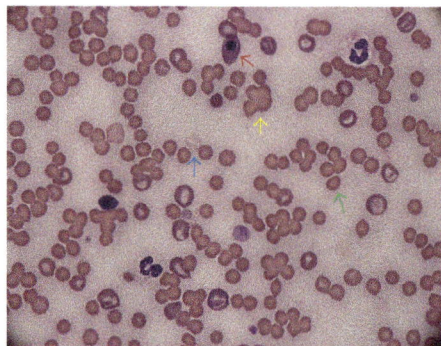

FIGURE 2: Peripheral blood smear. The orange arrow shows an agglutination that appears as irregular clusters of red blood cells. The blue arrow shows a ghost cell that appears as a very pale small blood cell. The green arrow shows a spherocyte that is a smaller cell that lacks central pallor. The red arrow shows a nucleated red blood cell with the round nucleus and condensed chromatin. Modified Wright ×50 objective.

No hemorrhages was observed by owners and thorax X-Ray and abdominal ultrasound were unremarkable.

CBC, serum chemistry, and urinary analysis were performed in a referenced laboratory. CBC was performed by automatic cell counter (ADVIA 120, Bayer) associated with the evaluation of blood smears stained with modified Wright technique (Aerospray slide stainer 7120, Delcon). Blood smears were evaluated by a board certified internist.

CBC revealed strongly regenerative anaemia, severe spherocytosis (Figure 2), a left shifted neutrophilia, and mild thrombocytopenia (Table 1). Serum chemistry showed slightly increased total bilirubin and increased C-reactive protein (CRP). The low level of haptoglobin despite inflammatory condition was consistent with hemorrhagic and/or hemolytic event. Serum protein electrophoresis revealed mild hypergammaglobulinemia (Table 1). Urinary analysis was unremarkable. Fibrinogen, D-Dimers, and fibrin/fibrinogen degradation products (FDPs) were increased (Table 1).

Based on haematological and physical findings IMHA associated with thrombocytopenia was suspected. Serology tests for Leishmania infantum (ELISA test), *Erlichia canis* (IFAT), and *Rickettsia conorii* (IFAT) were all negative.

Because of the suspected immune mediated condition a flow cytometry test for searching anti-platelets and anti-red blood cells antibodies was performed.

Although Coombs' test for the diagnosis of IMHS is available, its sensitivity is low in comparison with flow cytometry assays [2]. Actually flow cytometry is considered to provide more rapid, cost-effective, sensitive, objective method to determine erythrocytes-bound immunoglobulins [3–5] and PLT-bound immunoglobulins [1, 6–8] if compared with other assays.

CBC, serum chemistry, and urinary analysis were performed in a referenced laboratory. CBC was performed by automatic cell counter (ADVIA 120, Bayer) associated with the evaluation of blood smears stained with modified Wright technique (Aerospray slide stainer 7120, Delcon). Blood smears were evaluated by a board certified clinical pathologist.

Evaluation of anti-RBC antibodies and anti-PLT antibodies was performed by using the Epics XL-MCL (Beckman Coulter) FCI instrument throughout validated tests of a referenced laboratory [9, 10].

Blood samples were treated following the laboratory's guidelines and they were evaluated within 24 hours after the blood collection.

IgM-anti-platelets and IgG-anti-red blood cells antibodies were detected on blood samples by flow cytofluorometry (Figure 3). The lack of an evident or occult hemorrhage, together with the intense spherocytosis, intense reticulocytosis, and flow cytometric results, suggested IMHA as cause of the regenerative anemia. Although thrombocytopenia was mild and DIC and thrombosis may contribute to the lower thrombocyte count, the cytofluorometry result made IMT suspected too. Based on these findings of IMHA and IMT, Evans' syndrome was presumed and a treatment with prednisone (2 mg/kg/for day) was started. After 21 days no neurological abnormalities were noticed. Two months after the corticosteroid therapy, complete normalization of CBC, serum biochemistry parameters were present (Table 1). The dog remained stable for 7 months without therapy. Then he was one more time evaluated because of mild depression and lack of appetite. CBC revealed mild regenerative anemia, spherocytosis, and thrombocytopenia (Table 1) with normal D-Dimers. No other physical signs consistent with thrombotic events were noticed. Based on blood results and considering the outcome, thrombocytopenia in this dog was assumed as of immune mediated origin allowing a conclusive ES diagnosis. Suspecting a relapsed event, the dog was again treated with prednisone (2 mg/kg/for day) and cyclosporine (5 mg/kg/for day). After 4 months of treatment the dog was normal on owner's opinion and physical examination and CBC were unremarkable (Table 1).

2. Discussion

Ischemic stroke is a deprivation of blood flow leading to brain necrosis and most commonly occurs due to vascular occlusion by embolus or thrombus [11, 12]. These kinds of cerebrovascular accidents are commonly described in dogs [13–20] with few descriptions in cats [21, 22]. Although a large percentage of them have an unknown etiology, several underlying causes have been recognized including hypertension, endocrine, kidney, heart, and metastatic diseases [23].

In human being and dogs, IMHA and IMT have been associated with an increased incidence of thrombosis and seem to be a procoagulant condition [24–26].

ES is a pathological condition defined by the combination (either simultaneously or sequentially) of IMT and IMHA in the absence of known underlying aetiology [27].

The association of thrombosis and ES is extremely rare in human literature and the etiopathogenesis of thrombosis in these patients is not clear [28].

Cerebral venous thrombosis is reported in a man with ES probably not correlated with the therapeutic agent complications [28].

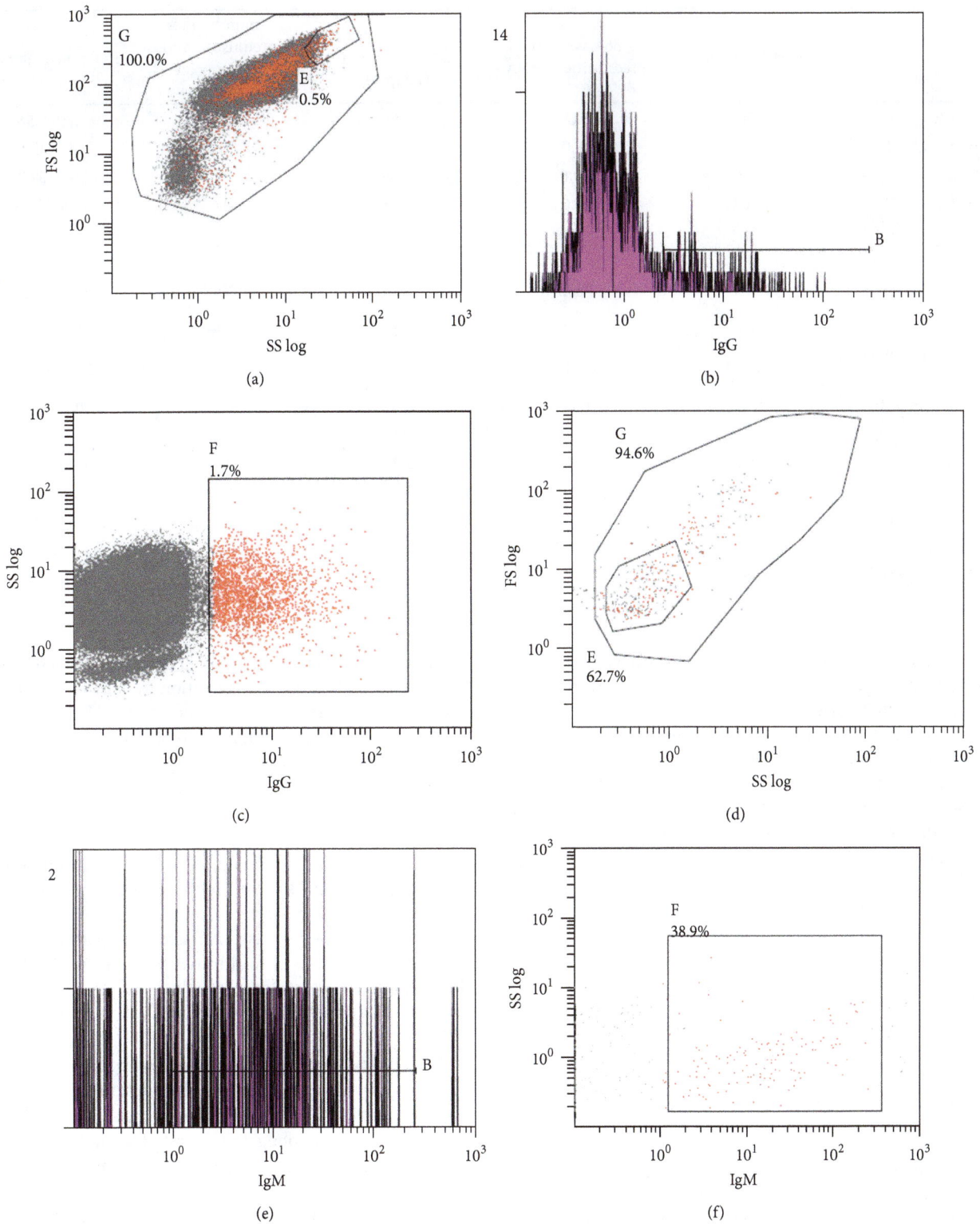

FIGURE 3: Cytofluorometric evaluation of anti-platelets and anti-red blood cells antibodies. (a) Forward versus side scatter plot showing the placement of the erythrocyte gate (E). (b) Fluorescence intensity histogram of the erythrocyte membrane-anti-RBC IgG bond. Negative and positive fluorescence peaks on the left and on the right, respectively. (c) Percentage of erythrocyte membrane binding IgG (F). (d) Forward versus side scatter plot showing the placement of the platelet gate (E). (e) Fluorescence intensity histogram of the platelet membrane-anti-PLT IgM bond. Negative and positive fluorescence peaks on the left and on the right, respectively. (f) Percentage of platelet membrane binding IgM (F).

TABLE 1: Cell blood count, serum chemistry, serum protein electrophoresis, and hemostatic profile: the first clinical evaluation and follow-up.

	The first evaluation	56 days after prednisone therapy	7 months after the first evaluation (relapse)	2 months after prednisone and cyclosporine suspension	Reference interval
RBC ($\times 10^6/\mu L$)	2.76	7.12	4.60	6.71	5.70–8.56
Hgb (gr/dL)	8.2	18.0	11.6	15.6	14.1–21.2
Hct (%)	27.2	60.6	36.8	50.3	39.0–59.2
WBC ($\times 10^3/\mu L$)	16.02	10.6	15.5	10.63	5.45–12.98
Band neutrophils ($\times 10^3/\mu L$)	139	0	0	0	0–286
Segmented neutrophils ($\times 10^3/\mu L$)	11954	7632	12710	8018	3555–9314
PLT ($\times 10^3/\mu L$)	146	339	121	396	176–479
Absolute reticulocytes count (/μL)	376464	15640	412620	76494	12320–100128
Bilirubin (mg/dL)	0.56	0.18	0.27	0.19	0.11–0.31
Haptoglobin (mg/dL)	1		98		1–96
RCP (mg/dL)	5.95	0.01	2.30	0.01	0.01–0.22
Gamma globulin (%)	21.3	14.4	14.9	13.9	6.4–14.5
Fibrinogen (mg/dL)	426		393		152–284
FDPs (μg/mL)	>20		<5		<5
D-Dimer (μg/mL)	0.61		0.23		0.01–0.34

In veterinary medicine few cases of ES have been documented in dogs [2, 29, 30]. In other reported cases of IMHA associated with thrombocytopenia in dogs the term "Evans' syndrome" is not used because of the difficulty to evaluate the immune mediated destruction of platelets [30], and the underlying mechanism of thrombocytopenia is suspected ruling out other causes of thrombocytopenia [30, 31]. In our dog diagnosis of ES was based on the presence of anti-platelets and anti-erythrocyte antibodies detected by cytofluorometric method [4, 5, 9, 10].

In both people and dogs it is well understood that IMHA per se is associated with a hypercoagulable state and the thrombosis is a frequent complication of hemolytic condition [24, 32, 33].

Clinical evidences suggestive of TE have been detected up to 35% of dogs with IMHA [34] and thromboembolic complications have been recognized as a clinically important factor for mortality [35–37], estimated up to 70% [37, 38] of cases. Pulmonary TE seems to be a common consequence of IHMA, but thrombi also can be found in heart, liver, spleen, kidney, and pituitary gland [26, 35, 36, 39].

Multiorgan TE was found from 32.2% up to 80% of dogs with IMHA after postmortem examination [26, 35, 36, 40].

It is often difficult to distinguish in patients with IMHA the predisposing factors due to treatment (immunosuppressant medication, blood product transfusion) from the real rule of the pathological condition, with several observations being made during medical treatment.

Several mechanisms have been investigated in human and dogs related to vascular complications of haemolytic anemia [33, 34, 41, 42].

There is increasing evidence that the products of haemolysis are vasculotoxic and coagulation system is principally involved in initiating the thrombotic events [24, 41].

The presence of free haemoglobin during haemolysis predisposes to hypercoagulability state by binding NO. The extracellular haemoglobin reacts with NO transforming it to nitrate and consequently reducing the bioavailability of NO [43].

NO is vital for vasodilatation, is a potent inhibitor of platelet aggregation [44], and inhibits releasing of procoagulant protein, inflammatory mediators, and proliferative factors [45]. A state of decreased NO availability as induced by haemolysis, predisposed to thrombus formations by means of vasoconstriction, endothelial adhesiveness, platelet activation, and aggregation and vessel wall cellular proliferation [45].

Reduced NO activity is also due to releasing of arginase-1 in plasma from erythrocytes destruction. This ectopic arginase activity converts arginine to ornithine, reducing plasma arginine, the obligate substrate for nitric oxide synthase [45] in human patients with hemolysis due to sickle cell disease or thalassemia [46].

Activated platelets have been identified in dogs with IMHA by measuring surface expression of P-selectin, an intercellular adhesion molecule, using a flow cytometric analyzer [34, 47, 48]. PMPs formation also occurs following platelet activation in human [49] and dogs [41] during haemolytic disorders. PMPs are membrane surrounded fragments of platelets [49] that have the potential to exhibit procoagulant activity.

Membrane of PMPs expresses binding sites for fibrinogen, PTS, P-selectin, and other adhesive receptors such as GPIIb/IIIa [47, 49].

PTS is a phospholipid with a negative charge that can be found primarily on the inner platelet membrane during a resting state [50]. As microparticles circulate, they can interact with coagulation factors through the exposed PTS, bind to leukocytes with P-selectin, or form platelet aggregates through their GPIIb/IIIa receptors. These interactions may contribute to inflammation and coagulation, possibly predisposing a patient to a thromboembolic event [47, 49].

Microparticles displaying PTS derived from erythrocytes [51], platelets [52], and endothelial cells [53] have been observed in association with human haemolytic condition such us sickle cell disease and thalassemia [54].

IMT, without a concomitant IMHA, is also considered a risk factor for ischemic stroke in human medicine [55–57].

A Danish study on human patients with primary chronic IMT suggested more than twofold higher risk of venous TE compared to the general population [58].

Heightened platelet activation in dogs with IMHA has been reported. In these patients a concurrent thrombocytopenia was found probably as a consequence of immune mediated platelet destruction, irrespective of IMHA [41].

Although in dogs the associations between IMHA, IMT, and increased risk of thromboembolic events have been described [25, 26] no reports exist about cerebrovascular complications of these immune-mediated disorders. Neurologic signs are rarely reported in dog with IMHA. There is only one report describing a dog that at the time of the initial evaluation had neurologic disease, characterized by head tilt and seizures [34].

In this paper we describe the onset of acute brain dysfunction with MRI lesions suggestive of ischemic strokes in a dog with ES.

To the authors' opinion IMHA and IMT should be considered in the list of possible underlying pathological conditions of the ischemic stroke in dogs.

Abbreviations

MRI: Magnetic resonance imaging
IMT: Immune-mediated thrombocytopenia
IMHA: Immune-mediated haemolytic anaemia
NO: Nitric oxide
PMPs: Platelet microparticles
PTS: Phosphatidylserine
ES: Evans' syndrome
TE: Thromboembolism.

Conflict of Interests

The authors declare that there is no conflict of interests regarding the publication of this paper.

Acknowledgments

The authors wish to thank Dr. Silvia Tasca and Dr. Ilaria Cerchiaro of the San Marco Veterinary Clinic, Padova, Italy, for their assistance with data collection.

References

[1] G. Terrazzano, L. Cortese, D. Piantedosi et al., "Presence of anti-platelet IgM and IgG antibodies in dogs naturally infected by Leishmania infantum," *Veterinary Immunology and Immunopathology*, vol. 110, no. 3-4, pp. 331–337, 2006.

[2] M. J. Wilkerson, "Principles and applications of flow cytometry and cell sorting in companion animal medicine," *Veterinary Clinics of North America: Small Animal Practice*, vol. 42, no. 1, pp. 53–71, 2012.

[3] K. R. Harkin, J. A. Hicks, and M. J. Wilkerson, "Erythrocyte-bound immunoglobulin isotypes in dogs with immune-mediated hemolytic anemia: 54 cases (2001–2010)," *Journal of the American Veterinary Medical Association*, vol. 241, no. 2, pp. 227–232, 2012.

[4] M. J. Wilkerson, E. Davis, W. Shuman, K. Harkin, J. Cox, and B. Rush, "Isotype-specific antibodies in horses and dogs with immune-mediated hemolytic anemia," *Journal of Veterinary Internal Medicine*, vol. 14, no. 2, pp. 190–196, 2000.

[5] K. A. Quigley, B. J. Chelack, D. M. Haines, and M. L. Jackson, "Application of a direct flow cytometric erythrocyte immunofluorescence assay in dogs with immune-mediated hemolytic anemia and comparison to the direct antiglobulin test," *Journal of Veterinary Diagnostic Investigation*, vol. 13, no. 4, pp. 297–300, 2001.

[6] B. H. Dircks, H.-J. Schuberth, and R. Mischke, "Underlying diseases and clinicopathologic variables of thrombocytopenic dogs with and without platelet-bound antibodies detected by use of a flow cytometric assay: 83 cases (2004–2006)," *Journal of the American Veterinary Medical Association*, vol. 235, no. 8, pp. 960–966, 2009.

[7] L. Chabanne, C. Bonnefont, J. Bernaud, and D. Rigal, "Clinical applications of flow cytometry and cell immunophenotyping to companion animals (dog and cat)," *Methods in Cell Science*, vol. 22, no. 2-3, pp. 199–207, 2000.

[8] A. Tomer, "Autoimmune thrombocytopenia: determination of platelet-specific autoantibodies by flow cytometry," *Pediatric Blood and Cancer*, vol. 47, no. 5, pp. 697–700, 2006.

[9] E. Carli, S. Tasca, M. Trotta, T. Furlanello, M. Caldin, and L. Solano-Gallego, "Detection of erythrocyte binding IgM and IgG by flow cytometry in sick dogs with *Babesia canis canis* or *Babesia canis vogeli* infection," *Veterinary Parasitology*, vol. 162, no. 1-2, pp. 51–57, 2009.

[10] *Proceedings of the 23th Meeting of European Society of Veterinary Clinical Pathology*, Napoli, 2005.

[11] S. T. Hecht, E. A. Eelkema, and R. E. Latchaw, "Cerebral ischemia and infarction," in *MR and CT Imaging of the Head and Neck*, R. E. Latchaw, Ed., Mosby Year Book, St. Louis, Miss, USA, 1991.

[12] R. D. Adams and M. L. Victor, "Cerebrovascular diseases," in *Principles of Neurology*, R. D. Adams and M. L. Victor, Eds., pp. 777–873, McGraw-Hill, New York, NY, USA, 6th edition, 1997.

[13] W. B. Thomas, D. C. Sorjonen, R. O. Scheuler, and J. N. Kornegay, "Magnetic resonance imaging of brain infarction in seven dogs," *Veterinary Radiology and Ultrasound*, vol. 37, no. 5, pp. 345–350, 1996.

[14] J. M. Berg and R. J. Joseph, "Cerebellar infarcts in two dogs diagnosed with magnetic resonance imaging," *Journal of the American Animal Hospital Association*, vol. 39, no. 2, pp. 203–207, 2003.

[15] J. F. McConnell, L. Garosi, and S. R. Platt, "Magnetic resonance imaging findings of presumed cerebellar cerebrovascular accident in twelve dogs," *Veterinary Radiology and Ultrasound*, vol. 46, no. 1, pp. 1–10, 2005.

[16] L. Garosi, J. F. McConnell, S. R. Platt et al., "Results of diagnostic investigations and long-term outcome of 33 dogs with brain infarction (2000–2004)," *Journal of Veterinary Internal Medicine*, vol. 19, no. 5, pp. 725–731, 2005.

[17] L. Garosi, J. F. McConnell, S. R. Platt et al., "Clinical and topographic magnetic resonance characteristics of suspected brain infarction in 40 dogs," *Journal of Veterinary Internal Medicine*, vol. 20, no. 2, pp. 311–321, 2006.

[18] A. Wessmann, K. Chandler, and L. Garosi, "Ischaemic and haemorrhagic stroke in the dog," *Veterinary Journal*, vol. 180, no. 3, pp. 290–303, 2009.

[19] A. C. Palmer, "Pontine infarction in a dog with unilateral involvement of the trigeminal motor nucleus and pyramidal tract," *Journal of Small Animal Practice*, vol. 48, no. 1, pp. 49–52, 2007.

[20] A. Negrin, L. Gaitero, and S. Añor, "Presumptive caudal cerebellar artery infarct in a dog: clinical and MRI findings," *Journal of Small Animal Practice*, vol. 50, no. 11, pp. 615–618, 2009.

[21] G. B. Cherubini, C. Rusbridge, B. P. Singh, S. Schoeniger, and P. Mahoney, "Rostral cerebellar arterial infarct in two cats," *Journal of Feline Medicine and Surgery*, vol. 9, no. 3, pp. 246–253, 2007.

[22] U. M. Altay, G. C. Skerritt, M. Hilbe, F. Ehrensperger, and F. Steffen, "Feline cerebrovascular disease: clinical and histopathologic findings in 16 cats," *Journal of the American Animal Hospital Association*, vol. 47, no. 2, pp. 89–97, 2011.

[23] L. S. Garosi, "Cerebrovascular disease in dogs and cats," *Veterinary Clinics of North America—Small Animal Practice*, vol. 40, no. 1, pp. 65–79, 2010.

[24] M. D. Cappellini, "Coagulation in the pathophysiology of hemolytic anemias," *Hematology*, pp. 74–78, 2007.

[25] A. R. Carr, D. L. Panciera, and L. Kidd, "Prognostic factors for mortality and thromboembolism in canine immune-mediated hemolytic anemia: a retrospective study of 72 dogs," *Journal of Veterinary Internal Medicine*, vol. 16, no. 5, pp. 504–509, 2002.

[26] M. K. Klein, S. W. Dow, and R. A. W. Rosychuk, "Pulmonary thromboembolism associated with immune-mediated hemolytic anemia in dogs: ten cases (1982–1987)," *Journal of the American Veterinary Medical Association*, vol. 195, no. 2, pp. 246–250, 1989.

[27] A. Norton and I. Roberts, "Management of Evans syndrome," *British Journal of Haematology*, vol. 132, no. 2, pp. 125–137, 2006.

[28] Ş. Yilmaz, H. Ören, G. Irken, M. Türker, E. Yilmaz, and E. Ada, "Cerebral venous thrombosis in a patient with Evans syndrome: a rare association," *Annals of Hematology*, vol. 84, no. 2, pp. 124–126, 2005.

[29] T. Michimoto, T. Okamura, K. Suzuki, T. Watari, R. Kano, and A. Hasegawa, "Thiazole orange positive platelets in a dog with Evans' syndrome," *Journal of Veterinary Medical Science*, vol. 66, no. 10, pp. 1305–1306, 2004.

[30] R. Goggs, A. K. Boag, and D. L. Chan, "Concurrent immune-mediated haemolytic anaemia and severe thrombocytopenia in 21 dogs," *Veterinary Record*, vol. 163, no. 11, pp. 323–327, 2008.

[31] E. S. Orcutt, J. A. Lee, and D. Bianco, "Immune-mediated hemolytic anemia and severe thrombocytopenia in dogs: 12 cases (2001–2008)," *Journal of Veterinary Emergency and Critical Care*, vol. 20, no. 3, pp. 338–345, 2010.

[32] R. K. Fenty, A. M. Delaforcade, S. P. Shaw, and T. E. O. Toole, "Identification of hypercoagulability in dogs with primary immune-mediated hemolytic anemia by means of thromboelastography," *Journal of the American Veterinary Medical Association*, vol. 238, no. 4, pp. 463–467, 2011.

[33] J. C. Scott-Moncrieff, N. G. Treadwell, S. M. McCullough, and M. B. Brooks, "Hemostatic abnormalities in dogs with primary immune-mediated hemolytic anemia," *Journal of the American Animal Hospital Association*, vol. 37, no. 3, pp. 220–227, 2001.

[34] D. J. Weiss and J. L. Brazzell, "Detection of activated platelets in dogs with primary immune-mediated hemolytic anemia," *Journal of Veterinary Internal Medicine*, vol. 20, no. 3, pp. 682–686, 2006.

[35] A. R. Carr, D. L. Panciera, and L. Kidd, "Prognostic factors for mortality and thromboembolism in canine immune-mediated hemolytic anemia: a retrospective study of 72 dogs," *Journal of Veterinary Internal Medicine*, vol. 16, no. 5, pp. 504–509, 2002.

[36] T. K. Weinkle, S. A. Center, J. F. Randolph, K. L. Warner, S. C. Barr, and H. N. Erb, "Evaluation of prognostic factors, survival rates, and treatment protocols for immune-mediated hemolytic anemia in dogs: 151 Cases (1993–2002)," *Journal of the American Veterinary Medical Association*, vol. 226, no. 11, pp. 1869–1880, 2005.

[37] M. E. Reimer, G. C. Troy, and L. D. Wamick, "Immune-mediated hemolitic anemia: 70 cases (1988–1996)," *Journal of the American Animal Hospital Association*, vol. 35, pp. 384–391, 1999.

[38] M. Ishihara, Y. Fujino, A. Setoguchi et al., "Evaluation of prognostic factors and establishment of a prognostic scoring system for canine primary immune-mediated hemolytic anemia," *Journal of Veterinary Medical Science*, vol. 72, no. 4, pp. 465–470, 2010.

[39] L. R. Johnson, M. R. Lappin, and D. C. Baker, "Pulmonary thromboembolism in 29 dogs: 1985–1995," *Journal of Veterinary Internal Medicine*, vol. 13, no. 4, pp. 338–345, 1999.

[40] M. F. Thompson, J. C. Scott-Moncrieff, and M. B. Brooks, "Effect of a single plasma transfusion on thromboembolism in 13 dogs with primary immune-mediated hemolytic anemia," *Journal of the American Animal Hospital Association*, vol. 40, no. 6, pp. 446–454, 2004.

[41] A. E. Ridyard, D. J. Shaw, and E. M. Milne, "Evaluation of platelet activation in canine immune-mediated haemolytic anaemia," *Journal of Small Animal Practice*, vol. 51, no. 6, pp. 296–304, 2010.

[42] R. P. Rother, L. Bell, P. Hillmen, and M. T. Gladwin, "The clinical sequelae of intravascular hemolysis and extracellular plasma hemoglobin: a novel mechanism of human disease," *The Journal of the American Medical Association*, vol. 293, no. 13, pp. 1653–1662, 2005.

[43] C. D. Reiter, X. Wang, J. E. Tanus-Santos et al., "Cell-free hemoglobin limits nitric oxide bioavailability in sickle-cell disease," *Nature Medicine*, vol. 8, no. 12, pp. 1383–1389, 2002.

[44] D. S. Houston, P. Robinson, and J. M. Gerrard, "Inhibition of intravascular platelet aggregation by endothelium-derived relaxing factor: reversal by red blood cells," *Blood*, vol. 76, no. 5, pp. 953–958, 1990.

[45] G. J. Kato and J. G. Taylor VI, "Pleiotropic effects of intravascular haemolysis on vascular homeostasis," *British Journal of Haematology*, vol. 148, no. 5, pp. 690–701, 2010.

[46] C. R. Morris, G. J. Kato, M. Poljakovic et al., "Dysregulated arginine metabolism, hemolysis-associated pulmonary hypertension, and mortality in sickle cell disease," *The Journal of the American Medical Association*, vol. 294, no. 1, pp. 81–90, 2005.

[47] T. B. Wills, K. J. Wardrop, and K. M. Meyers, "Detection of activated platelets in canine blood by use of flow cytometry," *American Journal of Veterinary Research*, vol. 67, no. 1, pp. 56–63, 2006.

[48] A. Piccin, W. G. Murphy, and O. P. Smith, "Circulating microparticles: pathophysiology and clinical implications," *Blood Reviews*, vol. 21, no. 3, pp. 157–171, 2007.

[49] E. V. Tocchetti, R. L. Flower, and J. V. Lloyd, "Assessment of in vitro-generated platelet microparticles using a modified flow cytometric strategy," *Thrombosis Research*, vol. 103, no. 1, pp. 47–55, 2001.

[50] B. R. Lentz, "Exposure of platelet membrane phosphatidylserine regulates blood coagulation," *Progress in Lipid Research*, vol. 42, no. 5, pp. 423–438, 2003.

[51] D. Allan, A. R. Limbrick, P. Thomas, and M. P. Westerman, "Release of spectrin-free spicules on reoxygenation of sickled erythrocytes," *Nature*, vol. 295, no. 5850, pp. 612–613, 1982.

[52] T. Wun, T. Paglieroni, A. Rangaswami et al., "Platelet activation in patients with sickle cell disease," *British Journal of Haematology*, vol. 100, no. 4, pp. 741–749, 1998.

[53] A. S. Shet, O. Aras, K. Gupta et al., "Sickle blood contains tissue factor-positive microparticles derived from endothelial cells and monocytes," *Blood*, vol. 102, no. 7, pp. 2678–2683, 2003.

[54] M. Westerman, A. Pizzey, J. Hirschman et al., "Microvesicles in haemoglobinopathies offer insights into mechanisms of hypercoagulability, haemolysis and the effects of therapy," *British Journal of Haematology*, vol. 142, no. 1, pp. 126–135, 2008.

[55] A. D. L. Peña, J. Fareed, I. Thethi, S. Morales-Vidal, M. J. Schneck, and D. Shafer, "Ischemic stroke in the setting of chronic immune thrombocytopenia in an elderly patient—a therapeutic dilemma," *Clinical and Applied Thrombosis/Hemostasis*, vol. 18, no. 3, pp. 324–326, 2012.

[56] J. Thachil, T. Callaghan, and V. Martlew, "Thromboembolic events are not uncommon in patients with immune thrombocytopenia," *British Journal of Haematology*, vol. 150, no. 4, pp. 496–497, 2010.

[57] S. Panzer, L. Höcker, R. Vormittag et al., "Flow cytometric evaluation of platelet activation in chronic autoimmune thrombocytopenia," *Pediatric Blood and Cancer*, vol. 47, no. 5, pp. 694–696, 2006.

[58] M. Nørgaard, "Thrombosis in patients with primary chronic immune thrombocytopenia," *Thrombosis Research*, vol. 130, no. 1, pp. S74–S75, 2012.

16

Localized Subcutaneous Acute Febrile Neutrophilic Dermatosis in a Dog

Karolin Schoellhorn,[1] Corinne Gurtner,[2] Petra J. Roosje,[3] Maja M. Suter,[2] Bernhard Schoellhorn,[1] Ulrich Rytz,[1] and Katrin Timm[3]

[1] Division of Small Animal Surgery and Orthopedics, Department of Clinical Veterinary Medicine, Vetsuisse Faculty, University of Berne, Laenggassstrasse 128, 3012 Berne, Switzerland
[2] Institute of Animal Pathology, Vetsuisse Faculty, University of Berne, Laenggassstrasse 122, 3012 Berne, Switzerland
[3] Division of Clinical Dermatology, Department of Clinical Veterinary Medicine, Vetsuisse Faculty, University of Berne, Laenggassstrasse 128, 3012 Berne, Switzerland

Correspondence should be addressed to Katrin Timm, katrin.timm@vetsuisse.unibe.ch

Academic Editors: J. Lakritz, C. Noli, and R. M. Santos

A two-year-old spayed female mixed-breed dog was presented with a five-day history of hemorrhagic gastroenteritis and fever. On physical examination, the dog was lethargic and clinically dehydrated. The skin of the entire ventral abdomen extending to both flanks was erythematous, swollen and painful on palpation. Histopathological examination of skin biopsies revealed a severe diffuse neutrophilic dermatitis and panniculitis, resembling the subcutaneous form of Sweet's syndrome in humans. A large part of the skin lesion developed full-thickness necrosis. After intensive care, three surgical wound debridements and wound adaptations, the wound healed by secondary intention within ten weeks. In the absence of infection of the skin or neoplasia, a diagnosis of neutrophilic dermatosis and panniculitis, resembling the subcutaneous form of acute febrile neutrophilic dermatosis, was made.

1. Introduction

Canine sterile neutrophilic dermatosis is a very rare disease. The reported clinical and histological features of the disorder in dogs are similar to those described in humans with acute febrile neutrophilic dermatosis (Sweet's syndrome (SS)) [1]. Clinical differential diagnoses in dogs include conditions characterized by erythematous papules, pustules, and plaques, such as erythema multiforme, canine eosinophilic dermatitis, sterile pustular erythroderma of Miniature Schnauzers, superficial pyoderma, pemphigus foliaceus, infectious dermatitides, adverse drug reactions, and toxic shock syndrome [1, 2]. Extracutaneous clinical signs described in previously reported cases in dogs include fever, arthritis, pneumonia, lameness, and peripheral neutrophilia and lymphadenomegaly [1–4]. As in humans, general malaise and extracutaneous signs often precede the cutaneous manifestations of this syndrome.

Sweet's syndrome in humans is associated with many diseases and divided into three categories depending on its associations: classical or idiopathic SS (often associated with upper respiratory tract or gastrointestinal tract infection, inflammatory bowel disease, or pregnancy), malignancy-associated or paraneoplastic SS (associated with acute leukemia and other neoplastic conditions), and drug-induced SS (associated with the administration of granulocyte colony stimulating factor, certain antibiotics, oral contraceptives, diuretics, and other medications) [5]. In addition, a fourth category, known as localized acute febrile neutrophilic dermatosis, has recently been described and is associated with cutaneous trauma [6]. The exact pathogenesis of SS in humans is not known but immune complexes, circulating autoantibodies and cytokines, as well as a hypersensitivity response to a bacterial, tumour or viral antigen are thought to play a role [5, 7–9].

In this paper, we describe new clinical and histological manifestations of canine neutrophilic dermatosis.

2. Case Presentation

A two-year-old, 7 kg, spayed female mixed-breed dog was presented to the referring veterinarian for acute febrile (40.3°C) gastrointestinal hemorrhage and had been treated for three days with different treatment protocols consisting of amoxicillin/clavulanic acid (Clavaseptin, Vetoquinol AG, Ittigen, Switzerland), marbofloxacin (Marbocyl, Vetoquinol AG, Ittigen, Switzerland), metronidazole (Metronidazol B. Braun, B. Braun Medical AG, Sempach, Switzerland), a combination of streptomycin and benzylpenicillin (Strepto-Penicillin, Vetoquinol AG, Ittigen, Switzerland), metamizole (Novalgin, Sanofi-Aventis, Meyrin, Switzerland), prednisolone (Prednisolon Streuli, G. Streuli & Co. AG, Uznach, Switzerland), ranitidine (Zantic, Glaxosmithkline, Muenchenbuchsee, Switzerland), metoclopramide (Paspertin, Abbott, Altishofen, Switzerland), and maropitant (Cerenia, Pfizer, Zuerich, Switzerland). Dosing regimens and frequency of administration were not available. The dog had been vaccinated six months prior to presentation against canine contagious hepatitis, parvovirosis, and distemper and had no previous history of illness.

On the fourth day of treatment, the dog was severely lethargic and was referred for further evaluation. At presentation, the dog was lethargic, dehydrated and had diarrhea which was no longer hemorrhagic. Physical examination revealed an increased heart rate (140 beats per minute), dry and pale mucous membranes, mild generalized peripheral lymphadenomegaly, and a rectal temperature of 39°C. A large tender erythematous patch with a deep purple- to black-colored center was present covering the entire ventral abdominal area from the caudal thorax to the inguinal region and extending up to both flanks. Ulcerations were seen in the center of the lesion from which a superficial layer could be further peeled off leaving a denuded, exudative surface (Figure 1). Furthermore, some small superficial vesicles were present. Nikolsky's sign was negative over the erythematous skin; the outer layer of skin was not rubbed off by applying pressure to it indicating no sign of poor cellular cohesion. In the darker colored part of the lesion; the skin did not blanche on diascopy. Differential diagnoses were a chemical or thermal burn, vasculitis, possibly associated with septicemia, cutaneous adverse drug reaction, and toxic epidermal necrolysis.

A complete blood count and serum chemistry profile revealed leukocytosis (24.8×10^9/L; reference range 6–12×10^9/L) with a left shift (band neutrophils 12.78×10^9/L; reference range 0–0.3×10^9/L) and hypoalbuminemia (12 g/L; reference range 29.7–40 g/L). The coagulation profile was within normal limits. Survey laterolateral and ventrodorsal thoracic radiographs and abdominal ultrasound were unremarkable.

Cytological examination of impression smears taken from an opened superficial vesicle showed numerous rod-shaped bacteria and neutrophils. Culture from this lesion

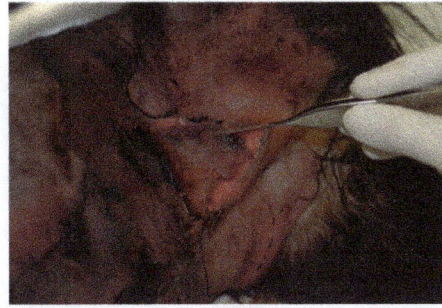

FIGURE 1: Photograph of skin lesions at the time of presentation: a large erythematous patch with a dark ulcerative center is visible extending across the entire ventral abdominal area up to both flanks. A superficial layer can be peeled off leaving a denuded surface.

subsequently revealed growth of *Pseudomonas aeruginosa*. Antibiotic sensitivity testing indicated the bacteria to be resistant to chloramphenicol, tetracycline, and trimethoprim sulfonamide but sensitive to ciprofloxacin and enrofloxacin as well as to ceftazidim.

Multiple skin punch biopsies were taken for histopathological examination which demonstrated a severe interstitial, neutrophilic deep dermatitis, and neutrophilic panniculitis. Analogous to the progression of the macroscopic skin lesions, histopathological findings varied in severity between those taken from areas with mild erythema to those taken in areas with necrosis. The dominating feature was an increasing perivascular-to-interstitial infiltration of neutrophils with a more intense infiltration of the subcutis than the dermis. In the mildly erythematous samples, the moderate infiltrate of mainly mature neutrophils was located in the septa of the subcutis and extended between the muscle fibers (Figure 2(a)), while the same cells were just sprinkled as single cells throughout the dermis. The blood vessels seemed to be free of changes. In more marked macroscopic lesions characterized by a dark-red skin color, a progression to a more severe perivascular-to-diffuse infiltration of the subcutis and the dermis with degenerate neutrophils, some round cells, and scattered karyorrhectic debris was seen (Figure 2(b)). Marked edema was present in the subepidermal dermis and in a lesser degree in the deep dermis. In some blood vessels there was leukocytostasis with neutrophils often attached to the vascular endothelium. The sample presenting a grossly visible vesicle showed severe diffuse interstitial infiltration of mainly degenerate neutrophils in the dermis and subcutis, in-between the muscle fibers, and in the fascia, and multifocal to coalescing necrosis with disseminated karyorrhectic debris and subcutaneous thrombosis of involved vessels (Figure 2(c)). The necrotic epidermis was either separated from the dermis leaving the dermis denuded or severely degenerate with hydropic and beginning ballooning changes with hypereosinophilic cytoplasm and multifocal nuclear pyknosis (Figure 2(d)). Sub- and intraepidermally, there was a severe infiltration with mainly degenerate neutrophils forming a pustule. In the sample with epidermal necrosis, the necrotic changes

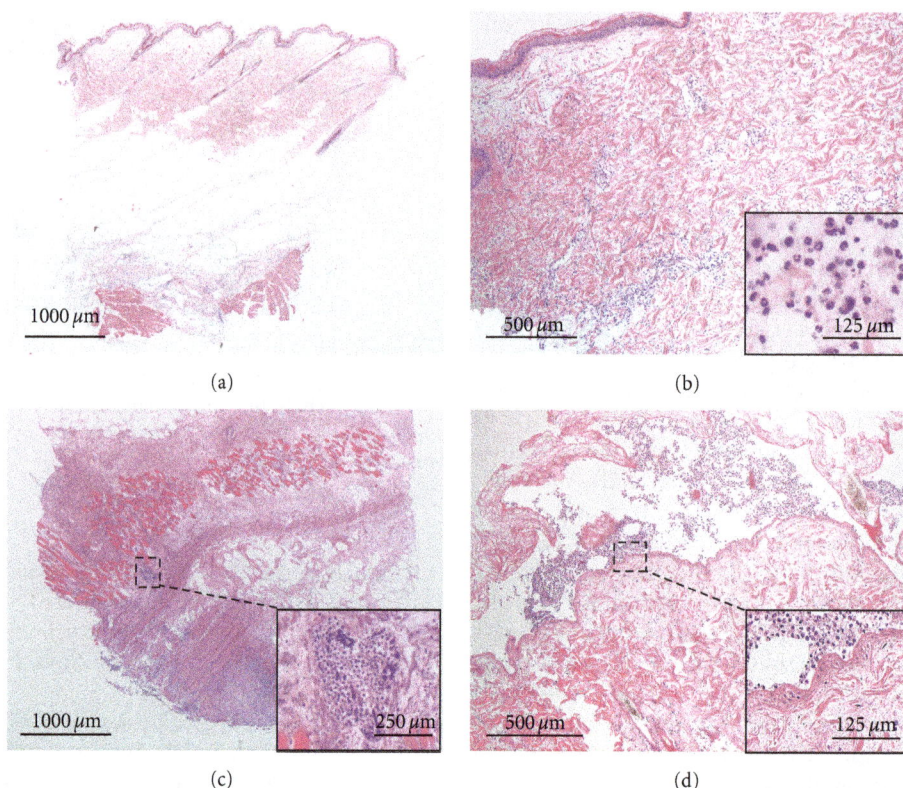

Figure 2: Histopathological images stained with hematoxylin and eosin (H&E) illustrating the histologic progression of severity analogous to the progression of macroscopic lesions. (a) Haired skin, the overview demonstrates a moderate infiltrate of neutrophils in the septa of the subcutis and extending between muscle fibers. Original magnification ×20. (b) Haired skin, epidermis and dermis: there is a perivascular to interstitial infiltrate of neutrophils (inset) in the dermis, giving the appearance of being sprinkled throughout the tissue. Original magnification ×100, inset ×400. (c) Haired skin, subcutis and muscle fibers: diffuse necrosis with disseminated karyorrhectic debris and subcutaneous thrombosis of involved vessels (inset). Original magnification ×40, inset ×400. (d) Haired skin, epidermis and dermis: the epidermis (inset) is hypereosinophilic and necrotic with severe infiltration with mainly degenerate neutrophils forming an intraepidermal pustule. The dashed line marks the border between dermis and necrotic epidermis. Original magnification ×100, inset ×400.

reached below the subcutis, affecting also the adnexa. The epidermis showed the same features as in the aforementioned sample but without the sub- and intraepidermal infiltrate. The dermis and subcutis were severely edematous, the collagen fibers were swollen and hyalinized, and there was widespread hemorrhage, all providing evidence for vascular damage. The inflammatory infiltration in the dermis was as described in the former samples.

The dog was treated with intravenous fluids, gastric protection therapy, analgesics, and antibiotics and dexamethasone (Table 1). On the third day, diarrhea had resolved, but the dog continued to vomit intermittently for three more weeks. By the seventh day, the dog's general condition had improved, the erythema at the margins of the patch resolved, and a large part of the darker colored center of the erythematous patch was demarcated (Figure 3). The necrotic skin was debrided, and partial closure of the defect was performed under general anesthesia. After 17 days of hospitalization, the leukocytes were within normal range, and the neutrophil left shift was absent after 33 days. Hypoalbuminemia normalized within 26 days.

Four weeks after initial presentation, an autologous full-thickness mesh graft was placed over a healthy bed of granulation tissue. A vacuum-assisted closure device was applied with continuous suction for five days, and the wound dressing was changed every three days [10]. The graft failed and was removed six days after surgery but multiple skin punch grafts, performed two weeks later, were successful. The remaining wound healed by secondary intention (Figure 4). Further wound treatment included daily wound irrigation with a full electrolyte solution (Plasma-Lyte A, Baxter AG, Volketswil, Switzerland) and a nonadhering wound dressing (Adaptic, Sytagenix Wound Management Limited, Gargrave, North Yorkshire, UK) until healing was complete.

The dog remained hospitalized for a total of ten weeks to ensure proper wound care. During this time the dog remained normothermic and was finally discharged from the hospital in good general condition and with a nearly resolved skin lesion. Complete healing of the lesion occurred after 12 weeks (Figure 5). On follow-up telephone consultation with the owner eight months after discharge, the dog was in excellent general condition and did not receive any further treatment.

TABLE 1: Protocol of the administered drugs during hospitalization of the dog. All listed drugs were administered from the day of presentation onwards, unless mentioned otherwise.

Drug ingredient	Dose and form of application	Duration of application
Antibiotics		
Enrofloxacin[a]	11 mg/kg *per os* (PO) *q* 12 hr	6 weeks
Amoxicillin/clavulanic acid[b]	20 mg/kg intravenously (IV) *q* 8 hr	5 weeks
Amoxicillin/clavulanic acid[c]	12.5 mg/kg PO *q* 12 hr	2 weeks (following IV administration)
Metronidazole[d]	15 mg/kg IV *q* 12 hr	1 week
Glucocorticoids		
Dexamethasone[e]	0.15 mg/kg IV *q* 12 hr	6 days
Prednisolone[f]	2 mg/kg PO *q* 24 hr	2 weeks (following dexamethasone), then gradually tapered over 4 weeks
Analgesics		
Fentanyl[g]	2.5–7.5 μg/kg/hr constant rate infusion (CRI)	10 days
Ketamine[h]	10 μg/kg/hr CRI	8 days
Buprenorphine[i]	0.01-0.02 mg/kg subcutaneously *q* 8 hr	3 weeks
Tramadol[j]	3 mg/kg PO *q* 8 hr	3 weeks
Gastric protection		
Omeprazole[k]	1 mg/kg PO *q* 24 hr	7 weeks
Sucralfate[l]	30 mg/kg PO *q* 12 hr	10 days
Metoclopramide[m]	0.2 mg/kg IV *q* 6 hr	10 days
Dolasetrone[n]	0.5 mg/kg *q* 24 hr	7 days
Fluid therapy		
Full electrolyte solution[o]	1–4 mL/kg/hr CRI	4 weeks

[a]Baytril 2.5%, Provet AG, Lyssach, Switzerland; [b]Augmentin Adult, Glaxosmithkline, Muenchenbuchsee, Switzerland; [c]Clavaseptin, Vetoquinol AG, Ittigen, Switzerland; [d]Metronidazol B. Braun, B. Braun Medical AG, Sempach, Switzerland; [e]Dexatat, Dr. E. Graeub AG, Bern, Switzerland; [f]Prednisolon Streuli, G. Streuli & Co. AG, Uznach, Switzerland; [g]Sintenyl i.v. 0.5 mg, Sintetica S.A., Mandrisio, Switzerland; [h]Ketasol, Dr. E. Graeub AG, Bern, Switzerland; [i]Temgesic, Essex Pharma GmbH, Munich, Germany; [j]Tramadol-Mepha 50 retard, Mepha Pharma AG, Aesch, Switzerland; [k]Omeprazol-Teva, Teva Pharma AG, Aesch, Switzerland; [l]Ulcogant Suspension, Merck Serono GmbH, Darmstadt, Germany; [m]Paspertin, Abbott, Altishofen, Switzerland; [n]Anzemet, Sanofi-Aventis; Meyrin, Switzerland; [o]Plasma-Lyte A, Baxter AG, Volketswil, Switzerland.

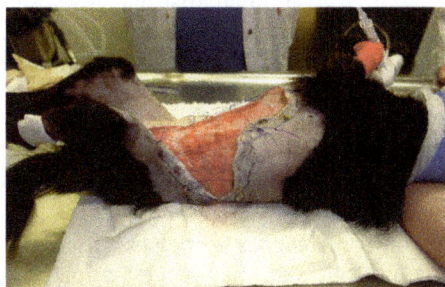

FIGURE 3: Photograph of skin lesions on day 7 after surgical debridement of necrotic areas: necrotic skin has been surgically resected after demarcation. Complete wound closure is not possible. The suture reduces the tension of the wound and holds the wound dressing in position.

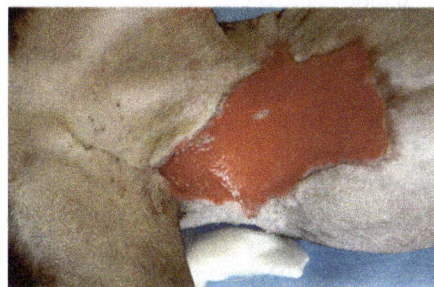

FIGURE 4: Photograph of skin lesions on day 38: granulation tissue is visible covering the wound.

3. Discussion

The cardinal features of SS in humans are an acute onset of general malaise, fever, marked leukocytosis, and the development of tender erythematous skin lesions with histological evidence of perivascular-to-interstitial dermal infiltrate of mature neutrophils [5, 8, 11]. In humans and in the five previously reported cases in dogs, multiple lesions including erythematous plaques, nodular, pustular, and papular lesions are described, unlike the single large lesion in the case reported herein [2–5, 8, 9, 11, 12]. It is also noteworthy that this dog survived whereas three of five previously described dogs died of the disease [2, 3]. Both surviving dogs were

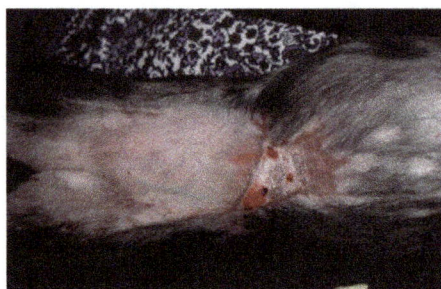

FIGURE 5: Photograph of skin lesions on day 84: almost complete wound healing is visible.

treated with corticosteroids soon after admission, as was the dog in this paper. In humans with classical SS, an excellent response to systemic corticosteroids is one of the criteria used to confirm diagnosis [5]. This positive effect of corticosteroids would seem to uphold the theory that SS is a sterile inflammatory process caused by an exaggerated immune response in otherwise immunocompetent patients.

The dog in this paper was initially presented to the referring veterinarian with signs of hemorrhagic gastroenteritis, which is consistent with the association with gastrointestinal disorders observed in some human classical SS cases [8, 11, 13–17]. However, it is unclear as to whether the inciting cause was a gastrointestinal disorder or the administration of drugs in this case. Drug-induced SS in people is associated with a large variety of drugs in humans, including nonsteroidal anti-inflammatory drugs and antibiotics [14, 16–22]. Moreover, carprofen was administered to three of the five previously reported dogs affected with SS, and firocoxib was administered to the fourth [2–4]. Although these drugs were not administered to the dog in the present paper, the COX inhibitor metamizole was, as well as a number of different antibiotics. Therefore a drug-induced etiology cannot be excluded. In contrast, a possible paraneoplastic etiology of SS was ruled out based on our diagnostic work-up and a follow-up time of several months. A previous local trauma could be excluded as there was no evidence for it in the history.

The common histological feature of SS is a uniform, dense, moderate-to-extensive infiltrate of neutrophils in the upper dermis. The epidermis is usually normal, although mild reactive changes may be seen [5, 8, 23]. Variable dermal edema is not uncommon, sometimes leading to subepidermal bulla formation which suggests the appearance of a vesicle. Based on the histopathological findings in the skin biopsies, a subcutaneous form of neutrophilic dermatosis is possible in the dog in this paper. A lobular or septal panniculitis or both are described features of subcutaneous SS in humans [5, 11, 24, 25]. In this variant of SS, the neutrophilic infiltrate may remain localized to the subcutaneous fat or extend secondarily to the overlying dermis, as seen in the present case [5, 24]. A neutrophilic septal panniculitis was also described in one previously reported dog with SS-like disease [2].

Vasculitis, which was observed in the dog in this paper, was initially a criterion for exclusion of a diagnosis of SS in humans. However, it is now recognized that leukocytoclastic vasculitis does occur in many SS patients, although it is unclear as to whether this represents a primary or secondary epiphenomenon in SS [5, 25, 26]. Vasculitis was also described in three of the five previously reported canine cases [3, 4]. Depending on the size, the number of involved vessels, and intensity of released cytokines, it is possible that necrosis developed as a result of vasculitis in the subcutis in the reported case, especially as necrosis was not observed in the areas in which vasculitis was not seen.

Some of the clinical and histological signs in the dog described herein are similar to those described in a dog with sterile neutrophilic nodular panniculitis in which a vasculitis was identified as well as those described in a dog with SS-like skin and extracutaneous lesions in which a neutrophilic septal panniculitis and vasculitis at extracutaeous sites were diagnosed histologically [2, 27]. Both conditions may represent part of a spectrum of signs of the same syndrome elicited by an immune response to an infection or other stimulus. The common features of the syndrome appear to include an acute onset, fever, a prodromal inflammatory process or drug history, and a range of lesions including vasculitis and panniculitis. The term canine acute febrile neutrophilic dermatosis may therefore be more appropriate than the currently used name canine sterile neutrophilic dermatosis, until more is understood about the pathophysiology of this condition in the dog. Furthermore, the role of bacteria as a primary or secondary agent is not evident in this particular case, as depicted below. Therefore the term "sterile" was avoided in the description of the diagnosis.

Although a favorable response to corticosteroids is reported in canine sterile nodular panniculitis, thus far only three reported dogs with SS-like disease survived, including our case. It is therefore unclear if treatment response may be used as a diagnostic criterion in dogs as in the human counterpart.

In the reported case differential diagnoses for the presenting clinical sign of an erythematous patch included a severe chemical or thermal burn but these were ruled out based on history and histopathology, in particular because a dense neutrophilic infiltrate in the subcutis with only few neutrophils in the dermis was found in less severely affected areas of the skin, suggesting an insult initiated in the deeper areas of the skin.

Culture of *Pseudomonas aeruginosa* from the surface swabs of the necrotic skin may suggest primary pyoderma or septicemia-induced cutaneous necrosis. However, bacteria were not observed on routine histopathology. Additionally, histopathological changes were not consistent with those expected in primary pseudomonal dermatitis, such as primary suppurative folliculitis and furunculosis with pyogranulomatous dermatitis and panniculitis, or sepsis characterized histologically by dermal necrosis associated with severe vascular fibrinoid necrosis and fibrin thrombi [28, 29]. Septicemia was also considered unlikely based on the results of hematology and coagulation profile. Blood cultures were not performed. With the information available, *Pseudomonas aeruginosa* was judged to be a secondary bacterial contaminant, probably restricted to the necrotic area without further impact on the etiology or pathogenesis of the disease.

In summary, this paper describes a dog with unusual clinical and histological signs of SS-like disease or acute febrile neutrophilic dermatosis with a favorable response to treatment.

Acknowledgments

The authors would like to thank Judith Howard and Thierry Francey for the critical reading of the paper.

References

[1] T. L. Gross, P. J. Ihrke, E. J. Walder et al., "Canine sterile neutrophilic dermatosis (Sweet's syndrome)," in *Skin Diseases of the Dog and Cat*, pp. 366–368, Blackwell Science, 2005.

[2] C. S. Johnson, E. R. May, R. K. Myers, and J. M. Hostetter, "Extracutaneous neutrophilic inflammation in a dog with lesions resembling Sweet's syndrome," *Veterinary Dermatology*, vol. 20, no. 3, pp. 200–205, 2009.

[3] C. B. Vitale, E. Zenger, and J. Hill, "Putative Rimadyl-induced neutrophilic dermatosis resembling Sweet's syndrome in two dogs," in *Proceedings of the 15th Annual Meeting of the American Academy of Veterinary Dermatology and American College of Veterinary Dermatology*, pp. 69–70, 1999.

[4] P. J. Mellor, A. J. A. Roulois, M. J. Day, B. A. Blacklaws, S. J. Knivett, and M. E. Herrtage, "Neutrophilic dermatitis and immune-mediated haematological disorders in a dog: suspected adverse reaction to carprofen," *Journal of Small Animal Practice*, vol. 46, no. 5, pp. 237–242, 2005.

[5] P. R. Cohen, "Sweet's syndrome—a comprehensive review of an acute febrile neutrophilic dermatosis," *Orphanet Journal of Rare Diseases*, vol. 2, no. 1, article 34, 2007.

[6] Y. S. Phua, S. A. Al-Ani, R. B. W. She, and T. M. de Chalain, "Sweet's syndrome triggered by scalding: a case study and review of the literature," *Burns*, vol. 36, no. 4, pp. e49–e52, 2010.

[7] N. P. Burrows, "Anti-neutrophil cytoplasmic antibodies in Sweet's syndrome," *Journal of the American Academy of Dermatology*, vol. 31, no. 5 I, pp. 825–826, 1994.

[8] P. R. Cohen and R. Kurzrock, "Sweet's syndrome: a neutrophilic dermatosis classically associated with acute onset and fever," *Clinics in Dermatology*, vol. 18, no. 3, pp. 265–282, 2000.

[9] P. R. Cohen, H. Hönigsmann, and R. Kurzrock, "Acute febrile neutrophilic dermatosis (Sweet syndrome)," in *Fitzpatrick's Dermatology in General Medicine*, K. Wolff, L. A. Goldsmith, S. I. Katz et al., Eds., pp. 289–295, McGraw-Hill Professional, New York, NY, USA, 2007.

[10] R. Ben-Amotz, O. I. Lanz, J. M. Miller, D. E. Filipowicz, and M. D. King, "The use of vacuum-assisted closure therapy for the treatment of distal extremity wounds in 15 dogs," *Veterinary Surgery*, vol. 36, no. 7, pp. 684–690, 2007.

[11] P. R. Cohen and R. Kurzrock, "Sweet's syndrome revisited: a review of disease concepts," *International Journal of Dermatology*, vol. 42, no. 10, pp. 761–778, 2003.

[12] M. J. Gains, A. Morency, F. Sauvé, M. C. Biais, and Y. Bongrand, "Canine sterile neutrophilic dermatitis (resembling Sweet's syndrome) in a Dachshund," *Canadian Veterinary Journal*, vol. 51, no. 12, pp. 1397–1399, 2010.

[13] O. Fain, E. Mathieu, N. Feton et al., "Intestinal involvement in Sweet's syndrome," *Journal of the American Academy of Dermatology*, vol. 35, no. 6, pp. 989–990, 1996.

[14] D. C. Walker and P. R. Cohen, "Trimethoprim-sulfamethoxazole-associated acute febrile neutrophilic dermatosis: case report and review of drug-induced Sweet's syndrome," *Journal of the American Academy of Dermatology*, vol. 34, no. 5, pp. 918–923, 1996.

[15] A. Vaz, K. Kramer, and R. A. Kalish, "Sweet's syndrome in association with Crohn's disease," *Postgraduate Medical Journal*, vol. 76, no. 901, pp. 713–714, 2000.

[16] K. H. Fye, E. Crowley, T. G. Berger, P. E. LeBoit, and M. K. Connolly, "Celecoxib-induced Sweet's syndrome," *Journal of the American Academy of Dermatology*, vol. 45, no. 2, pp. 300–302, 2001.

[17] B. K. Durani and U. Jappe, "Drug-induced Sweet's syndrome in acne caused by different tetracyclines: case report and review of the literature," *British Journal of Dermatology*, vol. 147, no. 3, pp. 558–562, 2002.

[18] C. Kaur, R. Sarkar, and A. J. Kanwar, "Fixed drug eruption to rofecoxib with cross-reactivity to sulfonamides," *Dermatology*, vol. 203, no. 4, article 351, 2001.

[19] J. Levang, P. Muller, P. Girardin, and P. Humbert, "Sweet's syndrome and phenylbutazone-induced sialadenitis," *Annales de Dermatologie et de Venereologie*, vol. 135, no. 4, pp. 291–294, 2008.

[20] C. R. Retief and F. D. Malkinson, "Nitrofurantoin-associated Sweet's syndrome," *Cutis*, vol. 63, no. 1–3, pp. 177–179, 2001.

[21] D. Aguiar-Bujanda, J. Aguiar-Morales, and U. Bohn-Sarmiento, "Sweet's syndrome associated with norfloxacin in a prostate cancer patient," *QJM: An International Journal of Medicine*, vol. 97, no. 1, pp. 55–56, 2004.

[22] D. Özdemir, U. Korkmaz, I. Şahin et al., "Ofloxacin induced Sweet's syndrome in a patient with Crohn's disease," *Journal of Infection*, vol. 52, no. 5, pp. e155–e157, 2006.

[23] R. L. Fitzgerald, "Review: Sweet's syndrome," *International Journal of Dermatology*, vol. 35, no. 1, pp. 9–15, 1996.

[24] P. R. Cohen, "Subcutaneous Sweet's syndrome: a variant of acute febrile neutrophilic dermatosis that is included in the histopathologic differential diagnosis of neutrophilic panniculitis," *Journal of the American Academy of Dermatology*, vol. 52, no. 5, pp. 927–928, 2005.

[25] G. Ratzinger, W. Burgdorf, B. G. Zelger, and B. Zelger, "Acute febrile neutrophilic dermatosis: a histopathologic study of 31 cases with review of literature," *American Journal of Dermatopathology*, vol. 29, no. 2, pp. 125–133, 2007.

[26] J. C. Malone, S. P. Slone, L. A. Wills-Frank et al., "Vascular inflammation (vasculitis) in Sweet syndrome: a clinicopathologic study of 28 biopsy specimens from 21 patients," *Archives of Dermatology*, vol. 138, no. 3, pp. 345–349, 2002.

[27] J. R. S. Dandrieux, K. Timm, P. J. Roosje et al., "Unusual systemic signs in a dog with sterile neutrophilic-macrophagic lymphadenitis and nodular panniculitis," *Journal of the American Animal Hospital Association*, vol. 47, no. 2, pp. 117–121, 2011.

[28] A. Hillier, J. R. Alcorn, L. K. Cole, and J. J. Kowalski, "Pyoderma caused by *Pseudomonas aeruginosa* infection in dogs: 20 cases," *Veterinary Dermatology*, vol. 17, no. 6, pp. 432–439, 2006.

[29] T. L. Gross, P. J. Ihrke, E. J. Walder et al., "Septic vasculitis," in *Skin Diseases of the Dog and Cat*, pp. 238–239, Blackwell Science, 2005.

17

Failure of Miltefosine Treatment in Two Dogs with Natural *Leishmania infantum* Infection

Daniela Proverbio, Eva Spada, Giada Bagnagatti De Giorgi, and Roberta Perego

Dipartimento di Scienze Veterinarie per la Salute, la Produzione Animale e la Sicurezza Alimentare, Università degli Studi di Milano, Via G. Celoria, 10-20133 Milano, Italy

Correspondence should be addressed to Daniela Proverbio; daniela.proverbio@unimi.it

Academic Editor: Katerina K. Adamama-Moraitou

Two dogs, with naturally acquired canine leishmaniasis, were treated orally with miltefosine (2 mg/kg q 24 hr) and allopurinol (10 mg/kg q 12 hr) for 28 days. Both dogs showed good initial response to therapy, with reduction in clinical signs and improvement of clinicopathological changes. However, in both dogs, clinical and clinicopathological abnormalities recurred 150 days after initial treatment and a second course of miltefosine and allopurinol was administered. One dog failed to respond to the 2nd cycle of miltefosine treatment and the other dog responded initially but suffered an early relapse. Treatment with meglumine antimoniate (100 mg/kg q 24 hr for a minimum of 4 weeks) was then started in both dogs. Both dogs showed rapid clinical and clinicopathological improvement and to date they have not received further treatment for 420 and 270 days, respectively. In view of the low number of antileishmanial drugs available and the fact that some of these are used in human as well as veterinary medicine, it is of paramount importance that drug resistance is monitored and documented.

1. Introduction

Canine leishmaniasis (CanL) caused by the protozoan *Leishmania infantum* is a life threatening zoonotic disease transmitted by insect vectors, sand flies (*Phlebotomus* spp.). CanL has a wide distribution in temperate and subtropical countries with a very wide prevalence covering both the old and new worlds. The dog is the main reservoir for human visceral leishmaniasis (VL) caused by *Leishmania infantum* [1] which is listed among the most important neglected tropical diseases by the WHO (http://www.who.int/neglected_disease/diseases; access April 2014).

The clinical features of CanL vary widely as a consequence of the numerous pathogenic mechanisms involved in the disease, the different organs affected, and the diverse nature of the immune responses mounted by individual hosts [2]. The main clinical findings include skin lesions (such as exfoliative dermatitis, papules, nodules, ulcerations, and alopecia), generalized lymphadenomegaly, splenomegaly, progressive weight loss, muscular atrophy, polyuria and polydipsia, ocular lesions, epistaxis, and onychogryphosis. Laboratory findings include nonregenerative anemia, serum hyperproteinemia, polyclonal beta and gamma hyperglobulinemia, hypoalbuminemia, decreased albumin/globulin ratio, renal azotemia, and persistent renal proteinuria [3].

The antileishmanial drugs currently used in dogs were originally developed to treat leishmaniasis in people, and most therapeutic protocols were developed through human clinical studies with subsequent adaption for use in dogs [4]. Many drugs (including amphotericin B, pentamidine, metronidazole, spiramycin, enrofloxacin, and ketoconazole) have been used, either alone or in combination, with variable results [4–7]. Currently, the first line treatment against CanL is meglumine antimoniate (MA), usually in combination with allopurinol [7]. This treatment protocol usually induces clinical remission, although it does not prevent relapses and in most cases does not completely eliminate parasites from the infected animal [8].

Recently, miltefosine (MLF) (in combination with allopurinol) has been suggested as an alternative to meglumine

TABLE 1: Case number 1: clinical score, therapy, and hematological and biochemical analysis of the first dog affected by canine leishmaniasis.

Followup	Clinical score	Therapy	RBC ×10³/μL	Hb g/dL	PCV%	PLT /uL	TP g/dL	ALB%	γG%	A/G	IFAT
D0	8/86	MLT + A 28/d	5220	12.6	34.8	37.000	9.3	31.7	42.7	0.46	1:1280
D30	3/86	A	5840	12.6	34.5	15.000	7.8	35.2	37.6	0.54	1:640
D60	2/86	A	6440	14.3	38.7	65.000	7.5	42.9	25.6	0.75	1:320
D90	0/86	A	6110	13.9	37.1	149.000	7.4	42.1	21.4	0.75	1:320
D150	11/86	MLT + A 28/d	6350	14.2	40.5	232.000	8.3	41	31.7	0.6	1:640
D 210	0/86	A	6220	13.9	43.3	138.000	7.6	49.3	11.4	0.97	1:160
D240	2/86	MA 28gg	6160	15	42.5	68.000	6.8	38.6	20.3	0.63	1:320
D270	0/86	A	5750	13.2	35.2	151.000	5.8	46.7	10.4	0.88	1:160
D330	0/86	A	6420	15.7	38.9	116.000	6.7	46.1	10	0.86	1:160
D390	0/86	A	6560	14	40.2	174.000	7.1	47.5	8.9	0.9	1:160
D660	1/86	—	6100	13.8	36.8	215.000	6.4	46.2	9.8	0.86	1:160

antimoniate for the treatment of CanL [9–13]. MLF is an alkyphospholipid originally developed as a topical and oral antineoplastic agent [8]. Multiple in vivo and in vitro trials have demonstrated the leishmanial killing activity of miltefosine [12] through disruption of both signaling pathways and cell membrane synthesis, which induces an apoptosis-like cell death. In people, MLF is an effective oral drug for the treatment of leishmaniasis although, in common with other antileishmanial drugs, some reports suggest possible development of resistance [14–16]. Some studies in dogs have reported the short-term efficacy of MLF therapy in association with allopurinol and suggest that this combination is a safe, convenient, and effective alternative treatment option for canine leishmaniasis which has only mild (and self-limiting) side effects [9–12]. Recent studies have reported cases where relapse of clinical CanL occurs between 3 and 6 months after cessation of treatment, in dogs treated with a combination of MLF and allopurinol, but no data has been provided on the outcome of further treatments in these cases [9, 11].

In this paper, we describe two dogs with naturally occurring CanL that, after an initially successful treatment with two cycles of MLF and allopurinol, relapsed, but subsequently responded to further treatment with meglumine antimoniate. These cases demonstrate that a failure of therapeutic response to MLT therapy, as has been reported in human patients, may also occur in dogs. Resistance surveillance is particularly important because the same drugs are used in dogs and human patients although, in Europe, miltefosine is not typically used to treat human visceral leishmaniasis.

2. Case Reports

Case Number 1. A 1-year-old, 10.7 kg, neutered female mixed-breed dog, adopted 4 months previously from a kennel in Sicily (a region in which canine leishmaniasis is endemic), fully vaccinated against canine distemper virus (CDV), canine parvovirus (CPV), leptospirosis, and infectious canine hepatitis (ICH), but not treated against endo- and ectoparasites. The dog was referred to the Internal Medicine Service of the Department of Health, Animal Science and Food Safety of the University of Milan, with a 30-day history of erythema and exfoliative dermatitis that had not responded to antibiotic therapy (cephalexin, ICF vet 20 mg/kg q 12 hr for 15 days).

Physical examination revealed a generalized lymphadenopathy, dry, nonpruritic dermatitis with generalized scaling and alopecia of the auricular pinna, eyelids, axilla, and groin. A provisional diagnosis of canine leishmaniasis was made. A blood count revealed a mild normochromic, anemia, and thrombocytopenia. Biochemical analysis showed hyperproteinemia with hypoalbuminemia and hypergammaglobulinemia. Serum protein electrophoresis showed a polyclonal gammopathy and a decreased albumin-globulin ratio (A/G) ratio (Table 1).

The serum indirect immunofluorescence antibody test (IFAT) for Leishmania infantum specific antibodies yielded a high positive titer of 1:1280 (reference range, <1:80) and conventional polymerase chain reaction (PCR) analysis of blood was positive for L. infantum. Indirect immunofluorescence assay (IFAT) for Ehrlichia canis was negative.

Diagnosis of CanL was made and the severity of clinical signs attributable to Leishmania infection was scored on a scale from 0 to 3 for a total of 86/86 (Table 2). The clinical score of the case 1 was 8/86 at diagnosis. Treatment was started with 2 mg/kg q 24 hr of MLF per os in combination with allopurinol at 10 mg/kg q 12 hr for 28 days. After the combined therapy, allopurinol was continued at the same dosage until the last follow-up (D390).

Complete clinical and blood examination was performed at 30, 60, 90, and 150 days from the start of treatment with MLF. Results of follow-up clinical scores, blood examinations, and biochemical analysis are shown in Table 2.

After the first cycle of therapy, the clinical score showed a gradual and constant decline. The anemia and the thrombocytopenia resolved during the first 90 days of followup and gamma globulin declined. At D150, the dog was presented

TABLE 2: Score for clinical parameters (on a scale from 0 to 86) used in dogs affected by canine leishmaniasis.

Clinical sign	0	1	2	3
Appetite	Normal	Slight decrease	Moderate decrease	Anorexia
Mentation	Normal	Slight depression	Depression	Prostration
Lethargy	No	Slight	Moderate	Refusal to move
Weight loss	No	Slight	Moderate	Severe
Polyuria	No	Slight	Moderate	Severe
Polydipsia	No	Slight	Moderate	Severe
Localized muscular atrophy (temporal muscles)	No	Slight	Moderate	Severe
Generalized muscular atrophy	No	Slight	Moderate	Severe
Lymphadenomegaly	No	1-2 nodes	2 > 4 nodes	Generalized
Splenomegaly	No		Yes	
Conjunctivitis and/or blepharitis	No	Unilateral and slight	Bilateral or unilateral severe	Bilateral and severe
Uveitis and/or keratitis	No	Unilateral and slight	Bilateral or unilateral severe	Bilateral and severe
Pale mucous membranes	No	Slight	Moderate	Severe
Epistaxis	Never presented	Sporadic	Frequent	Incoercible
Mouth ulcers or nodules	No	1 or 2 small ulcers or nodules	>2 small ulcers or nodules	>1/4 or oral mouth cover by ulcers or nodules
Vomiting	No	Sporadic	Frequent	Frequent with blood
Diarrhea	No	Sporadic	Frequent	Constant
Lameness	No	Sporadic	Frequent	Constant
Itching	No	Sporadic	Frequent	Constant
Erythema	No	<10% body surface or slight generalized erythema	10–25% body surface or moderate generalized erythema	>25% body surface
Dry exfoliative dermatitis	No	<10% body surface or slight generalized erythema	10–25% body surface or moderate generalized erythema	>25% body surface
Ulcerative dermatitis	No	1-2 ulcers	3–5 ulcers	>5 ulcers
Nodular dermatitis	No	1-2 nodules	3–5 nodules	>5 nodules
Sterile pustular dermatitis	No	1-2 pustules	3–5 pustules	>5 pustules
Alopecia	No	<10% body surface	10–25% body surface erythema	>25% body surface
Altered pigmentation	No	Localized	Multifocal	Generalized
Hyperkeratosis of nasal planum and pads	No	Slight	Moderate	Severe
Generalized hyperkeratosis	No	Slight	Moderate	Severe
Onychogryphosis	No	Slight	Moderate	Severe

with a clinical deterioration (clinical score 11/86) and worsening of hematological parameters. A relapse was diagnosed and a second 28-day cycle of MLF in combination with allopurinol at the same dose as in the first cycle was started.

Following the second treatment with MLF, clinical signs were resolved at D210 (clinical score 0/86) with improvement of clinicopathological abnormalities, but, at D240, the dog showed again clinicopathological signs (clinical score 2/86).

Following the classification by Oliva et al. (2010) [4], the dog was classified as "early relapse" and treatment with an alternative drug was initiated.

Therapy with meglumine antimoniate (100 mg/kg/sc) in combination with allopurinol (10 mg/kg/q 12 hr *per os*) for at least 4 weeks was started.

At D270, after 4 weeks of therapy, the dog had a clinical score of 0/86, biochemical analysis showed low total protein,

TABLE 3: Case number 2: clinical score, therapy, and hematological and biochemical analysis of the second dog affected by canine leishmaniasis.

Follow-up	Clinical score	Therapy	RBC $\times 10^3/\mu L$	Hb g/dL	PCV%	PLT /uL	TP g/dL	ALB%	γG%	A/G	IFAT
D0	11/86	MLT + A 28/d	5100	11.9	32	288.000	7.8	35.5	30.1	0.5	1:640
D30	7/86	A	5360	12.7	32.5	272.000	8.3	36.1	25.5	0.6	1:640
D90	3/86	A	6550	15.4	40.4	186.000	6.4	41.2	17.6	0.7	1:320
D150	7/86	MLT + A 28/d	5970	13.9	37.3	172.000	7.2	33.7	24.7	0.5	1:320
D180	11/86	MA 28/d	4280	8.9	26.3	295.000	8	37.6	26.4	0.6	1:320
D210	5/86	A	6470	15.3	41.2	197.000	5.9	32	19.8	0.5	1:320
D270	2/86	A	6700	14.6	40.2	307.000	7.4	38.6	14.7	0.63	1:160
D450	0/86	A	6760	14.5	42.7	230.000	6.9	46.3	13.9	0.7	1:160

RBC: red cells $\times 10/\mu L$ (reference range 5700–8800 $\times 10/\mu L$).
Hemoglobin: Hb (reference range: 12.9–18.4 g/dL).
Haematocrit: PCV (reference range: 37.1–57%).
Platelet: PLT (reference range: 143300–400000/uL).
Total protein: TP (reference range: 6–8 g/dL).
Albumine: ALB (reference range: 46.3–58.5%).
Gamma globuline: γG (reference range: 5.3–9.9%).
Albumine/globuline: A/G (reference rang: 0.8–1.7).
IFAT: immunofluorescence antibody test (reference range: <1:80).
Miltefosine: MLT.
Allopurinol: A.
Meglumine antimoniate: MA.
Days: d.

gamma globulin values were close to normal range, and the IFAT titer decreased at 1:160.

At examinations performed at D330, D390, and D660 (15 months after completing antimonial therapy), the dog was asymptomatic and no abnormalities were present on complete blood examination and urinalysis, whilst the IFAT titer was stable at 1:160. Allopurinol was discontinued 6 months after the end of antimonial therapy.

Case Number 2. A 10-year-old male Yorkshire terrier, 3.6 kg, was referred to the Internal Medicine Service of the Department of Health, Animal Science and Food Safety of the University of Milan with an 8-month history of weight loss, generalized scaling, and alopecia not responding to shampoo therapy. The dog had previously visited the south of Italy (Sicily Island), a region where canine leishmaniasis is endemic. Prophylaxis had been given for ectoparasites (fipronil and s-methoprene) but not for sandfly vectors of CanL. Physical examination revealed a poor body condition, depression, generalized lymphadenopathy, exfoliative, dry, nonpruritic dermatitis with alopecia and scales on the entire head, back and limbs, and onychogryphosis (clinical score 11/86). The presence of dermatophytosis or demodicosis was excluded by both negative hair culture and negative deep skin scrapings followed by antiparasitic treatment. A blood count revealed mild normocytic hypochromic anemia. Biochemical analysis showed polyclonal hypergammaglobulinemia and hypoalbuminemia (Table 3).

The serum indirect immunofluorescence antibody test (IFAT) for *L. infantum*-specific antibodies yielded a high positive titer of 1:640 (reference range, <1:80) and conventional polymerase chain reaction (PCR) analysis of blood was positive for *L. infantum*. Indirect immunofluorescence assays (IFAT) for *Ehrlichia canis* were negative.

Diagnosis of CanL was made and treatment with oral administration of 2 mg/kg q 24 hr of MLF in combination with allopurinol at 10 mg/kg q 12 hr for 28 days was started and follow-up examinations were performed at days 30, 60, 90, and 150. Results of follow-up clinical scores and blood biochemical examinations are shown in Table 3.

Following the initial treatment with MLF at D30, the dog showed weight gain and resolution of lymphadenopathy, although the alopecia, dry exfoliative dermatitis, and onychogryphosis persisted (clinical score 7/86). At D90, a general clinical improvement was seen (clinical score 3/86) and the only clinicopathological abnormality was hypergammaglobulinemia and an increase of A/G. At D150, the dog presented with recurrence of clinical signs (clinical score 7/86): extreme lethargy, dry and exfoliative dermatitis, and increased hypergammaglobulinemia. A relapse of CanL was diagnosed and a second cycle of MLF in combination with allopurinol was started.

Following the second treatment, with MLF, there was no clinical improvement by D180. The dog suffered further weight loss and showed lymphadenopathy, diffuse hair loss and crusting lesions (clinical score 11/86), and hematological abnormalities (Table 3). On the basis of the lack of improvement in both clinical score and laboratory tests, the dog was classified as "unresponsive" [3] and meglumine antimoniate therapy was started at a dose of 100 mg/kg/q 24 hr sc in combination with allopurinol at a dose of 10 mg/kg q 12 hr for at least 4 weeks.

At D210, following meglumine antimoniate treatment, the clinical status of dog was greatly improved with resolution of the dry, exfoliative dermatitis and of the alopecia (clinical score 5/86) and improvements in the clinicopathological abnormalities.

At D270 (from the start of therapy with MA), hair regrowth was almost complete and at D450 the dog was asymptomatic and the only clinicopathological abnormality was hypergammaglobulinemia and IFAT title at 1 : 80.

3. Discussion

We report the failure of therapeutic response in two dogs with CanL, following a second cycle of treatment with MFT in combination with allopurinol, which both responded promptly to a third therapeutic cycle using another leishmanicidal drug.

These reports draw attention to the need for close monitoring of the pharmacological activity of new molecules, such as MLT, against CanL in order to identify the best treatment protocol and monitor development of resistance in dogs.

It is important to emphasize that, although both dogs had travelled to areas where leishmaniasis is endemic, after diagnosis they remained in nonendemic areas and were treated using deltamethrin collars to prevent sandflies from feeding. It is therefore extremely unlikely that reinfection could have occurred between therapeutic cycles.

Several factors may have contributed to the failure of therapeutic response to MLF in the two cases described: these could be related to the parasite, the drug, or the host. It is known that differences in exposure to antigens, drug pharmacokinetics, doses, frequency of administrations of the therapy, and immune response of the host may affect outcome [17].

Following oral administration of MLF, there may have been a lack of, or incomplete, drug intake by the dogs or the incomplete absorption of the molecule from the intestine. Underdosing, due to poor owner compliance, is also a possibility and this is less likely to occur with a parenterally administered drug (such as salts of antimony) used for the third therapeutic cycle [4].

Dorlo et al. [18] established the first evidence for a drug exposure-effect relationship in human patients. When treating VL, it is essential to achieve sufficient miltefosine exposure for treatment success. In man, it has been recently reported that the cure rate of mucosal leishmaniasis is about 71% after 4 weeks of treatment with miltefosine (2.5 mg/kg/day) and the duration of therapy was increased in this study to try to increase the cure rate [19].

Development of resistance is one of the major concerns with the wide use of miltefosine [20], and one of the important factors contributing to drug resistance is the use of subtherapeutic doses and/or insufficient duration of therapy [14, 20]. Furthermore, miltefosine has a long half-life

(approximately 150 hours) which makes it highly susceptible to the development of resistance [21].

After early reports of therapeutic efficacy, there have been many reports in recent years of the failure of MLT therapy and the resistance to therapy with miltefosine against both visceral leishmaniasis (VL) and cutaneous leishmaniasis (CL) on the Indian subcontinent and new world [14–17, 22, 23]. Studies of in vitro susceptibility of Leishmania infantum isolated from cases in both people and dogs [24] highlight the possibility of cross-resistance to the drugs, including MLF, used in man for the treatment of leishmaniosis.

Clinical disease occurs in patients with a poor cell-mediated immune response. It is well known that the dog is a more sensitive host for L. infantum infection than human patients, but the therapeutic protocol used in the dog of MLT 2 mg/Kg/for 28 days is similar to that used for human beings (2.5 mg/Kg/for 28 days) [19]. In a study of 28 dogs treated with one cycle of 28 days with MLF and allopurinol, Pandey et al. [11] report that 4 dogs had a relapse and needed a second cycle of therapy which still failed to eradicate the parasite from lymph nodes.

In dogs, there is virtually no treatment that will completely eliminate parasites from the host and, even if temporary clinical remission is achieved, a relapse is to be expected in weeks to years after drug withdrawal [5, 8]. In this species, successful treatment is thought to depend, at least in part, on alterations in the host immune response to the parasite. This makes it difficult to distinguish whether a lack of treatment efficacy is attributable to the lack of immune surveillance that allows reactivation of the parasite or a true failure to respond to therapy. In animal models, T-cell-dependent immune mechanisms are not essential for miltefosine to be effective, suggesting that this agent may be useful in patients with depressed parasite-specific mediated immunity, such as sick dogs [12, 23].

This clinical report is limited by the fact that it was not possible to demonstrate the presence of a resistance to the drug, because we were not able to select the strain of Leishmania present in the two cases before and after treatment cycles. However, after an initial clinical improvement following the MLT treatment, both dogs relapsed or were unresponsive to the second therapeutic cycle.

Similar to findings in human medicine [19], it can be assumed that the cycle of therapy was insufficiently long to prevent the resumption of parasite replication and the activation of parasite-specific cell-mediated immunity in the host. It is also possible that the first cycle of MLF selected a resistant strain of Leishmania which was sensitive to the salts of antimony. Certainly, the therapeutic response to MLT was insufficient, whilst the two subjects responded readily to another molecule remaining disease-free for 420 and 270 days, respectively.

The importance of assessing whether treatment with miltefosine in dogs can lead to the selection of drug-resistant Leishmania strains has already been reported [3] and this is particularly relevant because of the sharing of drugs between human and canine medicine [23]. Therefore, in view of the relatively low number of antileishmanial drugs available and the fact that some of these are used in human as well as in veterinary medicine, vigilance of the clinical efficacy of MIL in dogs is crucial. Clinicians should be encouraged to try to isolate parasites collected from unresponsive dogs and submit these to a suitable laboratory so that the possible onset of drug resistance can be monitored.

Conflict of Interests

None of the authors (Daniela Proverbio, Eva Spada, Giada Bagnagatti De Giorgi, and Roberta Perego) declared any conflict of interests.

Acknowledgment

This research received no specific grant from any funding agency in the public, commercial, or nonprofit sectors.

References

[1] G. Baneth, "Canine leishmaniasis: bridging science, public health and politics," *Veterinary Journal*, 2013.

[2] G. Baneth, A. F. Koutinas, L. Solano-Gallego, P. Bourdeau, and L. Ferrer, "Canine leishmaniosis—new concepts and insights on an expanding zoonosis: part one," *Trends in Parasitology*, vol. 24, no. 7, pp. 324–330, 2008.

[3] P. Ciaramella, G. Oliva, R. de Luna et al., "A retrospective clinical study of canine leishmaniasis in 150 dogs naturally infected by Leishmania infantum," *Veterinary Record*, vol. 141, no. 21, pp. 539–543, 1997.

[4] G. Oliva, X. Roura, A. Crotti et al., "Guidelines for treatment of leishmaniasis in dogs," *Journal of the American Veterinary Medical Association*, vol. 236, no. 11, pp. 1192–1198, 2010.

[5] G. Baneth and S. E. Shaw, "Chemotherapy of canine leishmaniosis," *Veterinary Parasitology*, vol. 106, no. 4, pp. 315–324, 2002.

[6] E. Spada, D. Proverbio, D. Groppetti, R. Perego, V. Grieco, and E. Ferro, "First report of the use of meglumine antimoniate for treatment of canine leishmaniasis in a pregnant dog," *Journal of the American Animal Hospital Association*, vol. 47, no. 1, pp. 67–71, 2011.

[7] C. Noli and S. T. Auxilia, "Treatment of canine old world visceral leishmaniasis: a systematic review," *Veterinary Dermatology*, vol. 16, no. 4, pp. 213–232, 2005.

[8] L. Solano-Gallego, A. Koutinas, G. Miró et al., "Directions for the diagnosis, clinical staging, treatment and prevention of canine leishmaniosis," *Veterinary Parasitology*, vol. 165, no. 1-2, pp. 1–18, 2009.

[9] G. Miró, G. Oliva, I. Cruz et al., "Multicentric, controlled clinical study to evaluate effectiveness and safety of miltefosine and allopurinol for canine leishmaniosis," *Veterinary Dermatology*, vol. 20, no. 5-6, pp. 397–404, 2009.

[10] V. Woerly, L. Maynard, A. Sanquer, and H. Eun, "Clinical efficacy and tolerance of miltefosine in the treatment of canine leishmaniosis," *Parasitology Research*, vol. 105, no. 2, pp. 463–469, 2009.

[11] B. D. Pandey, K. Pandey, O. Kaneko, T. Yanagi, and K. Hirayama, "Short report: Relapse of visceral leishmaniasis after miltefosine treatment in a nepalese patient," *The American Journal of Tropical Medicine and Hygiene*, vol. 80, no. 4, pp. 580–582, 2009.

[12] M. Calvopina, E. A. Gomez, H. Sindermann, P. J. Cooper, and Y. Hashiguchi, "Relapse of new world diffuse cutaneous leishmaniasis caused by Leishmania (Leishmania) mexicana after

[13] V. N. R. Das, K. Pandey, N. Verma et al., "Short report: development of post-kala-azar dermal leishmaniasis (PKDL) in miltefosine-treated visceral leishmaniasis," *The American Journal of Tropical Medicine and Hygiene*, vol. 80, no. 3, pp. 336–338, 2009.

[14] L. Manna, F. Vitale, S. Reale et al., "Study of efficacy of miltefosine and allopurinol in dogs with leishmaniosis," *Veterinary Journal*, vol. 182, no. 3, pp. 441–445, 2009.

[15] M. Mateo, L. Maynard, C. Vischer, P. Bianciardi, and G. Miró, "Comparative study on the short term efficacy and adverse effects of miltefosine and meglumine antimoniate in dogs with natural leishmaniosis," *Parasitology Research*, vol. 105, no. 1, pp. 155–162, 2009.

[16] H. M. Andrade, V. P. C. P. Toledo, M. B. Pinheiro et al., "Evaluation of miltefosine for the treatment of dogs naturally infected with L. infantum (=L. chagasi) in Brazil," *Veterinary Parasitology*, vol. 181, no. 2-4, pp. 83–90, 2011.

[17] S. Rijal, B. Ostyn, S. Uranw et al., "Increasing failure of miltefosine in the treatment of kala-azar in nepal and the potential role of parasite drug resistance, reinfection, or noncompliance," *Clinical Infectious Diseases*, vol. 56, no. 11, pp. 1530–1538, 2013.

[18] T. P. Dorlo, S. Rijal, B. Ostyn et al., "Failure of miltefosine in visceral leishmaniasis is associated with low drug exposure," *Journal of Infectious Diseases*, vol. 210, no. 1, pp. 146–153, 2014.

[19] J. Soto, J. Rea, M. Valderrama et al., "Short report: efficacy of extended (six weeks) treatment with miltefosine for mucosal leishmaniasis in Bolivia," *American Journal of Tropical Medicine and Hygiene*, vol. 81, no. 3, pp. 387–389, 2009.

[20] H. C. Maltezou, "Drug resistance in visceral leishmaniasis," *Journal of Biomedicine and Biotechnology*, vol. 2010, Article ID 617521, 8 pages, 2010.

[21] J. Mishra, A. Saxena, and S. Singh, "Chemotherapy of leishmaniasis: past, present and future," *Current Medicinal Chemistry*, vol. 14, no. 10, pp. 1153–1169, 2007.

[22] S. Sundar and P. L. Olliaro, "Miltefosine in the treatment of leishmaniasis: clinical evidence for informed clinical risk management," *Therapeutics and Clinical Risk Management*, vol. 3, no. 5, pp. 733–740, 2007.

[23] S. Sundar and A. Singh, "What steps can be taken to counter the increasing failure of miltefosine to treat visceral leishmaniasis?" *Expert Review of Anti-Infective Therapy*, vol. 11, no. 2, pp. 117–119, 2013.

[24] C. Maia, M. Nunes, M. Marques, S. Henriques, N. Rolão, and L. Campino, "In vitro drug susceptibility of Leishmania infantum isolated from humans and dogs," *Experimental Parasitology*, vol. 135, no. 1, pp. 36–41, 2013.

18

Use of an Endobronchial Blocker and Selective Lung Ventilation to Aid Surgical Removal of a Lung Lobe Abscess in a Dog

Carl Bradbrook,[1] Louise Clark,[1] and Martina Mosing[2]

[1] *Davies Veterinary Specialists, Manor Farm Business Park, Higham Gobion, Hitchin SG5 3HR, UK*
[2] *Department of Anaesthesia, Vetsuisse Faculty, University of Zurich, Winterthurerstrasse 260, 8057 Zurich, Switzerland*

Correspondence should be addressed to Carl Bradbrook, carlbradbrook@gmail.com

Academic Editors: K. K. Adamama-Moraitou and C. Hyun

This paper documents use of an endobronchial blocker (EBB) to achieve selective lung ventilation (SLV) for the purpose of lung lobectomy with thoracoscopy. A 3-year-old female neutered Labrador Retriever, body mass of 18.5 kg, was presented for exploratory thoracoscopy. Acepromazine and methadone were administered as premedication, and anaesthesia was induced with propofol and maintained with isoflurane in 100% oxygen and continuous infusions of fentanyl and lidocaine. Mechanical ventilation of the dog's lungs was performed prior to placement of an Arndt EBB caudal to the right cranial bronchus to allow SLV. Successful SLV was achieved with this technique, allowing continued inflation of the right cranial lobe. A reduction in the arterial partial pressure of oxygen to fractional inspired oxygen ratio ($PaO_2 : FiO_2$) of 444 to 306 occurred after placement of the EBB, with no change in monitored cardiopulmonary variables. F-shunt increased from 17.4% to 23.7% with a reduction in oxygen content (CaO_2) of 20.0 to 18.7 mg dL^{-1}, remaining within the physiologic range. Due to lung adhesions to the diaphragm, conversion to thoracotomy was required for completion of the procedure. This technique is challenging to perform in the dog. Arterial blood gas analysis should be performed to allow adequate monitoring of ventilation.

1. Introduction

Thoracoscopic investigation of lung pathology is becoming a more widely used technique [1] with several advantages over the standard approach of lateral thoracotomy or sternotomy. Reduced requirement for analgesia postthoracoscopy compared to thoracotomy is evident in the human literature and has also been shown in dogs [2]. This may be due to the absence of requirement for rib retraction and a smaller incision when thoracoscopy is used.

To aid visualisation of structures within the thorax with an effectively closed chest, collapse of one lung or lung lobes is required by the surgeon. The use of either one lung ventilation (OLV) by placement of a double lumen endobronchial tube (DLT) [3], EZ-blocker [4], or an endobronchial blocker (EBB) [5, 6] placed proximal to the area of surgical interest are reported in humans and experimental dogs. In human

anaesthesia, selective lung ventilation is reported for blocking specific lung lobes, especially in trauma cases, but OLV is still used more commonly [7]. Currently, OLV has been performed in the dog with an EBB [5, 6], an endobronchial tube [8], and a DLT [3]. There are, however, no case reports of selective lung ventilation (SLV) in the literature that the authors are aware of.

This case report describes the clinical use of an EBB in a dog and the problems encountered whilst selectively blocking the caudal part of the right lung.

2. Case History

A 3-year-old female neutered Labrador Retriever with a body mass of 18.5 kg was presented for investigation of recurrent episodes of coughing, lethargy, and exercise intolerance. The dog had presented twice previously and on both occasions undergone general anaesthesia for computed tomography (CT) of the thorax. Changes between the subsequent CT scans had been suggestive of a migrating foreign body and revealed evidence of consolidation of the right caudal lung lobe. No improvement in this area of consolidation had been evident with antimicrobial therapy, and a decision was made to perform an exploratory thoracoscopy.

Clinical examination revealed a heart rate (HR) of 140 beats per minute (bpm) with a grade II out of VI left side systolic murmur, point of maximum intensity over the mitral valve. Peripheral pulses were strong and regular. Respiratory rate (f_R) was 16 breaths per minute with no increased effort. Auscultation revealed an area of dull lung sounds caudally on the right side of the thorax.

Echocardiography revealed a trivial mitral and tricuspid valve regurgitation, good systolic function, and no evidence of endocarditis.

Haematology and serum biochemistry were unremarkable.

2.1. *Anaesthetic Technique*. Preanaesthetic medication consisted of acepromazine (ACP $2 \, mg \, mL^{-1}$; Novartis AH, UK) $0.01 \, mg \, kg^{-1}$ and methadone (Methadone; Martindales, UK) $0.3 \, mg \, kg^{-1}$ given by the intramuscular route (IM). After preoxygenation, anaesthesia was induced with propofol $5.4 \, mg \, kg^{-1}$ (Propoflo; Abbott Animal Health, UK). The trachea was intubated with a 10 mm cuffed endotracheal tube, attached to a circle breathing system, and the lungs mechanically ventilated with intermittent-positive pressure ventilation (IPPV). Isoflurane was vaporised in 100% oxygen, and vaporiser settings were adjusted accordingly to maintain surgical depth of anaesthesia. IPPV was initially performed with a ventiPAC (Smiths Medical Pneupac, USA) volume/flow-regulated ventilator and in theatre with a Cato edition (Drager Medical AG & Co., Germany) volume-controlled ventilator. Initial ventilator settings was f_R 15 bpm, tidal volume (V_T) 185 mL, resulting in a peak inspiratory pressure (PIP) of $14 \, cm \, H_2O$.

Monitoring consisted of percentage haemoglobin saturation with oxygen (SpO$_2$, %), end tidal partial pressure of carbon dioxide (PE'CO$_2$), body temperature (°C), and lead II ECG (Datex Ohmeda S/5; GE Healthcare, UK). A 20-gauge catheter (Jelco; Smiths Medical, USA) was placed percutaneously into the left dorsalis pedis artery for arterial blood gas sampling and invasive blood pressure measurement (IBP). A 12 fr central venous catheter (Arrow International Inc., USA) was placed into the right jugular vein using the Seldinger technique to provide access for central venous pressure (CVP) measurement and fluid administration.

Fluid therapy consisted of Hartmanns solution (No. 11; Aquapharm, UK), $10 \, mL \, kg^{-1} \, hour^{-1}$ intravenously. Other drugs administered were amoxicillin and clavulanic acid (Augmentin; GlaxoSmithKline, UK) $20 \, mg \, kg^{-1}$ intravenously (IV) and meloxicam (Metacam; Boehringer Ingelheim, UK) $0.2 \, mg \, kg^{-1}$ IV. Fentanyl (Fentanyl citrate; Martindale Laboratories, UK) IV $10 \, mcg \, kg^{-1} \, hour^{-1}$ and lidocaine (Lidocaine HCl 2%; Hameln Pharmaceuticals, UK) IV $30 \, mcg \, kg^{-1} \, minute^{-1}$ were used during the surgical procedure.

2.2. *Surgery*. The dog was placed in left lateral recumbency to allow a right-sided approach to the thoracic cavity. An Arndt endobronchial blocker, 7 fr (Cook Medical, USA), was placed under endoscopic visualisation via the endotracheal tube adaptor (Cook Medical, USA) using the looped guide wire into the right caudal lobe bronchus, making sure it was caudal to the right cranial bronchus and the cuff inflated. The right medial, accessory, and caudal lobes were blocked using this technique. Ventilatory and respiratory parameters were f_R 15 bpm, V_T 185 mL resulting in a PIP of $12 \, cm \, H_2O$ and a dynamic lung compliance $35 \, mL \, cm \, H_2O^{-1}$. The thoracoscopic instrument portals were placed percutaneously in the right lateral thoracic wall and direct visualisation of the lung lobe abscess was possible. Arterial blood gas analysis taken 10 minutes after commencement of thoracoscopy and 30 minutes after the start of SLV showed a reduction in arterial oxygen partial pressure (PaO$_2$) from 400 mmHg to 275 mmHg corresponding to a reduction in PaO$_2$: FiO$_2$ from 444 to 306 and an increase in F-Shunt from 17.4 to 23.7%. f_R was increased to 17 bpm. Dynamic lung compliance had decreased to $20 \, mL \, cm \, H_2O^{-1}$.

Measured cardiovascular parameters during SLV remained stable, with HR 60 bpm and mean invasive blood pressure 70 mmHg. There was minimal sympathetic response to both thoracoscopy and thoracotomy.

After 20 minutes of thoracoscopy and 40 minutes of SLV, the surgeon made the decision that it would not be possible to remove the abscess by this approach due to adhesions of the lung to the diaphragm, and conversion to a standard lateral thoracotomy was made. The EBB cuff was deflated and two-lung ventilation initiated. The surgeon also felt the inflation of the cranial lung lobe reduced visibility within the thorax. On opening of the thoracic cavity, a positive end-expiratory pressure (PEEP) of $3 \, cm \, H_2O$ was applied. Arterial blood gas analysis showed a PaO$_2$ of 300 mmHg corresponding to a PaO$_2$: FiO$_2$ of 333. Cardiovascular parameters were within normal limits. No alterations to the ventilatory settings were made. The lung lobe abscess was successfully removed with this approach, and the dog made an uneventful recovery from anaesthesia.

Postoperatively, analgesia was provided with methadone $0.3 \, mg \, kg^{-1}$ IM as required, meloxicam $0.1 \, mg \, kg^{-1}$ per os, continuation of the lidocaine IV infusion for 24 hours, and intrapleural bupivacaine $1 \, mg \, kg^{-1}$ every 6 hours. Intercostal nerve blocks were performed in three rib spaces cranial and caudal to the incision. The dog progressed well and was discharged after 5 days.

3. Discussion

In this case, the EBB was successfully placed and used to achieve SLV. SLV cannot be achieved with any of the other techniques because the DLT, endobronchial tube, or EZ-blocker cannot easily be advanced distal enough to the carina to selectively block a specific lung lobe. In human anaesthesia, SLV has been shown to have beneficial effects not only during anaesthesia but also in the postoperative period compared to the use of OLV. Selective lung ventilation was associated with improved intra- and postoperative arterial oxygenation, a lower shunt fraction (Q_s/Q_t), and a shorter hospital stay [9].

Selective lung ventilation may be required for certain thorascopic procedures. In healthy dogs, the effect of OLV on PaO_2 and arterial oxygen content (CaO_2) was not deemed to be of any biological or clinical significance, although it does increase Q_s/Q_t due to nonventilation of a portion of lung in open chest thoracotomy [5]. These changes have been associated with a small increase in cardiac output [10]. The use of SLV may reduce the resultant Q_s/Q_t and have a lesser impact on oxygenation.

Selective lung ventilation was chosen in this case to minimise the reduction in PaO_2 associated with OLV [5] and because only the caudal lung lobe was diseased and required resection. A reduction in PaO_2 was observed after commencing SLV, reducing the $PaO_2:FiO_2$ ratio from 444 to 306 but with no resultant change in any monitored cardiovascular parameters including SpO_2. However, the reduction in PaO_2 in this case was 31% (444 to 306 mmHg) compared to 50% (361 to 184 mmHg) in a previous report of OLV [5]. The arterial oxygenation variables recorded in this case suggest SLV may be better at preserving PaO_2 than OLV. The oxygen indices recorded in this case are limited by the short duration of SLV, and we do not know what changes would occur if it was performed for a longer period of time.

In this case, we chose to use the oxygen index, F-shunt to illustrate changes associated with Q_s/Q_t during SLV because it can be easily calculated. For these calculations, there is no need to place a pulmonary artery catheter, only an arterial catheter is required to allow sampling for haemoglobin concentration, PaO_2 and $PaCO_2$. The usefulness of different oxygen tension indices to predict shunt fraction varies amongst studies. This is in direct contrast to another study in which F-Shunt and $PaO_2:FiO_2$ were good estimates of shunt fraction in sheep [11]. The human literature reports values for $PaO_2:FiO_2$ of less than 200 in acute respiratory distress syndrome and less than 300 in acute lung injury [12]; therefore, in this case the reduction in $PaO_2:FiO_2$ was not thought to be of clinical significance. This conclusion was also reached when we looked at the increase in calculated F-Shunt (17.4 to 23.7%), which was within the range reported by Araos et al. [11] and Briganti et al. [13] in sheep and horses, respectively. This is in comparison to the increase in Q_s/Q_t of 17 to 30% reported with OLV [5]. Therefore, we interpret this as not being of clinical significance. However, this increase in shunt most likely explains the reduction in PaO_2 observed.

Lung compliance (CL) reduced from 35 to 20 mL cm H_2O^{-1} after commencement of thoracoscopy. Unfortunately, we do not have a record of CL before SLV commenced. Lung compliance shortly after two-lung ventilation was restarted was 30 mL cm H_2O^{-1}.

Hypoxic pulmonary vasoconstriction (HPV) [10] is a process that aids in reducing pulmonary shunt. Its effect is reduced by a number of factors especially the use of volatile anaesthetic agents. Isoflurane was used in this case for maintenance of anaesthesia and is, therefore, likely to have reduced the HPV response. Isoflurane blocks HPV in a dose-dependent manner and in this case the adjunct analgesic agents, fentanyl and lidocaine, were utilised with the aim of reducing the end tidal isoflurane concentration. It may have been more appropriate to have used total intravenous anaesthesia to minimise both the blunting of HPV and the cardiorespiratory depressant effects of the volatile anaesthetic agents, but we still used isoflurane because of performing SLV and not OLV.

No change in $PE'CO_2$ was observed during this procedure with a marginal increase of $PaCO_2$. This can be explained by the small increase in alveolar dead space fraction (Vd/Vt) of 0.18 to 0.20 by SLV (Vd/Vt = ($PaCO_2$ − $PE'CO_2$)/$PaCO_2$), both though remaining within the reference range in the human literature [14].

Positive end expiratory pressure was not used in this case during SLV due to concern about possible reduction in cardiac output (Q'). This is particularly of concern in a closed chest situation, where it could cause overdistension of alveoli when the administered tidal volume remains as for two-lung ventilation. There was also a possibility that it would reduce visibility and surgical access. It was only initiated when the procedure was converted to a thoracotomy. The use of PEEP has been shown to have a beneficial effect on PaO_2, the resultant alveolar-arterial oxygen gradient and Q_s/Q_t in dogs undergoing closed chest thoracoscopy with OLV and no adverse effect on Q [8, 15]. It is, therefore, not known if the use of PEEP may have prevented the reduction in PaO_2 observed after commencing SLV in this case. After conversion to thoracotomy, the PaO_2 increased marginally, which could be accounted for by the use of PEEP, although no recruitment manoeuvre was performed.

Unfortunately in this case, the use of SLV did not provide the required surgical conditions for completion of the partial lung lobectomy, although no problems were encountered with its use. One of the most common reasons reported for conversion to a thoracotomy is poor visualisation within the thorax, primarily as a result of movement of the endobronchial cuff [7], which we did not observe in this case.

The nonsteroidal anti-inflammatory, meloxicam was also given as part of the multimodal approach to analgesia in this case. It may have been more appropriate to administer it after the procedure, especially as haemorrhage and periods of hypotension were possible, though not observed complications.

This paper documents the use of an EBB and SLV with continued ventilation of the right cranial lung lobe. EBB placement is a straightforward technique to learn, but due to problems with visualisation in this case further studies are required to show any benefits of SLV over OLV.

Conflict of Interests

All authors have no known conflict of interests.

References

[1] E. Monnet, "Interventional thoracoscopy in small animals," *Veterinary Clinics of North America—Small Animal Practice*, vol. 39, no. 5, pp. 965–975, 2009.

[2] P. J. Walsh, A. M. Remedios, J. F. Ferguson, D. D. Walker, S. Cantwell, and T. Duke, "Thoracoscopic versus open partial pericardectomy in dogs: Comparison of postoperative pain and morbidity," *Veterinary Surgery*, vol. 28, no. 6, pp. 472–479, 1999.

[3] C. Adami, S. Axiak, U. Rytz, and C. Spadavecchia, "Alternating one lung ventilation using a double lumen endobronchial tube and providing CPAP to the non-ventilated lung in a dog," *Veterinary Anaesthesia and Analgesia*, vol. 38, no. 1, pp. 70–76, 2011.

[4] K. Ruetzler, G. Grubhofer, W. Schmid et al., "Randomized clinical trial comparing double-lumen tube and EZ-Blocker for single-lung ventilation," *British Journal of Anaesthesia*, vol. 106, no. 6, pp. 896–902, 2011.

[5] S. T. Kudnig, E. Monnet, M. Riquelme, J. S. Gaynor, D. Corliss, and M. D. Salman, "Effect of one-lung ventilation on oxygen delivery in anesthetized dogs with an open thoracic cavity," *American Journal of Veterinary Research*, vol. 64, no. 4, pp. 443–448, 2003.

[6] S. T. Kudnig, E. Monnet, M. Riquelme, J. S. Gaynor, D. Corliss, and M. D. Salman, "Effect of positive end-expiratory pressure on oxygen delivery during 1-lung ventilation for thoracoscopy in normal dogs," *Veterinary Surgery*, vol. 35, no. 6, pp. 534–542, 2006.

[7] J. H. Campos, "An update on bronchial blockers during lung separation techniques in adults," *Anesthesia and Analgesia*, vol. 97, no. 5, pp. 1266–1274, 2003.

[8] M. Mosing, I. Iff, and Y. Moens, "Endoscopic removal of a bronchial carcinoma in a dog using one-lung ventilation," *Veterinary Surgery*, vol. 37, no. 3, pp. 222–225, 2008.

[9] J. Ye, M. N. Gu, C. Q. Zhang, K. C. Cai, and R. J. Cai, "Effects of selective left lower lobar blockade by Coopdech endobronchial blocker tube on intrapulmonary shunt and arterial oxygenation: a comparison with double-lumen endobronchial tube," *Nan Fang Yi Ke Da Xue Xue Bao*, vol. 29, no. 11, pp. 2244–2247, 2009.

[10] M. Riquelme, E. Monnet, S. T. Kudnig et al., "Cardiopulmonary changes induced during one-lung ventilation in anesthetized dogs with a closed thoracic cavity," *American Journal of Veterinary Research*, vol. 66, no. 6, pp. 973–977, 2005.

[11] J. Araos, M. P. Larenza, V. DeMonte et al., "Evaluation of different oxygenation indices for estimation of intrapulmonary venous admixture at different inspiratory oxygen fractions in anesthetized sheep," in *Proceedings of the Spring Meeting of the Association of Veterinary Anaesthetists*, p. 75, Bari, Italy, 2011.

[12] S. P. Pilbeam, "Oxygenation and acid-base evaluation," in *Mechanical Ventilation: Physiological and Clinical Applications*, S. P. Pilbeam and J. M. Cairo, Eds., pp. 1–13, Mosby Elsevier, 2006.

[13] A. Briganti, D. A. Portela, M. Sgorbini et al., "Comparison of different oxygenation indices for the estimation of intrapulmonary shunt in horses under general anaesthesia," in *Proceedings of the Spring Meeting of the Association of Veterinary Anaesthetists*, p. 129, Bari, Italy, 2011.

[14] S. P. Pilbeam, "Appendix B," in *Mechanical Ventilation: Physiological and Clinical Applications*, S. P. Pilbeam and J. M. Cairo, Eds., pp. 601–606, Mosby Elsevier, 2006.

[15] M. Riquelme, E. Monnet, S. T. Kudnig et al., "Cardiopulmonary effects of positive end-expiratory pressure during one-lung ventilation in anesthetized dogs with a closed thoracic cavity," *American Journal of Veterinary Research*, vol. 66, no. 6, pp. 978–983, 2005.

19

Canine Choroid Plexus Tumor with Intracranial Dissemination Presenting as Multiple Cystic Lesions

Trisha J. Oura,[1] Peter J. Early,[2] Samuel H. Jennings,[2] Melissa J. Lewis,[2] Jeremy R. Tobias,[2] and Donald E. Thrall[3]

[1] *Tufts Veterinary Emergency Treatment and Specialties, 525 South Street, Walpole, MA 02081, USA*
[2] *North Carolina State University Veterinary Teaching Hospital, 1052 William Moore Drive, Raleigh, NC 27607, USA*
[3] *Associate Dean for Research, Ross University School of Veterinary Medicine, P.O. Box 334, Basseterre, Saint Kitts, USA*

Correspondence should be addressed to Peter J. Early; pjearly@ncsu.edu

Academic Editors: S. C. Rahal, M. Santos, R. M. Santos, and S. Stuen

A Miniature Pinscher developed acute blindness and behavioral changes. On magnetic resonance imaging (MRI), there were multiple small intra-axial cystic lesions, and primary differential diagnoses included primary or metastatic neoplasia and neurocysticercosis. These cystic lesions were subsequently diagnosed histopathologically as disseminated choroid plexus carcinoma. This is only the second documented description of this diagnosis in a dog, but both patients had very similar MRI findings. This patient adds to the literature about the MRI characteristics of choroid plexus tumors and indicates that choroid plexus tumor should be considered as a possible cause of small multifocal intra-axial cystic brain lesions in dogs, regardless of whether a primary intraventricular lesion is visible.

1. Introduction

Choroid plexus tumors arise from the epithelium of the choroid plexus and account for approximately 10% of all primary intracranial tumors in dogs [1]. These predominantly benign tumors are found most commonly in the lateral, third, or fourth ventricles. Dogs are typically middle-aged at the time of presentation, and males and Golden Retrievers may be overrepresented [1]. Clinical signs, which can include ataxia, circling, blindness, and behavior changes, are often due to hydrocephalus as ventricular lesions may cause cerebrospinal fluid (CSF) accumulation due to obstruction and/or overproduction [1, 2].

Definitive diagnosis of choroid plexus tumors is by histopathologic evaluation; however, there are often distinctive findings on magnetic resonance imaging (MRI), such as well-differentiated, irregularly margined, intraventricular masses. These masses are typically hyperintense on T2 and proton density (PD) sequences with strong, homogeneous contrast enhancement [3]. Perilesional edema may be present or absent, and primary choroid plexus tumors may contain foci of hemorrhage or mineralization [3].

Both choroid plexus papillomas and carcinomas can metastasize, often to the spinal subarachnoid space, creating the so-called drop metastases. Rarely, tumor dissemination and meningeal carcinomatosis of choroid plexus tumors have been documented, with spread of neoplastic cells within the leptomeninges [4, 5]. Although documented histologically [5], there has been only one prior report of the MRI findings of a dog with choroid plexus carcinoma and secondary leptomeningeal metastases [4, 5]. The purpose of this report is to add information from one additional patient with this interesting and unusual manifestation of choroid plexus tumor.

2. Case Presentation

A 9-year-old neutered male Miniature Pinscher developed acute-onset blindness and possible seizure activity. When examined, the patient was anxious, vocalizing, and exhibiting compulsive behaviors. Both pupils were mydriatic with absent menace response, absent dazzle, and absent direct and indirect papillary light reflexes. Mild to moderate cervical pain was elicited on palpation and during range of motion.

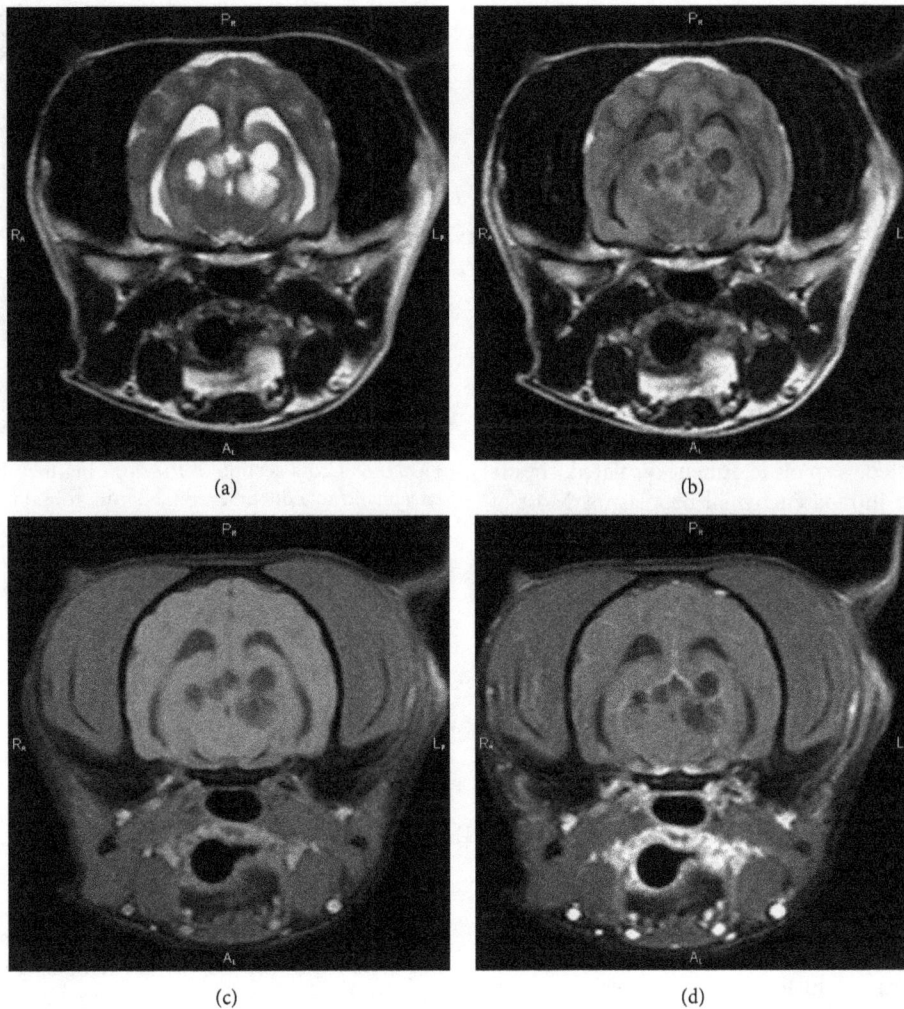

FIGURE 1: Transverse magnetic resonance images (MRIs) at the level of the mesencephalic aqueduct. (a) T2W image (TE/TR, 104/4440 ms) with several round lesions within the caudal thalamus that are isoattenuating to cerebrospinal fluid within the lateral ventricles. (b) These lesions null on FLAIR sequences (TR/TE, 78/9000 ms) with mild perilesional hyperintensities representing edema. (c) The lesions are isoattenuating to CSF on T1W images (TE/TR, 12/53 ms) and have mild contrast enhancement of the lesion wall (d).

The neuroanatomic localization was multifocal involving the prosencephalon and brainstem and or possible cervical involvement.

Magnetic resonance imaging of the brain was performed using a 1.5 T magnet (Symphony 1.5 T; Siemens Medical Solutions USA, Inc., Malvern, PA, USA). Caudal to the interthalamic adhesion, there were numerous small, ~1.0–10.0 mm diameter, intra-axial, thin-walled, T2 hyperintense (TE/TR, 104/4440 ms), T1-hypointense (TE/TR, 12/53 ms) nodules within the thalamus, colliculi, and hippocampus. The T2-signal of these nodules was nulled in FLAIR images (TR/TE, 78/9000 ms) indicating a cystic nature, and the wall of the nodules enhanced following intravenous administration of gadoversetamide contrast medium (Optimark; Mallinkrodt Inc., St. Louis, MO, USA). Based on the FLAIR sequences, there was also mild perilesional edema (Figure 1). There was mild obstructive hydrocephalus due to mesencephalic aqueduct compression by the more caudal nodules, mild transtentorial herniation causing compression of the rostral

aspect of the cerebellum, and syrinx formation in the cranial aspect of the cervical spinal cord. Additional smaller nodules were present in the ventral aspect of the cerebellum. Based on the MRI findings, differential diagnoses for the cystic lesions included atypical cystic metastatic neoplasia or neural cysticercosis, though the latter was considered much less likely as the animal was not known to have lived in or travelled to an area endemic for cysticercosis.

Differential diagnoses for the cystic lesions included atypical cystic metastatic neoplasia or neural cysticercosis. Obstructive hydrocephalus and compression of the lateral geniculate nuclei by the cystic lesions were thought to be possible causes of the blindness.

On CSF analysis, there was a mild mononuclear pleocytosis (21 cells/uL) and an elevated total protein (54.5 mg/dL). No etiologic agents or neoplastic cells were identified.

The patient was discharged with prednisone 5 mg tablet given orally once every 24 hours, omeprazole 10 mg capsule given orally once every 24 hours, aspirin 5 mg capsule given orally once every 24 hours, enalapril 3.75 mg tablet orally given every 12 hours, albendazole 227 mg oral suspension given orally every 12 hours for 3 days, and praziquantel/pyrantel pamoate/febantel 54.4 mg tablet given orally once.

Within four days of discharge, the patient had an improved mental status with decreased compulsive behavior. However, within one week the patient exhibited generalized seizure activity, and anticonvulsant therapy was initiated. Approximately three weeks after discharge, the patient developed cluster seizures and was euthanized.

At postmortem examination, the cystic lesions and mild hydrocephalus were confirmed. There were also several additional pinpoint to 0.1 cm cystic foci within the cerebral leptomeninges (Figure 2). On histopathology, approximately 20% of the left thalamus was replaced by scattered, variably sized, well-demarcated, expansile, unencapsulated, cystic intraventricular, and intraparenchymal neoplasms. Most of the clear cystic cavities were often lined by a relatively uniform population of cuboidal to columnar cells arranged in a single layer with a few, simple to complex, intraluminal papillary projections supported by thin fibrovascular cores. These cells had well-defined cell borders with small to moderate amount of eosinophilic cytoplasm with an oval, basal nucleus with finely stippled chromatin and an indistinct nucleolus. The cells exhibited minimal anisocytosis and anisokaryosis. Occasionally, however, the cysts and papillary projections were lined by up to eight layers of jumbled epithelial cells with more variably sized, shaped, and located nuclei with more open chromatin. There was rare single cell necrosis within the neoplastic population. The mitotic rate varied regionally from zero to seven mitotic figures in 10 high magnification (400x) fields. The cysts occasionally contained small amounts of laminated, mineralized material. The adjacent neuropil was compressed and vacuolated with mild gliosis and, rarely, a few perivascular lymphocytes and plasma cells. Similar cystic neoplasms were present within sections of brainstem bilaterally adjacent to the fourth ventricle, presumed to be in the lateral apertures, and throughout the cerebral and cerebellar meninges. The final diagnosis was choroid plexus carcinoma with multifocal intracranial metastasis and mild, secondary hydrocephalus.

3. Discussion

Presently there is only one other description of the MRI findings associated with intracranial dissemination of a choroid plexus tumor in a dog. Given the rarity of this condition, it is important that additional patients be described as they are discovered. Similar clinical finding between both dogs included blindness and behavioral changes. On MRI, both patients had mild hydrocephalus and similar sized intra-axial cystic lesions which, in our patient, were located primarily in the caudal thalamus, colliculi and hippocampus, while in the previously reported patient, additional lesions were also found throughout the temporal and frontal lobes [4]. The cystic lesions in our patient were also associated with mild perilesional edema and mild contrast enhancement of the cyst walls which was not observed previously. This difference

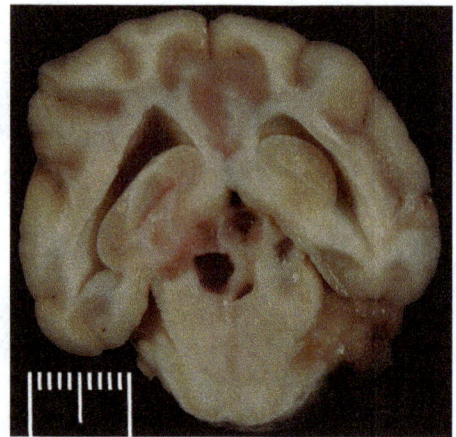

FIGURE 2: Cross-section of the dog's brain at the level of the mesencephalic aqueduct. Several 2-3 mm, round to oval, cystic lesions multifocally expand and replace the dorsal thalamic parenchyma and compress the mesencephalic aqueduct. Histopathologically, these corresponded to choroid plexus tumors.

may be due to the fact that the previous patient received glucocorticoids prior to MRI acquisition [4]. The primary tumor could not be identified in either patient.

Meningeal carcinomatosis is uncommon in animals but has been documented with metastatic mammary carcinoma and carcinoma without an identified primary tumor [6, 7]. Specifically, intraparenchymal dissemination of choroid plexus tumors is documented rarely [4, 5]. Intracranial dissemination of choroid plexus tumors is also uncommon in people, with few reports of neoplasia involving the leptomeninges or seeding of the subarachnoid space [8–10]. One human patient had multiple, nonenhancing, cystic subarachnoid lesions of the cerebellum, brainstem, and frontal lobe on MRI, an appearance very similar to our findings [9].

4. Conclusion

Multiple intra-axial cystic lesions are an unusual manifestation of choroid plexus tumors in both people and animals. More commonly, choroid plexus tumors are typically solitary, lobulated, strongly contrast-enhancing lesions within the ventricular system [3]. This case report of a canine patient adds to the available literature regarding choroid plexus tumors and indicates that disseminated choroid plexus tumor should be considered as a differential diagnosis for multiple small intra-axial cysts in dogs, regardless of whether a primary intraventricular tumor is visible.

References

[1] D. R. Westworth, P. J. Dickinson, W. Vernau et al., "Choroid plexus tumors in 56 dogs (1985–2007)," *Journal of Veterinary Internal Medicine*, vol. 22, no. 5, pp. 1157–1165, 2008.

[2] F. A. Zaki and L. A. Nafe, "Choroid plexus tumors in the dog," *Journal of the American Veterinary Medical Association*, vol. 176, no. 4, pp. 328–330, 1980.

[3] S. L. Kraft, P. R. Gavin, C. DeHaan, M. Moore, L. R. Wendling, and C. W. Leathers, "Retrospective review of 50 canine intracranial tumors evaluated by magnetic resonance imaging," *Journal of Veterinary Internal Medicine*, vol. 11, no. 4, pp. 218–225, 1997.

[4] D. Lipsitz, R. E. Levitski, and A. E. Chauvet, "Magnetic resonance imaging of a choroid plexus carcinoma and meningeal carcinomatosis in a dog," *Veterinary Radiology and Ultrasound*, vol. 40, no. 3, pp. 246–250, 1999.

[5] A. K. Patnaik, R. A. Erlandson, and P. H. Lieberman, "Choroid plexus carcinoma with meningeal carcinomatosis in a dog," *Veterinary Pathology*, vol. 17, no. 3, pp. 381–385, 1980.

[6] M. Pumarola and M. Balasch, "Meningeal carcinomatosis in a dog," *Veterinary Record*, vol. 138, no. 21, pp. 523–524, 1996.

[7] I. Mateo, V. Lorenzo, A. Muñoz, and J. Molín, "Meningeal carcinomatosis in a dog: magnetic resonance imaging features and pathological correlation," *Journal of Small Animal Practice*, vol. 51, no. 1, pp. 43–48, 2010.

[8] R. Leblanc, S. Bekhor, D. Melanson, and S. Carpenter, "Diffuse craniospinal seeding from a benign fourth ventricle choroid plexus papilloma. Case report," *Journal of Neurosurgery*, vol. 88, no. 4, pp. 757–760, 1998.

[9] T. McCall, M. Binning, D. T. Blumenthal, and R. L. Jensen, "Variations of disseminated choroid plexus papilloma: 2 case reports and a review of the literature," *Surgical Neurology*, vol. 66, no. 1, pp. 62–67, 2006.

[10] F. Doglietto, L. Lauretti, T. Tartaglione, M. Gessi, E. Fernandez, and G. Maira, "Diffuse craniospinal choroid plexus papilloma with involvement of both cerebellopontine angles," *Neurology*, vol. 65, no. 6, p. 842, 2005.

aspartate aminotransferase activity (7437 U/L; reference interval 15–50 U/L), and creatine kinase activity (452,500 U/L; reference interval 92–357) remained above the reference interval and were increased compared to the previous day.

A recheck urinalysis collected via cystocentesis had slightly cloudy dark yellow urine with a specific gravity of 1.012, a pH of 7.5, proteinuria (114.8 mg/dL), and 3+ blood. Sediment examination contained 0–5 erythrocytes per high power field. Urine protein to creatinine ratio was 5.5.

On evaluation of a coagulation panel, the dog was thrombocytopenic ($146 \times 10^3/\mu$L; reference interval $164–510 \times 10^3/\mu$L) with increased mean platelet volume (13.3 fL; reference interval 8.4–13 fL), prolonged activated partial thromboplastin time (16.0 s; reference interval 8–14.4 s), shortened thrombin time (3.3 s; reference interval 7.6–22 s), and hyperfibrinogenemia (780 mg/dL; reference interval 100–300 mg/dL). D-dimers (500–1000 ng/mL; reference interval 0–250 ng/mL) and fibrin degradation products (>20,000 μg/mL; reference interval 0–5 μg/mL) were increased. Antithrombin activity was decreased (62%; reference interval 85–100%).

After one episode of vomiting, metoclopramide (0.4 mg/kg subcutaneously every 6 hours) and famotidine (1 mg/kg intravenously once daily) were added to his drug regimen. He remained on the previous doses of heparin constant rate infusion, acetylsalicylic acid, and crystalloid with KCl. He was given multiple small meals throughout the afternoon and experienced no further episodes of nausea, regurgitation, or vomiting. His food was removed overnight.

The patient remained stable the following morning and was premedicated with acepromazine (0.05 mg/kg intravenously) and hydromorphone (0.1 mg/kg intravenously). General anesthesia was induced with propofol (6 mg/kg intravenously) and maintained with isoflurane (1.5–2% in 100% O_2) for an abdominal exploratory surgery. The ventral aspect of the abdomen was prepared aseptically, and a standard celiotomy was performed. White to translucent 2-3 cm long fibrin sheets were attached to the visceral and retroperitoneal surfaces of both kidneys. Portions were removed and submitted for culture. Multifocal, 3-4 mm firm, flat, white to tan plaques were visualized on the pancreas. A section of the right limb of the pancreas containing these lesions was biopsied using the guillotine method with 4-0 polydioxanone (PDS, Ethicon, Cornelia, GA). The left kidney was biopsied using a biopsy needle (TruCut, CareFusion, San Diego, CA) and the liver was biopsied using the guillotine method with 4-0 polydioxanones (PDS, Ethicon). The abdominal aorta was identified and traced caudally to the bifurcation. Umbilical tape was placed around the aorta and both external iliac arteries, and bulldog clamps were placed across the aorta immediately proximal to the thrombus and on both external iliac arteries distal to the thrombus. A full thickness, 1 cm incision was made on the ventral surface of the aorta (Figure 2). Atraumatic microforceps and a nerve hook were used to remove three to four pieces of thrombus approximately 1-2 cm in diameter (Figure 3). The bifurcation was subsequently flushed with sterile saline to ensure removal of all pieces of the thrombus. The defect was sutured using 6-0 polypropylene (Prolene, Ethicon) in

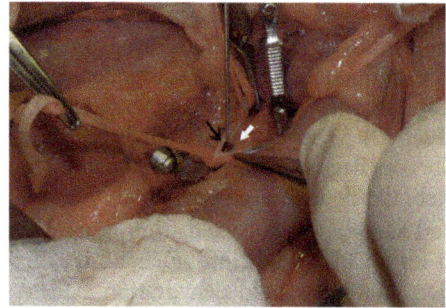

FIGURE 2: Intraoperative photograph of the aortotomy (black arrow). The cranial portion of the dog is to the left of the image. The thrombus is seen within the lumen of the aorta, just cranial to the aortic bifurcation (white arrow).

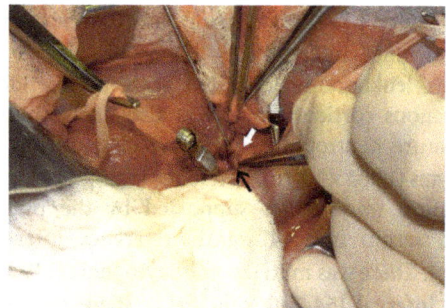

FIGURE 3: Intraoperative photograph of thrombus removal. The cranial portion of the dog is to the left of the image. The thrombus (black arrow) is removed from the aorta, at the level of the aortic bifurcation (white arrow).

a simple interrupted pattern. Prior to complete closure, the proximal vascular clamp was temporarily released to allow flooding of the operated aortic segment with blood, to prevent an air embolism. After the final sutures were placed in the aorta, the vascular clamps were carefully released and the aortotomy was observed for hemorrhage. Minor hemorrhage was controlled with gentle pressure. A Foley catheter was passed through the penis and into the urethra for retropulsion of the urethral stones into the bladder lumen. Stay sutures were placed in the urinary bladder and a cystotomy was performed. The contents of the bladder were examined and no stones were found. The bladder was closed using 4-0 polydioxanone (PDS, Ethicon), in a simple continuous pattern. The celiotomy was closed in a routine manner, and a jugular catheter was placed. All biopsy samples and the thrombus were submitted for histopathology.

The dog had an uneventful recovery from anesthesia. Postoperatively, the femoral pulse quality was immediately noted to have improved, and the distal limbs were warm to the touch. Postoperative analgesia was provided by hydromorphone (0.1 mg/kg intravenously every 6 hours) and a constant rate infusion of lidocaine (1.5 mg/kg/h intravenously). The dog experienced one mild episode of vomiting, associated with hydromorphone administration.

Histopathologic examination of the surgical biopsies confirmed the formation of a thrombus and identified changes in

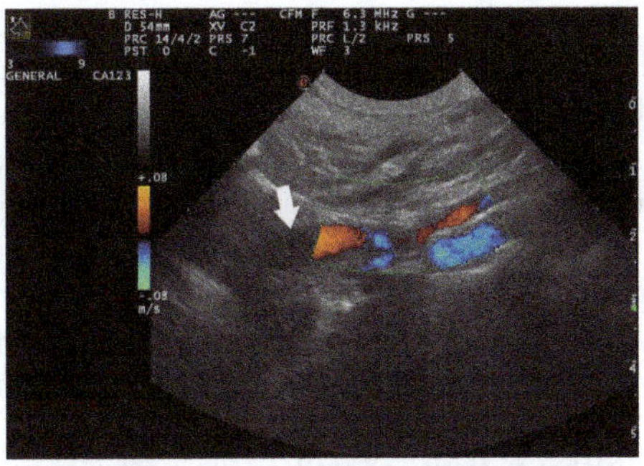

FIGURE 4: Recheck abdominal ultrasound at the level of the aortic bifurcation. The cranial portion of the dog is to the left of the image. The aorta is anechoic (arrow), and Color-flow Doppler application indicates blood flow within the aorta and external iliac arteries.

the pancreas consistent with necrotizing pancreatitis. There was moderate renal tubular and hepatocellular vacuolation, suggestive of lipidosis.

Over the next several days in the hospital, the dog was weaned off of hydromorphone, lidocaine, metoclopramide, famotidine, heparin, and intravenous fluids. Tramadol (5 mg/kg *per os* every 8 hours) was instituted for continued analgesia, and acetylsalicylic acid was continued. The vomiting episodes decreased, and appetite gradually improved.

The patient was discharged on acetylsalicylic acid (0.5 mg/kg *per os* once daily), famotidine (1 mg/kg *per os* once daily for 7 days), and sucralfate (0.5 g/dog *per os* every 8 hours) after 10-day hospitalization. At the time of discharge, the dog displayed ambulatory paraparesis. His owners were instructed to continue feeding a bland diet (Hill's Prescription Diet i/d, Hill's Pet Nutrition Inc.) and restrict his activity when unsupervised.

The dog was presented 6 weeks later for a recheck examination. His physical examination revealed rectal euthermia (38.2°C) and a grade II/VI left-sided systolic heart murmur. His femoral pulses were strong bilaterally, and his distal pelvic limbs felt warm to the touch. Neurologic examination revealed no abnormalities. A recheck abdominal ultrasound showed a normal abdominal aorta (Figure 4) and pancreas. The previously noted bilateral renal diverticular mineralization and hyperechoic debris within the urinary bladder were still present; there was no evidence of cystolithiasis. The dog was discharged with instructions to wean off of oral acetylsalicylic acid over the ensuing 6 weeks. Follow-up phone call 5 years after the incident confirmed that the dog continues to do well. He ambulates normally and has not had any further bouts of pancreatitis.

3. Discussion

Though it frequently occurs in cats with hypertrophic cardiomyopathy, ATE is relatively uncommon in dogs. Rare cases of canine ATE have been associated with underlying conditions, such as hyperadrenocorticism, hypothyroidism,

diabetes mellitus, cardiac arrhythmias and structural cardiac disease, various neoplasms, protein-losing nephropathy, protein-losing enteropathy, gastric dilatation/volvulus, and trauma [1–8]. In contrast to feline ATE, affected dogs have a better prognosis, owing to collateral circulation [8]. Dogs also differ from cats in that they can present with acute or chronic signs. Dogs presenting with an acute onset of ATE tend to have more severe neurologic dysfunction, such as paraparesis or paraplegia, while dogs with a chronic onset tend to have milder signs, such as exercise intolerance [6]. The patient in this case had moderately to markedly increased muscle enzyme concentrations that corresponded with the acute presentation and ongoing ischemic necrosis. Some of the electrolyte changes such as the high normal phosphorous and hypocalcemia could be attributed to acute rhabdomyolysis as described in foals and people [9–12]. In addition, acute aortic thrombosis is associated with moderate to marked increase in activity of serum muscle enzymes (AST and CK), while patients with chronic lesions often have normal to mild increased activity of muscle enzymes [10, 12].

Clinical laboratory data in this case strongly suggested a hypercoagulable state. There are numerous underlying conditions that result in a hypercoagulable state with formation of a thrombus. These conditions affect one of the main factors of coagulation that were originally outlined by Virchow: blood flow, endothelial integrity, and the balance between coagulation and fibrinolysis [13]. The valvular disease noted on echocardiography was not thought to be the cause of the thrombus, due to the lack of spontaneous echocardiographic contrast or thrombus noted within the left atrium [14].

Clinical findings (blood work, history, and physical examination) made other causes of hypercoagulability, such as hyperadrenocorticism, hypothyroidism, immune-mediated hemolytic anemia, sepsis or other systemic infection, polycythemia vera, and lipemia, less likely; however, endocrine disease such as hypothyroidism and hyperadrenocorticism could not be ruled out without specific testing. The decreased antithrombin activity led to the consideration of hepatic or glomerular disease as etiologies for thromboembolic disease. Although the liver and kidneys were judged to be normal on abdominal ultrasound, histopathologic evaluation revealed mild to moderate vacuolation of the kidneys and liver. Pancreatitis was not originally a consideration because of the lack of history and clinical signs of pancreatitis and the lack of identifiable pancreatic lesions on ultrasound.

In this case, there were three potential factors that may have contributed to formation of the thrombus. The first and most significant contributor is local vasculitis secondary to necrotizing pancreatitis. Vasculitis mediates thrombus formation through exposure of subendothelial components such as collagen, tissue factor, and fibronectin [15]. These are all potential stimuli for platelet aggregation and coagulation [15]. Pancreatitis induces disseminated intravascular coagulation (DIC) via release of active pancreatic enzymes into circulation. These enzymes normally are inactivated by α-macroglobulin [16]. Once α-macroglobulin is depleted, the enzymes are capable of activating the coagulation cascade and initiating DIC [16]. Systemic inflammation induces the production of fibrinogen, an acute phase protein. In situations where there is imbalance of fibrin formation and degradation, hyperfibrinogenemia may promote thrombosis by increasing fibrin formation and clot stabilization [17, 18]. In addition, hyperfibrinogenemia along with increased concentrations of fibrin degradation products and d-dimers are considered risk factors for thrombotic events [17]. In this case, the dog had all three risk factors, moderate to marked hyperfibrinogenemia, mild to moderate increase in d-dimers, and marked increase in fibrin degradation products.

The patient also had a protein-losing nephropathy (urine protein:creatinine ratio of 5.5). Antithrombin was likely lost in the urine and contributed to an imbalance in coagulation and fibrinolysis. Routine histopathologic examination of the kidney did not identify glomerular disease but did suggest moderate tubular lipidosis which may have inhibited protein resorption. Glucosuria in the face of hypoglycemia and trace ketonuria also support renal tubular disease. Because antithrombin was not measured until after the clot was formed, it was possibly decreased due to consumption during thrombus formation. An additional test which may have been helpful in determining this patient's global hemostatic condition would be thromboelastography (which was not available at the time).

Lastly, the patient also had underlying cardiovascular disease that altered systemic blood flow. There was no evidence of a thrombus or spontaneous echocardiographic contrast; however, even slight alternations in blood flow because of valvular disease can lead to stasis or turbulence and development of thrombi [8, 13]. While structural heart disease may have contributed to systemic alteration in blood flow, inflammation associated with pancreatitis may have also altered blood flow locally.

Acute therapeutic options described for ATE in the short term include thrombolytic drug therapy and rheolytic thrombectomy. Rheolytic thrombectomy for ATE has been mentioned in the veterinary literature, but its use has not been fully described in dogs [3, 19, 20]. In a recent feline study, thrombi were successfully dissolved in 5/6 cats, using a commercially available rheolytic thrombectomy system, but only 3/6 cats survived till discharge [19]. There are few reports regarding the use of thrombolytic drug therapy, such as tissue plasminogen activator (t-PA), for dissolution of an ATE in cats and dogs [2, 4, 5, 21–23]. Though t-PA can reportedly improve functional neurologic outcome in cats, it is also associated with severe adverse side effects, including fatal hyperkalemia and hemorrhage, and its use is not widely recommended [19, 21]. Catheter-directed thrombolysis, in which thrombolytic drugs are applied directly to the thrombus, has been described [22, 24]. Side effects include hemorrhage, pulmonary embolism, and reperfusion injury. While catheter-directed thrombolysis has been shown to improve outcome and have fewer complications in people, such studies in animals are lacking. Balloon dilation and angioplasty present problems, such as pulmonary embolism and reocclusion, although this technique has shown some promise when combined with endovascular stents in people [22]. Studies on this technique are lacking in veterinary patients.

Long-term treatment options include anticoagulant and antiplatelet medications, such as heparin, acetylsalicylic acid, and clopidogrel [25]. In this case, heparin was given immediately not to lyse the thrombus but to reduce its expansion/extension [26]. Heparin interrupts coagulation in both the intrinsic and extrinsic pathways. At a low dose, heparin prevents further thrombosis by inactivating factor Xa and preventing the conversion of prothrombin to thrombin through the enhancement of antithrombin activity [25, 26]. Given the decreased antithrombin activity reported in this patient, as well as the presence of pancreatitis, the overall effect of the heparin therapy cannot be determined. Acetylsalicylic acid reduces platelet aggregation by inhibiting cyclooxygenase-1, which decreases synthesis of prostaglandins and thromboxanes (TXA2) [25]. However, antiplatelet activity of acetylsalicylic acid in diseased canine patients has not been fully elucidated [25].

Thrombectomy for canine ATE has been mentioned in the literature, but methods for open aortic thrombus removal have not been previously described [2]. Surgical removal of thrombi has reportedly been met with mixed results and is considered to be a risky procedure in cats with ATE [21, 22], but to the authors' knowledge there are no reports describing open surgical thrombectomy in dogs. Feline ATE is usually caused by underlying cardiac disease, specifically hypertrophic or restrictive cardiomyopathy. The long-term prognosis for cats presenting with ATE and underlying cardiac disease is poor, with mean and median survival times reported at 51 and 350 days [27, 28]. Even if the ATE can be removed or dissolved, recurrence rates range within 17–50% with treatment of the cardiac disease [27, 28]. Aortic thromboembolism in dogs is more rarely seen than in cats, and it may not be due to cardiac disease. The dog in this report had evidence of structural cardiac disease, but there was no evidence that this was directly contributing to the development of thromboembolism [14]. The cause for this dog's ATE was unknown at the time of work-up. Due to the significant neurologic dysfunction and the lack of information about rheolytic thrombectomy in dogs, the decision to perform a surgical thrombectomy was made. It was also speculated that this patient's ATE was an isolated incident, decreasing the risk of recurrence after thrombectomy that often occurs in feline patients. Surgical thrombectomy may be warranted in dogs that do not have the underlying risk factors for ATE recurrence, primarily cardiac disease, and that are considered good anesthetic candidates.

Ischemia-reperfusion injury is a concern after ATE [29]. After a period of decreased or absent tissue oxygenation, reactive oxygen species (ROS), such as the hydroxyl radical, are formed [29, 30]. Reactive oxygen species interact with cells in many deleterious ways, including protein, DNA, and RNA damage, lipid peroxidation of cell membranes, and loss of cell membrane permeability [29, 30]. Neutrophils are recruited into the area of tissue damage, become activated, and release their own ROS. After addressing the occluded vessel, reperfusion of the damaged tissue allows release of these reactive oxygen species into systemic circulation, which may cause myocardial and lung damage [29].

Additionally, during ischemia there is lack of aerobic cellular respiration, leading to decreased adenosine triphosphate (ATP). This causes failure of ATP-dependent cell membrane pumps, such as Na^+/K^+ and Na^+/Ca^{++}. As a result of pump failure and direct damage to cell membranes, sodium and calcium are allowed to accumulate within cells, leading to cytoplasmic swelling and lysis and the initiation of the proapoptotic caspase and calpain cascades [29]. Massive cell death can be the end result. Additionally, potassium is allowed to accumulate extracellularly, leading to systemic hyperkalemia. This, in turn, can have deleterious effects on the patient, causing cardiac arrhythmias and further neuromuscular dysfunction [31, 32]. In this case, the dog was not hyperkalemic. A possible explanation for this finding may be associated with decreased dietary intake secondary to the pancreatitis or increased renal excretion. Fortunately, the thrombus in this report caused an incomplete blockage of the arterial supply to the patient's pelvic limbs, and the ischemic damage was mild and incomplete. Postoperative blood work and monitoring did not reveal evidence of clinically significant ischemia/reperfusion damage. Lidocaine has been purported to be helpful in prevention of ischemia/reperfusion injury. Its mechanisms of action are inhibiting intracellular calcium, decreasing neutrophil accumulation, activation and release of ROS, and scavenging the hydroxyl radical [30].

Though pancreatitis has been associated with splenic vein thrombosis, it has not yet been documented as an inciting cause of ATE in the dog [33]. Arterial thromboembolism is a known complication of pancreatitis in humans [34], and rare cases of ATE are documented in the human medical literature [35, 36]. Pancreatitis was an unexpected finding in this case, as the dog had no historical findings which would indicate that diagnosis, such as nausea, vomiting, or abdominal pain, though he did begin regurgitating/vomiting once hospitalized. Abdominal ultrasound did not show evidence of pancreatitis, though it has been shown that ultrasound is not a sensitive indicator of pancreatitis, nor hepatic or presumably renal histologic disease [37, 38].

Development of thromboembolic disease is a common complication of other primary disease processes. Prognosis for acute thromboembolism in cats is poor to grave when seen with underlying cardiac conditions; however, in dogs, the prognosis is often more favorable, dependent upon the underlying disease processes. A proposed explanation for the more favorable prognosis is better potential for the development of collateral circulation in dogs [8]. In cats, there is inhibition of collateral vessel development with experimental thrombotic occlusion [39]. This finding is thought to be associated with effects of vasoactive agents such as serotonin and prostaglandins that are released from platelets. To the authors' knowledge, these findings have not been evaluated in dogs.

This case presents new and interesting findings for canine ATE. Pancreatitis, alone or in combination with other systemic causes for hypercoagulability, should be considered as an etiology for canine ATE. Additionally, surgical aortic thrombectomy can have an excellent functional outcome and should be considered for patients without a terminal primary diagnosis.

Disclosure

This paper was presented in abstract form at the Auburn University College of Veterinary Medicine Annual Conference, Auburn, AL, April 2009.

Conflict of Interests

The authors declare that there is no conflict of interests regarding the publication of this paper.

Acknowledgments

The authors thank Sharron Barney for the intraoperative photographs and Dr. Judy Hudson for guidance with ultrasound interpretation.

References

[1] A. Boswood, C. R. Lamb, and R. N. White, "Aortic and iliac thrombosis in six dogs," *Journal of Small Animal Practice*, vol. 41, no. 3, pp. 109–114, 2000.

[2] R. L. Winter, C. D. Sedacca, A. Adams, and E. Christopher Orton, "Aortic thrombosis in dogs: presentation, therapy, and outcome in 26 cases," *Journal of Veterinary Cardiology*, vol. 14, no. 2, pp. 333–342, 2012.

[3] G. A. Lake-Bakaar, E. G. Johnson, and L. G. Griffiths, "Aortic thrombosis in dogs: 31 cases (2000–2010)," *Journal of the American Veterinary Medical Association*, vol. 241, no. 7, pp. 910–915, 2012.

[4] M. F. Thompson, J. Scott-Moncrieff, and D. F. Hogan, "Thrombolytic therapy in dogs and cats," *Journal of Veterinary Emergency and Critical Care*, vol. 11, pp. 111–121, 2001.

[5] A. C. Clare and B. J. Kraje, "Use of recombinant tissue-plasminogen activator for aortic thrombolysis in a hypoproteinemic dog," *Journal of the American Veterinary Medical Association*, vol. 212, no. 4, pp. 539–543, 1998.

[6] R. Gonçalves, J. Penderis, Y. P. Chang, A. Zoia, J. Mosley, and T. J. Anderson, "Clinical and neurological characteristics of aortic thromboembolism in dogs," *Journal of Small Animal Practice*, vol. 49, no. 4, pp. 178–184, 2008.

[7] W. O. Carter, "Aortic thromboembolism as a complication of gastric dilatation/volvulus in a dog," *Journal of the American Veterinary Medical Association*, vol. 196, no. 11, pp. 1829–1830, 1990.

[8] A. de Laforcade, "Diseases associated with thrombosis," *Topics in Companion Animal Medicine*, vol. 27, no. 2, pp. 59–64, 2012.

[9] S. L. Stockham and M. A. Scott, "Calcium, phosphorus, magnesium and their regulatory hormones," in *Fundamentals of Veterinary Clinical Pathology*, S. L. Stockham and M. A. Scott, Eds., pp. 593–638, Blackwell, Ames, Iowa, USA, 2nd edition, 2008.

[10] S. L. Stockham and M. A. Scott, "Monovalent electrolytes and osmolality," in *Fundamentals of Veterinary Clinical Pathology*, S. L. Stockham and M. A. Scott, Eds., pp. 495–545, Blackwell Publishing, Ames, Iowa, USA, 2nd edition, 2008.

[11] G. Perkins, S. J. Valberg, J. M. Madigan, G. P. Carlson, and S. L. Jones, "Electrolyte disturbances in foals with severe rhabdomyolysis," *Journal of Veterinary Internal Medicine*, vol. 12, no. 3, pp. 173–177, 1998.

[12] W. H. Bagley, H. Yang, and K. H. Shah, "Rhabdomyolysis," *Internal and Emergency Medicine*, vol. 2, no. 3, pp. 210–218, 2007.

[13] D. R. Kumar, E. R. Hanlin, I. Glurich, J. J. Mazza, and S. H. Yale, "Virchow's contribution to the understanding of thrombosis and cellular biology," *Clinical Medicine & Research*, vol. 8, no. 3-4, pp. 168–172, 2010.

[14] S. Beppu, Y. Nimura, H. Sakakibara, S. Nagata, Y. D. Park, and S. Izumi, "Smoke-like echo in the left atrial cavity in mitral valve disease: its features and significance," *Journal of the American College of Cardiology*, vol. 6, no. 4, pp. 744–749, 1985.

[15] D. A. Mosier, "Vascular disorders and thrombosis," in *Pathologic Basis of Veterinary Disease*, J. F. Zachary and M. D. McGavin, Eds., pp. 63–99, Elsevier, St. Louis, Mo, USA, 4th edition, 2007.

[16] D. A. Williams and J. M. Steiner, "Canine exocrine pancreatic disease," in *Textbook of Veterinary Internal Medicine*, S. J. Ettinger and E. C. Feldman, Eds., pp. 1482–1488, Saunders Elsevier, St. Louis, Mo, USA, 6th edition, 2005.

[17] D. Davalos and K. Akassoglou, "Fibrinogen as a key regulator of inflammation in disease," *Seminars in Immunopathology*, vol. 34, no. 1, pp. 43–62, 2012.

[18] B. Hoppe, "Fibrinogen and factor XIII at the intersection of coagulation, fibrinolysis and inflammation," *Thrombosis and Haemostasis*, vol. 112, no. 4, pp. 649–658, 2014.

[19] S. B. Reimer, M. D. Kittleson, and A. E. Kyles, "Use of rheolytic thrombectomy in the treatment of feline distal aortic thromboembolism," *Journal of Veterinary Internal Medicine*, vol. 20, no. 2, pp. 290–296, 2006.

[20] M. E. Dunn, "Thrombectomy and thrombolysis: the interventional radiology approach," *Journal of Veterinary Emergency and Critical Care*, vol. 21, no. 2, pp. 144–150, 2011.

[21] P. D. Pion, "Feline aortic thromboemboli and the potential utility of thrombolytic therapy with tissue plasminogen activator," *Veterinary Clinics of North America: Small Animal Practice*, vol. 18, no. 1, pp. 79–86, 1988.

[22] V. L. Fuentes, "Arterial thromboembolism: risks, realities and a rational first-line approach," *Journal of Feline Medicine and Surgery*, vol. 14, no. 7, pp. 459–470, 2012.

[23] K. E. Moore, N. Morris, N. Dhupa et al., "Retrospective study of streptokinase administration in 46 cats with arterial thromboembolism," *Journal of Veterinary Emergency and Critical Care*, vol. 10, pp. 245–257, 2000.

[24] H. Koyama, H. Matsumoto, R.-U. Fukushima, and H. Hirose, "Local intra-arterial administration of urokinase in the treatment of a feline distal aortic thromboembolism," *Journal of Veterinary Medical Science*, vol. 72, no. 9, pp. 1209–1211, 2010.

[25] S. A. Smith, "Antithrombotic therapy," *Topics in Companion Animal Medicine*, vol. 27, no. 2, pp. 88–94, 2012.

[26] D. C. Plumb, "Heparin sodium," in *Plumb's Veterinary Drug Handbook*, D. C. Plumb, Ed., pp. 494–496, Wiley-Blackwell, Ames, Iowa, USA, 7th edition, 2011.

[27] N. J. Laste and N. K. Harpster, "A retrospective study of 100 cases of feline distal aortic thromboembolism—1977-1993," *Journal of the American Animal Hospital Association*, vol. 31, no. 6, pp. 492–500, 1995.

[28] J. P. Schoeman, "Feline distal aortic thromboembolism: a review of 44 cases (1990-1998)," *Journal of Feline Medicine and Surgery*, vol. 1, no. 4, pp. 221–231, 1999.

[29] M. McMichael and R. M. Moore, "Ischemia-reperfusion injury pathophysiology, part I," *Journal of Veterinary Emergency and Critical Care*, vol. 14, no. 4, pp. 231–241, 2004.

[30] B. H. Cassutto and R. W. Gfeller, "Use of intravenous lidocaine to prevent reperfusion injury and subsequent multiple organ dysfunction syndrome," *Journal of Veterinary Emergency and Critical Care*, vol. 13, no. 3, pp. 137–148, 2003.

[31] H. Haimovici, "Muscular, renal, and metabolic complications of acute arterial occlusions: myonephropathic-metabolic syndrome," *Surgery*, vol. 85, no. 4, pp. 461–468, 1979.

[32] D. J. Hall, J. E. Rush, and E. A. Rozanski, "ECG of the month," *Journal of the American Veterinary Medical Association*, vol. 236, no. 3, pp. 299–301, 2010.

[33] M. P. Laurenson, K. Hopper, M. A. Herrera, and E. G. Johnson, "Concurrent diseases and conditions in dogs with splenic vein thrombosis," *Journal of Veterinary Internal Medicine*, vol. 24, no. 6, pp. 1298–1304, 2010.

[34] V. Kolar, S. Verma, B. Karthikeyan, A. Kishore, and T. Dutta, "Cerebral infarction leading to hemiplegia: a rare complication of acute pancreatitis," *Indian Journal of Critical Care Medicine*, vol. 17, no. 5, pp. 308–310, 2013.

[35] A. Bhalla, S. Gupta, A. P. Jain, U. N. Jajoo, O. P. Gupta, and S. P. Kalantri, "Blue toe syndrome: a rare complication of acute pancreatitis," *Journal of the Pancreas*, vol. 4, no. 1, pp. 17–19, 2003.

[36] S. Y. Lee, K. H. Ng, and M. G. Sebastian, "Arterio-pancreatic syndrome," *Case Reports in Gastroenterology*, vol. 5, no. 1, pp. 17–21, 2011.

[37] C. G. Ruaux, "Diagnostic approaches to acute pancreatitis," *Clinical Techniques in Small Animal Practice*, vol. 18, no. 4, pp. 245–249, 2003.

[38] C. M. R. Warren-Smith, S. Andrew, P. Mantis, and C. R. Lamb, "Lack of associations between ultrasonographic appearance of parenchymal lesions of the canine liver and histological diagnosis," *Journal of Small Animal Practice*, vol. 53, no. 3, pp. 168–173, 2012.

[39] R. G. Schaub, K. M. Meyers, R. D. Sande, and G. Hamilton, "Inhibition of feline collateral vessel development following experimental thrombolic occlusion," *Circulation Research*, vol. 39, no. 5, pp. 736–743, 1976.

21

Mitral Valve Replacement with a Mechanical Valve for Severe Mitral Regurgitation in a Small Dog

Daisuke Taguchi,[1,2] Isamu Kanemoto,[1] Satoko Yokoyama,[1,3] Masashi Mizuno,[1,4] and Makoto Washizu[5]

[1] *Chayagasaka Animal Hospital, 1-1-5 Shinnishi, Chikusa, Nagoya, Aichi 464-0003, Japan*
[2] *Green Animal Hospital, 179 Tamakake-maeda, Nanbu, Sannohe, Aomori 039-0101, Japan*
[3] *Miyashita Animal Hospital, 5-8-29 Keigoya, Kure, Hiroshima 737-0012, Japan*
[4] *Veterinary Internal Medicine of Nihon University, 1866 Kameino, Fujisawa, Kanagawa 252-8510, Japan*
[5] *Animal Teaching Hospital of Gihu University, 1-1 Yanagido, Gifu 501-1193, Japan*

Correspondence should be addressed to Isamu Kanemoto; kanemoto@ta2.so-net.ne.jp

Academic Editor: Paola Roccabianca

A seven-year-old Shih Tzu with refractory repeated pulmonary edema and syncope was presented for surgical operation. From the results of cardiovascular examinations, the dog was diagnosed as severe mitral regurgitation (ACVIM consensus class D) and mild tricuspid regurgitation. The dog first underwent surgery with mitral valve plasty; however, the results were unsatisfactory due to severe damage of the whole mitral valve. The operation was quickly changed to mitral valve replacement using a mechanical valve (19 mm). The dog survived surgery and lived for 2 years and one month after operation using long-term anticoagulant (warfarin) therapy in spite of several thrombosis-related events.

1. Introduction

Mitral regurgitation (MR) caused by degenerative valve disease is quite common in small breed dogs [1]. There are two methods of surgical operation for MR [2, 3]: mitral valvuloplasty (MVP) which is the repair of the valve itself and mitral valve replacement (MVR) which entails an exchange with an artificial valve, either mechanical or bioprosthetic. Although MVR using a mechanical heart valve is excellent in its durability, it needs to be maintained with lifetime anticoagulant therapy because of the foreign body response. In contrast, although MVR using a bioprosthetic valve does not require long-term anticoagulant therapy, it is less durable [2, 3].

There are a few clinical case reports of MVR using a mechanical valve [4–6], and there are some clinical [7, 8] and experimental [9] reports of MVR using a bioprosthetic valve in medium-size or large breed dogs. However, there is only one clinical case report of MVR using a mechanical valve in

a small breed dog and of the postoperative long-term result of anticoagulant therapy in such dogs [6].

This report presents the first successful case of MVR using a mechanical valve in a small breed dog, which survived 2 years and one month after operation using long-term anticoagulant (warfarin) therapy in spite of several thrombosis-related events.

2. Case Presentation

The dog was a male Shih Tzu, 7 years old, weighing 5.3 kg. It was diagnosed with MR and treatment had begun 1 year 3 months earlier. Dyspnea occurred 2 months before the first visit and then recently recurred every few days. Syncope occurred 1 month and 8 days before the first visit. Although the dog's prognosis was considered to be very poor, he was presented to our hospital for surgery at the owner's strong wish. On physical examination, auscultation revealed Levine 3-4/6 systolic murmur (SM) at the apex, 2/6 SM at

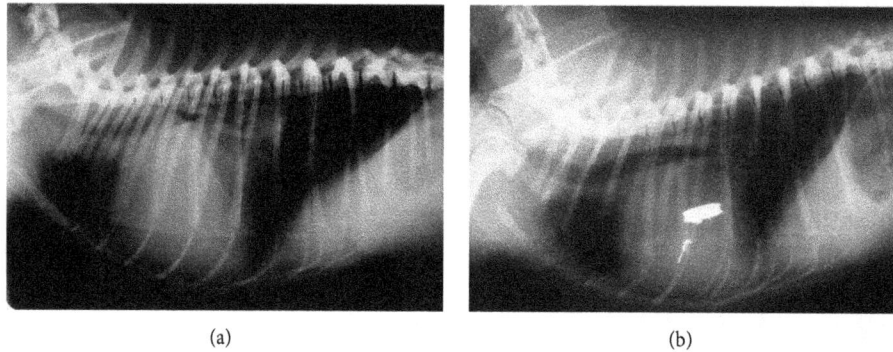

(a)   (b)

FIGURE 1: (a) Preoperative and (b) postoperative L-R X-ray photographs. Preoperative VHS 12.0 v decreased to 10.1 v 3.5 months after operation, and a mechanical valve is recognized in (b).

the tricuspid valve area, and crackle in the lung area. On chest X-ray examination, elevation of trachea and enlargement of cardiac size (VHS 12.0 v, CTR 89%), especially in the left atrium and ventricle, were recognized (Figure 1(a)).

Echocardiogram revealed dilation of left atrium (LA/Ao: 3), enlargement of mitral valve ring size (diameter 28.4 mm), prolapsed chordae of the anterior leaflet, and ruptured chorda of the posterior one. Color Doppler showed severe mitral regurgitation from the posterior commissure to the posterior side of the left atrium. Fractional shortening (FS) showed a normal range (35–45%) which means the presence of impaired myocardial cell contraction. The left ventricular end diastolic internal dimension (LVIDd) distended remarkably 49.5 mm, and mild tricuspid regurgitation was recognized. Severe (ACVIM consensus class D) MR with mild TR was diagnosed. Although the prognosis was considered poor, open heart surgery was performed as a last measure.

Open Heart Assist Method. This entails surface-cooling hypothermia (sHT) combined with low-flow cardiopulmonary bypass (CPB) [10]. In this case, the lowest esophageal temperature (ET) was 20.1°C, the aortic cross-clamp (ACC) time was 79 minutes, the lowest pump flow was 60 mL/kg/minute, and the recorded CPB time was 2 hours and 53 minutes. Anesthesia: the dog was administered acepromazine (0.05 mg/kg SC), atropine (0.025 mg/kg SC), and hydroxyzine (1 mg/kg SC) at 30 minutes and 15 minutes before induction, respectively. Anesthesia was induced with thiamylal (12.5 mg/kg IV) and maintained with inhalation of isoflurane in oxygen and intermittent administration of pancuronium (0.06 mg/kg IV). After administration of heparin (400 IU/kg IV), a 12 Fr venous cannula was inserted from the left jugular vein into the right atrium. A 2.0 mm diameter metal arterial cannula was then inserted through the left carotid artery toward the heart and connected with the CPB circuit (NAPS III and Mera S-circuit, Senko Ika Kogyo). Deep hypothermia was slowly induced by surface-cooling with ice bags. At ET 30°C, the left 5th intercostal space was opened and the surgical field was distended by cutting the costal cartilage of the 6th rib. The pericardium was opened by cutting parallel under the left phrenic nerve and sutured to the chest wall to create a pericardial cradle. An aortic root

cannula for cardioplegia was inserted in the aortic root. A two-stage (18–24 F) venous tube was additionally inserted from the right appendage into the posterior vena cava and connected with CPB. At ET 25°C, CPB was started. After both the ascending aorta and main pulmonary artery were cross-clamped together, cold (4°C) cardioplegia solution (10/mL/kg St Thomas II solution) was immediately injected antegrade through an aortic root cannula. The left atrium was cut transversely above the coronary groove. The whole mitral valve was hypertrophied with mucous degeneration, and many portions of the anterior and posterior leaflets prolapsed widely like a yacht sail, and one chorda of the posterior leaflet ruptured near the posterior commissure.

Surgical Method. At first, MVP was performed. The prolapsed anterior leaflet and ruptured posterior leaflet were sutured with the triangular plication (McGoon) method [11] and the posterior commissural valve ring was sutured with the mattress (JH Kay) method [12], as we reported previously [13]. However, the leak test showed a great volume of regurgitation. Therefore, the MVR method was performed instead of MVP. After the whole mitral valve with chordae tendineae was cut off leaving the base of the valve annulus, a 19 mm diameter Bjork-Shiley oblique valve for aortic valve was attached there conversely with three 5-0 prolines and the continuous suture method (Figure 2(a)). After the left atrium was closed and intracardiac air removed completely, the aortic cross-clamp (ACC) was removed. Immediately, a spontaneous beat occurred from ventricular fibrillation with one DC shock. The patient was weaned from CPB 40 minutes after removing the ACC, and also from controlled ventilation 15 hours after operation.

Postoperative Course. Anticoagulant therapy using warfarin was started on the second day after surgery. Appetite and vigor recovered on the 4th day after operation, and the patient was discharged 12 days after surgery. Since then, warfarin therapy was controlled by the attending doctor. On 3.5-month postoperative chest X-ray examination, VHS decreased from preoperative 12.0 v to 10.1 v (Figure 1(b)). The echocardiogram revealed disappearance of MR, reduced LVIDd from preoperative 49.5 mm to 32.6 mm, and slightly persisting TR.

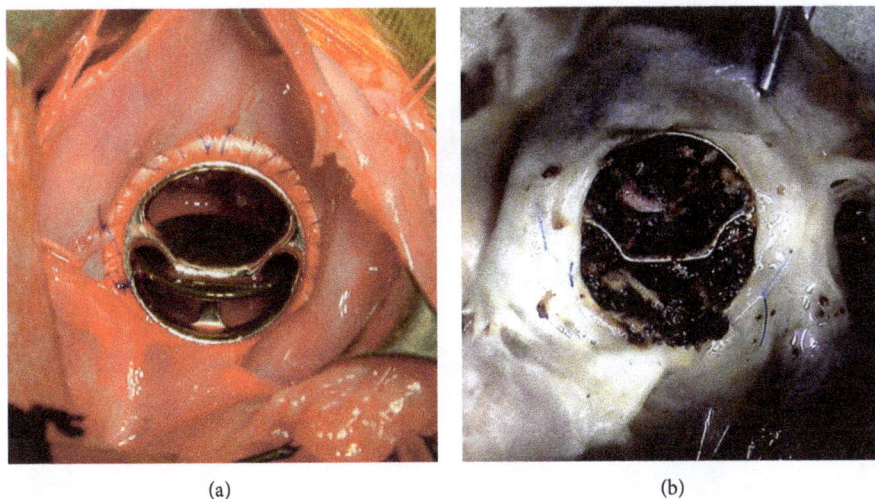

FIGURE 2: (a) An intraoperative photograph shows Bjork-Shiley oblique valve for aortic valve attached conversely at the mitral valve position. (b) An autopsy photograph (surgeon view) shows the artificial valve covered with a great amount of thrombi.

After discharge from our hospital, warfarin was administered at 0.25–0.55 mg/kg/day (almost 0.35 mg/kg/day) by the attending doctor. Six events associated with the artificial valve reported by the attending doctor and owner were a swelling of the right leg and bleeding from the nail root 3.5 months after operation, mild paralysis of the left leg 8 months after operation, and mild seizure at 1 year, 1 year 9 months, and 2 years after operation, nearly all of which seemed to be associated with blood clot formation except for bleeding from the nail root. Two years after operation, prosthetic valve dysfunction due to thrombus was suspected because the opening and closing sounds of the artificial valve became suddenly inaudible. After warfarin administration was increased, the opening and closing sounds of the artificial valve were again auscultated. One month after the event, however, the dog had an abrupt onset of severe coughing and dyspnea during the night, although he acted normally during daytime. On auscultation, sounds of the artificial valve were not audible, but severe lung rales were heard in both lung fields. The dog was finally euthanized because of symptomatic worsening as time advanced, despite various rescue treatments (Figure 3).

Autopsy Findings. The artificial valve was covered with a large amount of thrombi (Figure 2(b)). Trachea was filled with a large amount of pink bubbly fluid.

3. Discussion

In human [2, 3] and veterinary medicine [13–17], MVP is currently preferred over MVR for providing good QOL. However, it is difficult to completely repair severely damaged valves with MVP in a terminal stage case. In human medicine, there are many reports related to MVR [2, 3]. However, in veterinary literature, to our knowledge, there are only three reports of MVR using a mechanical valve in clinical cases which were operated in medium-size to large breed dog

[4–6]. There is only one reported case of surgery with MVR using a mechanical valve (19 mm) in a small dog (4.3 kg) [6], but the dog died during surgery due to oversized valve prosthesis. In our small dog (5.3 kg), we first attempted to use MVP [13] (McGoon [11] combined with the JH Kay [12] method), but the results were unsatisfactory due to severe damage of the entire mitral valve. Therefore, we quickly switched from MVP to MVR with a mechanical valve (19 mm diameter for aortic valve; the smallest available valve prosthesis). The dog survived surgery and after discharge remained alive for 2 years.

In this case, sHT was combined with CPB. Deep sHT can be easily performed in a small dog, and CPB can assist the systemic circulation during ACC and rewarming using a heat-exchanger. CPB using peripheral vessels improves cardiac access in small dogs, although HT is needed because of low-flow CPB due to decreased venous return volume. A combination of deep sHT with low-flow CPB enhances the benefits and minimizes the disadvantages of both techniques in small dogs [10].

Regarding postoperative anticoagulant therapy, there is only one report [6] from 3 clinical reports [4–6] of MVR using a mechanical valve in dogs. Orton and colleagues [6] reported administration of warfarin at the same dosage in 6 dogs as in the guideline for humans; but all died of thrombosis-related causes, 5 dogs within one year and 1 dog at 5.25 years (median survival after surgery: 4.5 months). The same warfarin dosage as used in the guideline for humans is recommended to maintain the prothrombin time-based INR of 2.5–3.5 [2, 3, 18]. According to an experimental study using Hall-Haster mitral valves [19], warfarin dosage of a thrombotest aimed at 20–25% normal coagulation activity was ineffective in preventing thrombosis, and a more intensive antithrombotic prophylaxis was required.

In the case under study, the warfarin dosage was 0.25–0.55 mg/kg/day, but mainly 0.35 mg/kg/day was administered. However, 6 thrombosis-related events occurred in spite

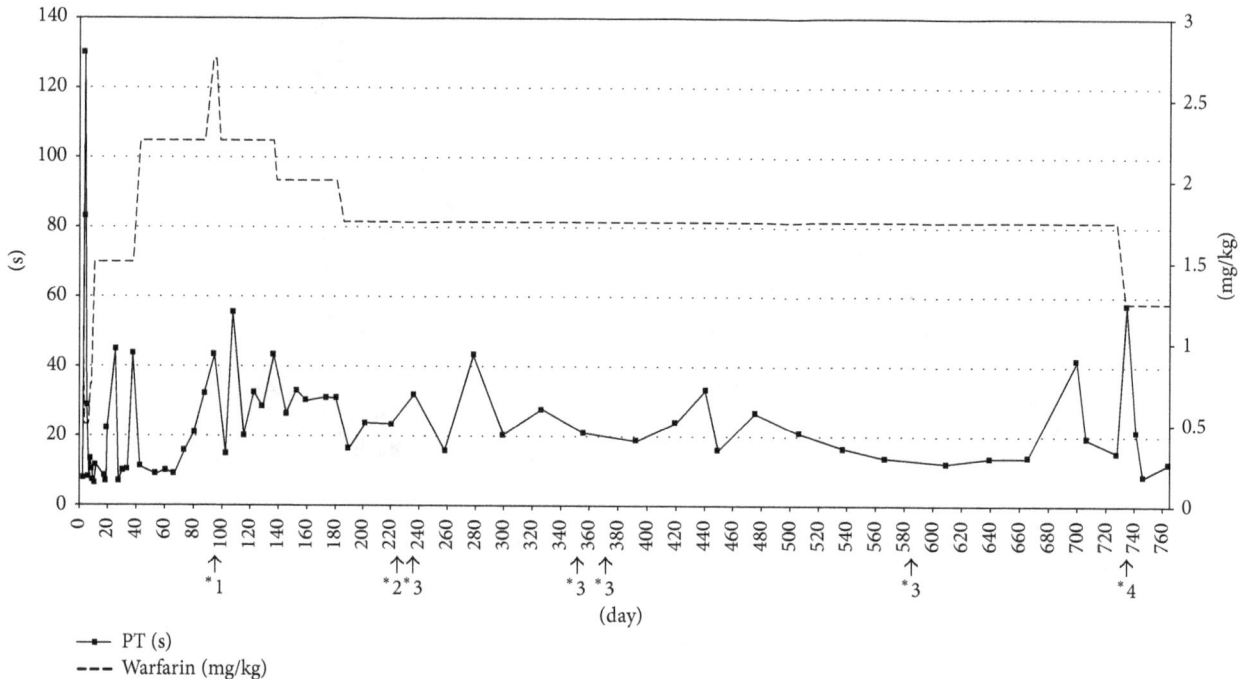

FIGURE 3: Changes of prothrombin time (PT) and dosage of warfarin administered after operation. *1 swelling of the right leg and bleeding from the nail root (95 days after operation). *2 mild paralysis of left leg and mild seizure (226 days after operation). *3 mild seizure (229, 348, 370, 585 days after operation). *4 prosthetic valve dysfunction due to thrombus (733 days after operation).

of prothrombin time (PT) 7.5–24 sec or <24 sec, except for swelling of the right leg and bleeding from the nail root 3.5 months after operation; the PT underwent great changes in spite of the same warfarin dosage. Unfortunately, the dog died of prosthetic valve thrombosis 2 years and one month after operation. From our experience with this case, it seemed that oral administration of warfarin only was not suitable for controlling the prothrombin time in a dog, unlike in a human. Klement and colleagues [20] reported MVR using the same Bjork-Shiley Monostat valve in large experimental dogs for which anticoagulation was started 48 hours postoperatively by giving warfarin and adjusted on a daily basis to maintain the prothrombin time at 1.5 to 2 times the preoperative value. However, wide variations of prothrombin time were controlled by adding aspirin and dipyridamole to warfarin. Unfortunately, a follow-up survey was not conducted until 3 weeks after operation. Still another problem with dogs is that the normal prothrombin time varies widely (6–10 sec [21], 9–14 sec [22], and 14–18 sec [23]) at each facility. Thus, each facility should have its own prothrombin time or use the prothrombin time-based INR.

Recently, new anticoagulant drugs (Purazakisa, Izagureru, Erikyusu) have become available, and in the future, their effects are expected to serve well in the anticoagulant therapy for MVR in dogs.

4. Conclusions

We experienced the first successful case of MVR using a mechanical valve in a small breed dog, which survived 2 years

and one month after operation using long-term anticoagulant (warfarin) therapy in spite of several thrombosis-related events. Anticoagulant therapy using only warfarin makes it very difficult to control PT for MVR in dog.

Conflict of Interests

The authors declare that there is no conflict of interests regarding the publication of this paper.

Acknowledgment

This paper was presented at the 13th Federation Asian Veterinary Association (FAVA) Congress, October 25–28, 2004, in Seoul, Korea, and as a case in the paper in Open Heart Surgery with Deep Hypothermia and Cardiopulmonary Bypass in Small and Toy Dogs, Vet. Surg., 39: 674–679, 2010.

References

[1] M. D. Kittleson and R. D. Kienle, "Myxomatous atrioventricular valvular degeneration," in Small Animal Cardiovascular Medicine, M. D. Kittleson and R. D. Kienle, Eds., pp. 297–318, Mosby, Kimberton, Pa, USA, 1998.

[2] R. P. Gallegos, T. Gudbjartsson, and S. Aranki, "Mitral valve replacement," in Cardiac Surgery in the Adult, L. H. Cohn, Ed., pp. 849–876, McGraw-Hill Medical, New York, NY, USA, 4th edition, 2012.

[3] N. T. Kouchoukos, E. H. Blackstone, F. L. Hanley, and J. K. Kirklin, "Mitral valve disease," in Kirklin/Barratt-Boyes Cardiac Surgery, N. T. Kouchoukos, E. H. Blackstone, F. L. Hanley, and

J. K. Kirklin, Eds., pp. 484–536, Elsevier Saunders, Philadelphia, Pa, USA, 4th edition, 2013.

[4] G. E. Eyster, W. Weber, S. Chi et al., "Mitral valve prosthesis for correction of mitral regurgitation in a dog," *Journal of the American Veterinary Medical Association*, vol. 168, no. 12, pp. 1115–1118, 1976.

[5] E. M. Breznock, "Tricuspid and mitral valvular disease: valve replacement," *Seminars in Veterinary Medicine and Surgery (Small Animal)*, vol. 9, no. 4, pp. 234–239, 1994.

[6] E. C. Orton, T. B. Hackett, K. Mama, and J. A. Boon, "Technique and outcome of mitral valve replacement in dogs," *Journal of the American Veterinary Medical Association*, vol. 226, no. 9, pp. 1508–1511, 2005.

[7] R. N. White, R. L. Stepien, R. A. Hammond et al., "Mitral valve replacement for the treatment of congenital mitral dysplasia in a bull terrier," *The Journal of Small Animal Practice*, vol. 36, no. 9, pp. 407–410, 1995.

[8] L. Behr, V. Chetboul, C. C. Sampedrano et al., "Beating heart mitral valve replacement with a bovine pericardial bioprosthesis for treatment of mitral valve dysplasia in a bull terrier," *Veterinary Surgery*, vol. 36, no. 3, pp. 190–198, 2007.

[9] K. Takashima, A. Soda, R. Tanaka, and Y. Yamane, "Long-term clinical evaluation of mitral valve replacement with porcine bioprosthetic valves in dogs," *Journal of Veterinary Medical Science*, vol. 70, no. 3, pp. 279–283, 2008.

[10] I. Kanemoto, D. Taguchi, S. Yokoyama, M. Mizuno, H. Suzuki, and T. Kanamoto, "Open heart surgery with deep hypothermia and cardiopulmonary bypass in small and toy dogs," *Veterinary Surgery*, vol. 39, no. 6, pp. 674–679, 2010.

[11] D. C. McGoon, "Repair of mitral insufficiency due to ruptured chordae tendineae," *Journal of Thoracic Cardiovascular Surgery*, vol. 39, pp. 357–362, 1960.

[12] J. H. Kay and W. S. Egerton, "The repair of mitral insufficiency associated with ruptured chordae tendineae," *Annals of Surgery*, vol. 157, no. 3, pp. 351–360, 1963.

[13] I. Kanemoto, S. Shibata, H. Noguchi, S. Chimura, M. Kobayashi, and Y. Shimizu, "Successful mitral valvuloplasty for mitral regurgitation in a dog," *Japanese Journal of Veterinary Science*, vol. 52, no. 2, pp. 411–414, 1990.

[14] L. S. Boggs, S. J. Dewan, and S. E. Ballard, "Mitral valve reconstruction in a toy-breed dog," *Journal of the American Veterinary Medical Association*, vol. 209, no. 11, pp. 1872–1876, 1996.

[15] I. Kanemoto, H. Suzuki, D. Taguchi, S. Yokoyama, M. Mizuno, and T. Kanamoto, "Successful surgical repair for severe mitral regurgitation in five small-breed dogs," *Veterinary Surgery*, vol. 33, no. 5, p. 435-E12, 2004.

[16] L. G. Griffiths, E. C. Orton, and J. A. Boon, "Evaluation of techniques and outcomes of mitral valve repair in dogs," *Journal of the American Veterinary Medical Association*, vol. 224, no. 12, pp. 1941–1945, 2004.

[17] M. Uechi, "Mitral valve repair in dogs," *Journal of Veterinary Cardiology*, vol. 14, no. 1, pp. 185–192, 2012.

[18] P. D. Stein, J. S. Alpert, J. E. Dalen, D. Horstkotte, and A. G. G. Turpie, "Antithrombotic therapy in patients with mechanical and biological prosthetic heart valves," *Chest*, vol. 114, no. 5, pp. 602S–610S, 1998.

[19] J. Dale, A. O. Aasen, F. Resch, B. Semb, K. Stadskleiv, and P. Lilleaasen, "Mitral disc valve implantation in the dog: early and late valve thrombosis and its prevention," *European Surgical Research*, vol. 15, no. 5, pp. 249–255, 1983.

[20] P. Klement, C. M. Feindel, H. E. Scully et al., "Mitral valve replacement in dogs. Surgical technique and postoperative management," *Veterinary Surgery*, vol. 16, no. 3, pp. 231–237, 1987.

[21] *Kirk and Bistner's Handbook of Veterinary Procedures and Emergency Treatment*, p. 888, WB Saunders, Philadelphia, Pa, USA, 7th edition, 2000.

[22] R. M. Jacobs, J. H. Lumsden, and J. A. Taylor, "Canine and feline reference values," in *Kirk's Current Veterinary Therapy XIII, Small Animal Practice*, p. 1221, W. B. Saunder, Philadelphia, Pa, USA, 2000.

[23] M. B. Brooks, "Coagulation disease," in *Saunders Manual of Small Animal Practice*, S. J. Birchard and R. G. Sherding, Eds., pp. 256–264, Saunders Elsevier, St. Louis, Mo, USA, 3rd edition, 2006.

22

Ventricular Habronemiasis in Aviary Passerines

Jennifer N. Niemuth,[1] Joni V. Allgood,[1,2] James R. Flowers,[1] Ryan S. De Voe,[1,3] and Brigid V. Troan[1,3]

[1] College of Veterinary Medicine, North Carolina State University, 1060 William Moore Drive, Raleigh, NC 27607, USA
[2] Happy Tails Veterinary Emergency Clinic, Greensboro, NC 27418, USA
[3] North Carolina Zoological Park, 4401 Zoo Parkway, Asheboro, NC 27205, USA

Correspondence should be addressed to Jennifer N. Niemuth; jennifer_niemuth@ncsu.edu

Academic Editors: C. Gutierrez, F. Mutinelli, and I. Pires

A variety of Habronematidae parasites (order Spirurida) have been described as occasional parasites of avian species; however, reports on passerines are relatively uncommon. From 2007 to 2008, 11 passerine deaths at The North Carolina Zoological Park in Asheboro, NC, USA, were associated with ventricular habronemiasis, which was determined to be the cause of death or a major contributing factor in 10 of the 11 individuals. The number and species affected were 5 Red-billed Leiothrix (*Leiothrix lutea*), 2 Japanese White-eye (*Zosterops japonicus*), 2 Golden-headed Manakin (*Pipra erythrocephala*), 1 Blue-grey Tanager (*Thraupis episcopus*), and 1 Emerald Starling (*Coccycolius iris*). Affected animals displayed nonspecific clinical signs or were found dead. The ventricular nematodes were consistent in morphology with *Procyrnea* sp. Koilin fragmentation with secondary bacterial and fungal infections was the most frequently observed pathologic lesion. Secondary visceral amyloidosis, attributed to chronic inflammation associated with nematodiasis, was present in 4 individuals. An insect intermediate host is suspected but was not identified. Native passerine species within or around the aviary may be serving as sylvatic hosts.

1. Introduction

Habronemiasis is used to describe infection by any of the genera of the family Habronematidae within the order Spirurida. The most well-known Habronematidae parasites, *Draschia megastoma*, *Habronema muscae*, and *Habronema microstoma*, are of minimal clinical significance as equine stomach parasites [1]. However, many members of the family Habronematidae (*Odontospirura*, *Sicarius*, *Exsica*, *Procyrnea*, *Cyrnea*, and *Metacyrnea*) are found in birds [2].

In nonpasserines, a variety of habronemes have been described as occasional parasites found within the proventriculus, ventriculus, and/or intestine. Reports are predominantly from Africa, Asia, and Australia and include buzzard, eagle, egret, falcon, fowl, hawk, hummingbird, kite, kiwi, owl, parrot, pigeon, tinamou, vulture, and woodpecker species [3–22]. With the exception of a lethal case in a black-backed woodpecker (*Picoides arcticus*), no host morbidity, mortality,

or significant pathology is reported with habronemiasis in nonpasserines.

Reports on habronemiasis in passerines appear to be much less common. *Habronema hyderabadensis* was found in the proventriculus and ventriculus of *Gracula* (*religiosa*) *intermedia* in India [11], while habronemes from the genera *Viguiera* and *Cyrnea* have been reported in the ventriculus of Australian passerines [12]. Neither described any clinical significance. A case report from Germany [23] describes a series of cases of ventricular habronemiasis causing morbidity and mortality in Red-billed Leiothrix (*Leiothrix lutea*) and Bali Myna (*Leucopsar rothschildi*). A survey of American robins (*Turdus migratorius*) appears to be the only published record of North American passerine habronemiasis. *Habronema* sp. were recovered from the esophagus and proventriculus of 6 adult birds (3 males, 3 females) out of 62 surveyed [24].

This report describes two outbreaks of ventricular habronemiasis occurring in 2007 and 2008, which resulted in

TABLE 1: Passerine deaths associated with habronemiasis at the North Carolina Zoological Park, Asheboro, NC, USA.

Date	Species	Sex	Age	Cause of death	Other/associated lesions
3/28/2007	L. lutea	M	10 yrs	Hepatic amyloidosis	Ventricular habronemiasis
6/18/2007	L. lutea	F	7 yrs	Hepatic amyloidosis	Ventricular habronemiasis with secondary bacterial ventriculitis; ovarian amyloidosis
6/19/2007	T. episcopus	F	2 yrs	Trauma	Ventricular habronemiasis with secondary bacterial ventriculitis
7/23/2007	Z. japonicus	M	7 yrs	Ventricular habronemiasis	Secondary fungal ventriculitis
7/23/2007	P. erythrocephala	N/A	13 days	Ventricular habronemiasis	Secondary bacterial and fungal ventriculitis
7/23/2007	L. lutea	F	2 yrs	Ventricular habronemiasis	Secondary bacterial and fungal ventriculitis
8/13/2007	P. erythrocephala	N/A	40 days	Ventricular habronemiasis	Secondary bacterial ventriculitis
10/5/2007	L. lutea	F	7 yrs	Ventricular habronemiasis	Secondary bacterial ventriculitis; hepatic amyloidosis
5/10/2008	C. iris	M	4 yrs	Ventricular habronemiasis	Secondary bacterial ventriculitis; hepatic, splenic, and renal amyloidosis
8/16/2008	L. lutea	M	11 yrs	Ventricular habronemiasis	Secondary bacterial and fungal ventriculitis
9/2/2008	Z. japonicus	F	8 yrs	Ventricular habronemiasis	Secondary bacterial and fungal ventriculitis; pulmonary aspergillosis; polyoma nephritis; and myocarditis

morbidity and mortality in passerines at The North Carolina Zoological Park, Asheboro, NC, USA.

2. Cases

2.1. Affected Animals. The R. J. Reynolds Forest Aviary at the North Carolina Zoological Park simulates tropical forest and displays approximately 36 species of exotic birds from Africa, Asia, Australia, Indonesia, and South America. The aviary sporadically houses native, rehabilitated, unreleasable passerine species. All birds complete at least a 30-day quarantine prior to introduction into the exhibit. While considered a closed system, native insects, reptiles, amphibians, and occasional birds have entered the habitat.

From March to October 2007 and May to September 2008, 11 passerine deaths were associated with habronemiasis. Five of the individuals were hatched at the North Carolina Zoological Park, while 6 were obtained from other institutions over time and had passed through quarantine. The number and species affected were 5 Red-billed Leiothrix (*Leiothrix lutea*), 2 Japanese White-eye (*Zosterops japonicus*), 2 Golden-headed Manakin (*Pipra erythrocephala*), 1 Blue-grey Tanager (*Thraupis episcopus*), and 1 Emerald Starling (*Coccycolius iris*). Gender and age of each individual are presented in Table 1.

2.2. Clinical Examination, Gross Pathology, and Microscopy. The deaths of 10 individuals were spontaneous: 8 were found dead, 1 individual died in-hand during examination, and 1 individual died en route to treatment. The eleventh individual was humanely euthanized because of declining quality of life.

Before death, a majority of affected individuals (*n* = 7) displayed nonspecific clinical signs associated with illness in birds, such as depression or lethargy, perching low or on the ground, and/or a fluffed appearance. After death, 7 individuals (5 with other clinical signs) were noted to be

in thin to emaciated body condition (body condition scores ranging from 1 to 2 out of 5 for the 6 individuals given a score).

All individuals were stored at 4°C until postmortem examination and necropsy by a veterinarian. On gross examination, 8 individuals were found to have visible nematodes associated with the koilin layer or within the lumen of the ventriculus or intestinal tract. Four individuals had gross hepatomegaly. Thickened, irregular, or friable koilin was noted in 3 individuals.

Nematodes were preserved in 70% ethanol for identification. Representative specimens were cleared and temporarily mounted in an alcohol and glycerine solution. Habronematidae taxonomy and identification follow those of Chabaud [2].

Whole nematode specimens recovered from the ventriculus of a *C. iris* were consistent in morphology with *Procyrnea* sp. As with Chabaud's [2] key, our specimen had weakly developed teeth near the anterior border of the pseudolabia. Median teeth and a cylindrical, chitinous buccal cavity (Figure 1(a)) were present. The male had a distinct copulatory spicule (Figure 1(b)) and a tail of the spirurid type with 9 preanal papillae, 4 postanal papillae, and a terminal group of papillae and phasmids. The uteri of females were filled with thick-shelled, larvated eggs (Figure 1(c)). Although the quality and number of specimens examined for identification were not adequate for confident speciation, our specimens were similar in appearance and measurement to *Procyrnea mansioni* [16, 23].

2.3. Histopathology. Samples of brain, lung, kidney, liver, and gastrointestinal tract were collected for histopathology from each individual. Spleen, heart, skeletal muscle, gonads, pancreas, and thyroid were collected from some individuals. The samples were fixed in 10% neutral buffered formalin. Fixed samples were embedded in paraffin wax; 5 μm serial sections were made and then stained with hematoxylin and eosin (H&E) stain. When applicable, additional staining

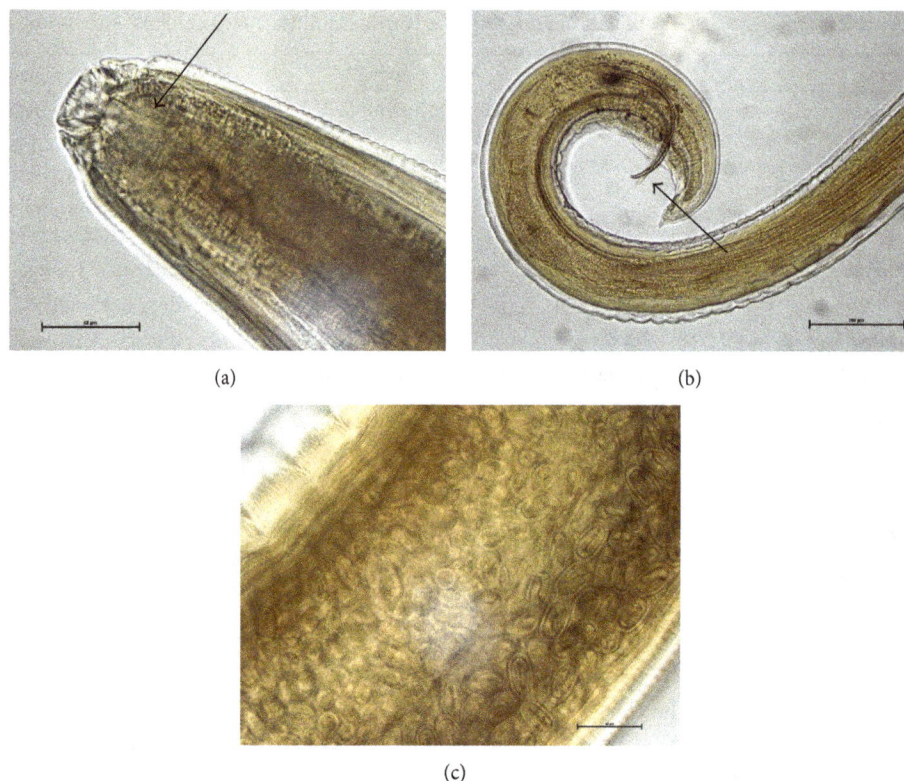

(a)

(b)

(c)

FIGURE 1: Whole mount of *Procyrnea* sp. nematodes from ventriculus of *C. iris*. (a) Anterior showing lips and cylindrical, chitinous buccal cavity (arrow). Scale bar = 50 μm. (b) Posterior aspect of male with copulatory spicule (arrow). Scale bar = 200 μm. (c) Uterus filled with thick-shelled, larvated eggs. Scale bar = 50 μm.

with acid fast, trichrome, Sirius red, periodic acid Schiff, Grocott's methenamine silver stain, or Congo red (pre- and post-acid digestion with 0.5% potassium permanganate and 0.3% sulfuric acid) was performed. Board-certified veterinary pathologists performed histopathologic examinations.

Histologically, *Procyrnea* sp. parasites were found between the koilin and mucosal layers of the ventriculus (Figure 2(a)) and occasionally within the lumen of the proventriculus, ventriculus, or intestinal tract. A thin cuticle, polymyarian, coelomyarian musculature, lateral cords, complete digestive tract, pseudocoelom, and a tripartite esophagus were identified on cross-section. Numerous oval, thick-shelled, embryonated eggs were present within the uterus (Figure 2(c)).

The associated koilin layer was frequently fragmented and admixed with aggregates of fibrin, necrotic cell debris, and inflammatory cells (Figure 2(b)). Ventriculitis was severe in 5 individuals, moderate in 2 individuals, and mild in 4 individuals. In 10 of the 11 affected individuals, secondary bacterial infections and/or fungal infections (consistent with *Candida albicans*) were identified. Mucosal ulceration was occasionally noted.

Four of the adult animals, including 3 of the 5 *L. lutea* and the single *C. iris*, also had visceral amyloidosis verified by Congo red staining (Figure 2(d)). Amyloidosis in the 3 *L. lutea* was moderate to severe, while the amyloidosis in the *C. iris* was mild. Amyloid deposits were most commonly found

within hepatic sinusoids but were also identified in ovarian, splenic, and renal tissue. Loss of Congo red staining after acid digestion with 0.5% potassium permanganate and 0.3% sulfuric acid was consistent with reactive, serum amyloid-associated (SAA) secondary amyloidosis.

Severe ventricular habronemiasis was determined to be the cause of death in 8 of the 11 individuals (Table 1) and a major contributing factor in the death of 2 individuals with severe hepatic amyloidosis. A single individual died of trauma.

3. Discussion

Unlike the low pathogenicity often seen with equine gastric and nonpasserine avian habronemiasis, increased morbidity and mortality were associated with ventricular habronemiasis of passerines at the North Carolina Zoological Park. Ventricular habronemiasis in these individuals caused chronic ventriculitis and resulted in poor body condition and death. Disruption of the protective koilin layer of the ventriculus led to inflammation and increased susceptibility to secondary bacterial and fungal infections. Similar koilin disruption and large bacterial colonies were noted in the black-backed woodpecker [20], but no inflammatory reaction or change in the koilin layer was reported by Ehrsam et al. [23] for German cases of ventricular habronemiasis in *L. lutea* and *L. rothschildi*.

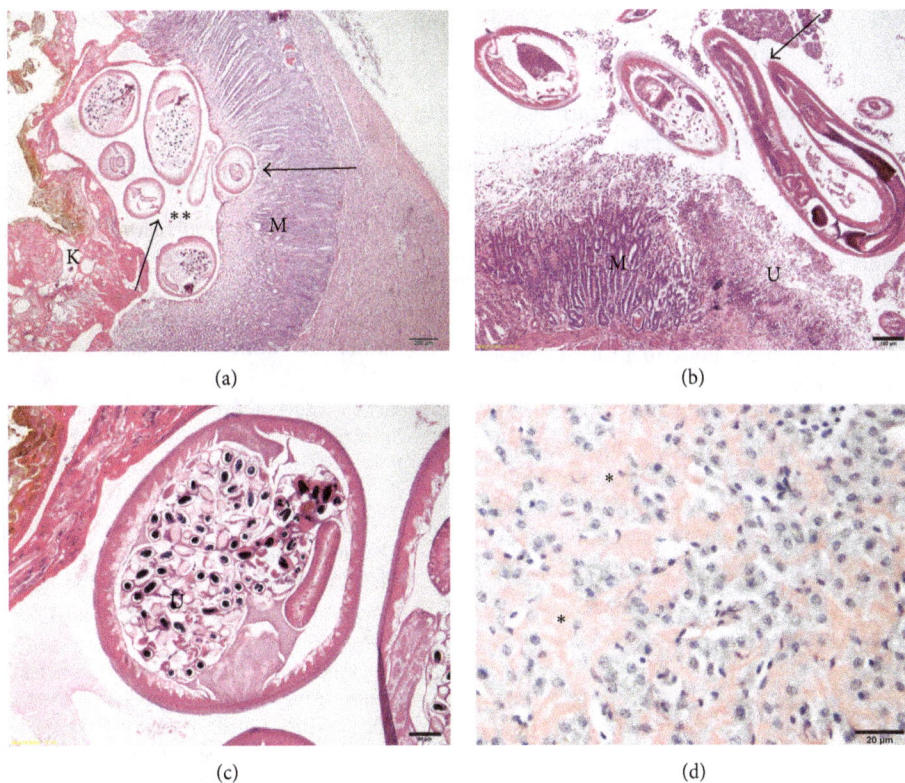

(a)

(b)

(c)

(d)

FIGURE 2: (a) Lower power view of ventriculus from *L. lutea*. Multiple cross-sections of *Procyrnea* sp. nematodes (asterisks) with lateral alae (arrows) are visible between the mucosa and fragmented koilin layer (H&E stain). M: mucosa; K: koilin layer. Scale bar = 200 μm. (b) Higher power view of the ventriculus from a more severely affected *Z. japonicus*. The koilin layer above the *Procyrnea* sp. nematodes is largely absent and there is regionally extensive mucosal ulceration which is covered with a mat of fungal hyphae admixed with fibrin and cell debris. The posterior spicule from a male nematode (arrow) is captured in longitudinal section (H&E stain). M: mucosa; U: ulceration. Scale bar = 100 μm. (c) Cross-section through a female *Procyrnea* sp. nematode from a *Z. japonicus* containing large numbers of larvated, thick-shelled eggs (H&E stain). U: uterus. Scale bar = 50 μm. (d) Large sinusoidal accumulations of brightly eosinophilic amyloid (asterisks) compress the adjacent hepatocytes in a liver from a *L. lutea* (Congo red stain). Scale bar = 20 μm.

Amyloidosis in birds usually occurs in the liver, spleen, and/or kidneys [25]. It is typically of the SAA type and is associated with chronic infectious disease [25]. Given the absence of other inflammatory lesions, amyloidosis was attributed to chronic ventriculitis caused by nematode infestation. The overrepresentation of *L. lutea* in cases of amyloidosis could denote species-specific variation in amyloid formation in response to chronic inflammation.

Antemortem direct fecal smears and sodium nitrate fecal flotations had been negative for spirurid nematodes. The eggs of the equine *Habronema* and *Draschia* spp. tend not to float well in fecal flotation solutions and are fragile, thus making them hard to find [1]. A combination filtration and centrifugation method is described by Ehrsam et al. [23] and could be attempted in the future.

Given the use of fly intermediates by equine habronememes, the clustering of cases during warm months, and the omnivorous habits of the species affected, an insect intermediate is suspected in this case. Maggots used in diets in the aviary were unlikely to be the intermediate as they are obtained from a commercial source and have been analyzed by a parasitologist and were negative for nematode larvae. Rehabilitated, unreleasable, native passerines introduced to

the aviary undergo the same quarantine procedures as exotic aviary species prior to introduction to the general population including prophylactic deworming, typically with a single dose of ivermectin. However, while the aviary is technically a closed environment, native insects, reptiles, amphibians, and occasional birds still get into the exhibit. Efforts to identify an insect intermediate have been unsuccessful and collection and necropsy of native passerines found dead within the zoological park have not identified a sylvatic host. Reported intermediate hosts of *Procyrnea pileata* include pillbugs (*Armadillidium vulgare*) and earwigs (*Euborellia annulipes*) [20], while the German cockroach (*Blattella germanica*) has been experimentally infected with *Cyrnea colini* [23]. These insect species or close relatives could be foraged by birds within the aviary. If an intermediate host is identified, xenodiagnosis may be an effective antemortem diagnostic tool and biologic control using parasitoid wasps could be considered if the insect intermediate is *Musca* sp. [1, 26].

For companion and aviary birds, treatment with oral fenbendazole given daily for 3–5 days, pyrantel pamoate given orally and repeated after 14 days, or ivermectin has been successful at eliminating nematode infections [27]. Treatment with oral fenbendazole, repeated after 14 days, has been reported to be an effective option in raptors [4]. Equine cases are typically treated with a single dose of ivermectin or moxidectin [1, 26, 28, 29].

After the initial diagnosis of habronemiasis, four of the affected *L. lutea* and the *C. iris* were treated symptomatically or prophylactically with either pyrantel pamoate (22 mg/kg by mouth repeated every 10 days for 2-3 doses) or fenbendazole (50 mg/kg by mouth every 24 hours for 1–6 days repeated at variable intervals). These treated birds died within 2 months after their last anthelminthic treatment. However, the small sample size, variation in dosing regimes, and lack of regular repeated dosing preclude any conclusions about anthelminthic efficacy or parasite resistance.

In future outbreaks, prophylactic deworming of all affected species with single doses of ivermectin or moxidectin during the summer months may prove to be more efficacious and practical for the free-flight aviary setting. Increased insect pest control and preventing entry of native avian species into the habitat may also help in the reduction or management of outbreaks.

Acknowledgment

The authors thank Judy Hunt for her assistance in compiling medical records.

References

[1] D. D. Bowman, *Georgis' Parasitology for Veterinarians*, Elsevier/Saunders, St. Louis, Mo, USA, 9th edition, 2009.

[2] A. G. Chabaud, "Spirurida," in *Keys to the Nematode Parasites of Vertebrates: Archival Volume*, R. C. Anderson, A. G. Chabaud, and S. Willmott, Eds., pp. 334–382, CABI, Cambridge, Mass, USA, 2009.

[3] A. C. Chandler, "A new spiruroid nematode, *Habronema americanum*, from the Broad-Winged Hawk, *Buteo platypterus*," *Journal of Parasitology*, vol. 27, no. 2, pp. 184–185, 1941.

[4] J. C. Chebez and R. F. Aguilar, "Order falconiformes (Hawks, Eagles, Falcons, Vultures)," in *Biology, Medicine, and Surgery of South American Wild Animals*, M. E. Fowler and Z. S. Cubas, Eds., pp. 115–124, Iowa State University Press, Ames, Iowa, USA, 2001.

[5] S. A. Smith, "Parasites of birds of prey: their diagnosis and treatment," *Seminars in Avian and Exotic Pet Medicine*, vol. 5, no. 2, pp. 97–105, 1996.

[6] M. P. Illescas Gomez, M. Rodriguez Osorio, and F. Aranda Maza, "Parasitation of falconiform, strigiform and passeriform (Corvidae) birds by helminths in Spain," *Research and Reviews in Parasitology*, vol. 53, no. 3-4, pp. 129–135, 1993.

[7] A. A. Kocan and L. N. Locke, "Some helminth parasites of the American bald eagle," *Journal of wildlife diseases*, vol. 10, no. 1, pp. 8–10, 1974.

[8] V. Agrawal, "On a new avian nematode, *Habronema (Aviabronema) hrishii* sp. nov. from the intestine of *Milvus migrans* (Kite)," *Transactions of the American Microscopical Society*, vol. 84, no. 4, pp. 573–576, 1965.

[9] E. Gendre, "Sur quelques espèces d'*Habronema* parasites de oiseaux," *Actes de la Société Linnéenne de Bordeaux*, vol. 74, pp. 112–133, 1922.

[10] R. Ortlepp, "On *Habronema murrayi* n. sp. from the barn owl, *Tyto alba*," *Onderstepoort Journal of Veterinary Science and Animal Industry*, vol. 3, pp. 351–355, 1934.

[11] S. M. Ali, "On some new nematodes (Habronematinae) from birds in hyderabad, India, and the relationships of the genus *Habronema*," *Journal of Helminthology*, vol. 35, no. 1-2, pp. 1–48, 1961.

[12] P. M. Mawson, "Habronematinae (Nematoda: Spiruridae) from Australian birds," *Parasitology*, vol. 58, no. 4, pp. 745–767, 1968.

[13] R. M. Pinto, J. J. Vicente, and D. Noronha, "Nematode parasites of Brazilian accipitrid and falconid birds (Falconiformes)," *Memorias do Instituto Oswaldo Cruz*, vol. 89, no. 3, pp. 359–362, 1994.

[14] W. C. Clark, "*Procyrnea kea* sp. nov. (Habronematidae: Spirurida: Nematoda) from the New Zealand Kea (*Nestor notabilis* Gould, 1865) (Aves: Psittaciformes)," *Journal of the Royal Society of New Zealand*, vol. 8, no. 3, pp. 323–328, 1978.

[15] S. Zhang, J. Song, and L. Zhang, "Three species of Procyrnea Chabaud, 1958 (Nematoda: Habronematoidea: Habronematidae) from raptors in Beijing, China, with descriptions of two new species," *Journal of Natural History*, vol. 45, no. 47-48, pp. 2915–2928, 2011.

[16] J. C. Quentin, C. Seureau, and C. Railhac, "Biological cycle of *Cyrnea (Procyrnea) mansoni* Seurat, 1914, a habronemid nematode parasite of birds of prey in Togo," *Annales de Parasitologie Humaine et Comparee*, vol. 58, no. 2, pp. 165–175, 1983.

[17] J. Vercruysse, E. A. Harris, R. A. Bray, M. Nagalo, M. Pangui, and D. I. Gibson, "A survey of gastrointestinal helminths of the common helmet guinea fowl (*Numida meleagris galeata*) in Burkina Faso," *Avian Diseases*, vol. 29, no. 3, pp. 742–745, 1985.

[18] E. A. Harris, "Two new nematodes parasitic in the kiwi in New Zealand," *Bulletin of the British Museum of Natural History*, vol. 28, no. 5, pp. 199–205, 1975.

[19] L. Zhang, D. R. Brooks, and D. Causey, "*Procyrnea chabaud*, 1958 (Nematoda: Habronematoidea: Habronematidae) in birds from the Area de Conservación Guanacaste, Costa Rica, including descriptions of 3 new species," *Journal of Parasitology*, vol. 90, no. 2, pp. 364–372, 2004.

[20] R. B. Siegel, M. L. Bond, R. L. Wilkerson et al., "Lethal *Procyrnea* infection in a black-backed woodpecker (*Picoides arcticus*) from California," *Journal of Zoo and Wildlife Medicine*, vol. 43, no. 2, pp. 421–424, 2012.

[21] W. R. Davidson, L. T. Hon, and D. J. Forrester, "Status of the genus *Cyrnea* (Nematoda: Spiruroidea) in wild Turkeys from the southeastern United States," *Journal of Parasitology*, vol. 63, no. 2, pp. 332–336, 1977.

[22] G. W. Foster, J. M. Kinsella, E. L. Walters, M. S. Schrader, and D. J. Forrester, "Parasitic helminths of red-bellied woodpeckers (*Melanerpes carolinus*) from the Apalachicola National Forest in Florida," *Journal of Parasitology*, vol. 88, no. 6, pp. 1140–1142, 2002.

[23] H. Ehrsam, S. K. Spillmann, and K. Wolff, "Nematodes (*Procyrnea mansioni*, Spirurida) as a cause of stomach changes in Chinese nightingales (*Leiothrix lutea*) and Rothschild's mynah birds (*Leucopsar rothschildi*)," *Schweizer Archiv für Tierheilkunde*, vol. 127, no. 10, pp. 665–670, 1985.

[24] R. L. Slater, "Helminths of the Robin, *Turdus migratorius* Ridgway, from Northern Colorado," *The American Midland Naturalist*, vol. 77, no. 1, pp. 190–199, 1967.

[25] K. E. Roertgen and K. H. Johnson, "Amyloidosis," in *Noninfectious Diseases of Wildlife*, A. Fairbrother, L. N. Locke, and G. L.

Hoff, Eds., pp. 194–202, Iowa State University Press, Ames, Iowa, USA, 1996.

[26] R. K. Schuster and S. Sivakumar, "A xenodiagnostic method using *Musca domestica* for the diagnosis of gastric habronemosis and examining the anthelmintic efficacy of moxidectin," *Veterinary Parasitology*, vol. 197, no. 1-2, pp. 176–181, 2013.

[27] I. Langlois, "The anatomy, physiology, and diseases of the avian proventriculus and ventriculus," *Veterinary Clinics of North America*, vol. 6, no. 1, pp. 85–111, 2003.

[28] A. A. Cutolo, A. T. D. Santos, and S. M. Allegretti, "Field study on the efficacy of an oral 2% ivermectin formulation in horses," *Revista Brasileira de Parasitologia Veterinaria*, vol. 20, no. 2, pp. 171–175, 2011.

[29] A. J. Costa, O. F. Barbosa, F. R. Moraes et al., "Comparative efficacy evaluation of moxidectin gel and ivermectin paste against internal parasites of equines in Brazil," *Veterinary Parasitology*, vol. 80, no. 1, pp. 29–36, 1998.

23

A Case of Bilateral Auricular Chondritis in a Heifer

Hibret A. Adissu,[1,2] John D. Baird,[3] and Geoffrey A. Wood[1]

[1] Department of Pathobiology, Ontario Veterinary College, University of Guelph, Guelph, ON, Canada N1G 2W1
[2] Centre for Modeling Human Disease, Toronto Centre for Phenogenomics, 25 Orde Street, Toronto, ON, Canada M5T 3H7
[3] Department of Clinical Studies, Ontario Veterinary College, University of Guelph, Guelph, ON, Canada N1G 2W1

Correspondence should be addressed to Hibret A. Adissu; adissu@lunenfeld.ca

Academic Editor: Maria Teresa Mandara

Auricular chondritis is an extremely rare condition in cattle and other domestic animals. A 13-month-old Jersey heifer was presented with cutaneous papillomatosis and bilaterally droopy ears. Histopathology revealed bilateral auricular chondritis characterized by lymphoplasmacytic infiltrate and extensive destruction and fibrosis of the auricular cartilage.

1. Introduction

Auricular chondritis, also known as auricular chondropathy, is an inflammatory condition of the cartilaginous tissues of the pinna rarely reported in human beings and animals. In human beings, it manifests as part of relapsing polychondritis complex, a rare systemic autoimmune disease characterized by episodic destructive inflammation of cartilaginous tissues throughout the body especially those of the ear, nose, joints, and respiratory tract [1–3]. In animals, auricular chondritis has been reported in rats [4–6], mice [2, 7], cats [8–10], and a horse [11]. It is extremely rare in cattle and, to the authors' knowledge, there is only a single case report involving two heifers [12]. In this report, we describe the pathological findings in a case of auricular chondritis in a Jersey heifer.

2. Case Description

A 13-month-old Jersey heifer was presented to the Ontario Veterinary College Teaching Hospital with extensive cutaneous papillomatosis and bilaterally droopy ears (Figure 1). Previously, the heifer had dermatophytosis due to *Trichophyton mentagrophytes* that responded to topical enilconazole (Elanco Animal Health, Guelph, Ontario, Canada) and terbinafine HCl (LAMISIL, Novartis Pharmaceuticals Canada Inc., Quebec, Canada), supplied as emergency drug

release. The proportion of different populations of blood lymphocytes as determined by flow cytometry was within normal limits. Mild neutrophilia and lymphocytosis were present on complete blood count. Lymphocytes were of unremarkable morphology on blood smear analysis. Urinalysis and blood biochemistry findings were unremarkable. Real time PCR on ear-notch sample was negative for Bovine Viral Diarrhoea Virus type 1 and type 2. The cow was euthanized based on the extensive papillomatosis and recurrent dermatophytosis.

At necropsy, the pinnae were soft, thickened, and flabby. The skin and hair of the pinnae were unremarkable. Numerous multifocal to coalescing round to irregular exophytic hyperkeratotic nodules from 0.5 to 6 cm in diameter were present on the skin of the cranial thorax, neck, and head, including the face. The nodules were more numerous and larger on the cranial aspect of the neck. In the intervening cutaneous tissue, notably in the caudal neck region, there were occasional round pale and scaly foci (interpreted as resolving dermatophytic lesions). Some of these foci had central small (0.5 cm diameter) hyperkeratotic nodules resembling those described above. The skin nodules have grey exterior cut surfaces with adjacent light pink tissue. Macroscopic diagnoses of cutaneous papillomatosis, dermatophytosis, and auricular chondropathy were made.

Blocks of various tissues including the skin, the pinna, nasal planum, trachea, lungs, lymph nodes, and spleen

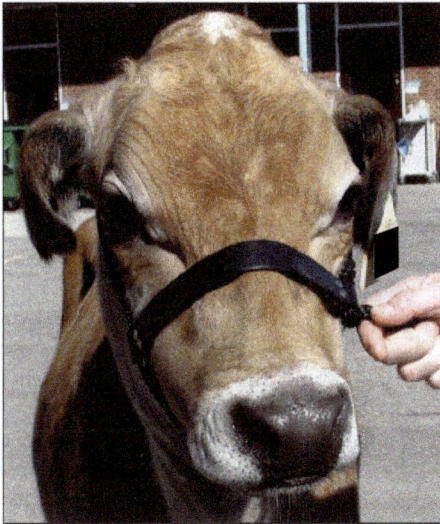

FIGURE 1: Jersey heifer presented with bilateral droopy ears.

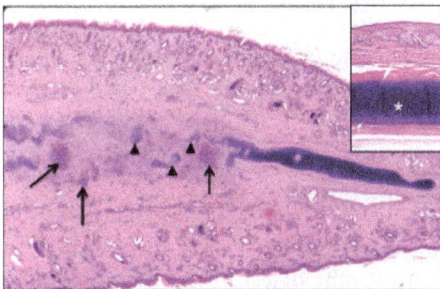

FIGURE 2: Histopathological features of auricular chondritis. The pinna is markedly expanded and the cartilage plate is disrupted (arrow heads) by multifocal to coalescing inflammatory infiltrates (arrows). Inset shows a section of pinna from an unaffected cow with normal cartilage plate (∗). Hematoxylin and eosin: 1.25x.

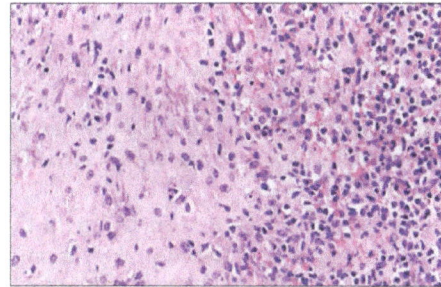

FIGURE 3: The auricular cartilage plate is disrupted by aggregates of lymphocytes and other mononuclear inflammatory cells. Hematoxylin and eosin: 40x.

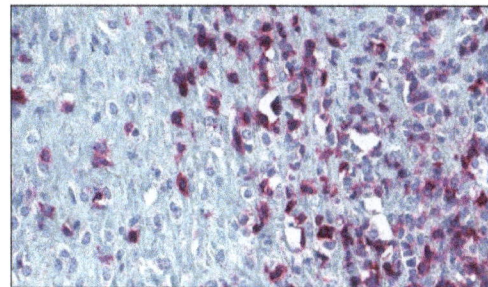

FIGURE 4: T-lymphocytes (red) predominate in the inflammation. Immunohistochemistry for CD3; avidin-biotin-peroxidase method with NovaRed chromogen and hematoxylin counterstain 40x.

were fixed in 10% neutral-buffered formalin and routinely processed and stained with hematoxylin and eosin (HE). Multiple longitudinal and cross sections along the entire length of the middle aspect of the pinna were made. Similar sections of the pinna, obtained from a cow with grossly normal ear, were made for comparison. Sections of the ear were also evaluated immunohistochemically to detect CD3 (T cells) and CD79a (B cells) using polyclonal rabbit anti-human CD3 and monoclonal mouse anti-human CD79a antibodies, respectively (DakoCytomation, Mississauga, ON). Primary antibodies were omitted for negative controls. Sections of the pinna were also stained with Brown and Brenn gram stain and periodic acid-Schiff (PAS) to rule out bacterial and fungal infection, respectively.

Microscopically, multifocal to coalescing aggregates of numerous lymphocytes, plasma cells, and a few macrophages were present along the whole length of the perichondrium and within the cartilaginous plate of the pinna, notably towards the base of the ear (Figures 2 and 3). The cartilaginous plate was expanded by multiple basophilic cartilaginous

nodules, vascularization, and perivascular fibrosis. Chondrocytes found in the centre of the cartilaginous nodules were swollen with pale round or oval nuclei; rare clusters of chondrocytes were present within a lacuna (interpreted as proliferation). In rare foci, streams of thick dense collagen bundles were present within the disorganized cartilage; low numbers of spindle cells surrounded by lacuna were present within these dense collagenous bundles (interpreted as early osseous metaplasia). A section of the pinna from an unaffected cow showed a regular narrow band of elastic cartilage (Figure 2, inset). On IHC, 60–70% of the lymphocytes within the auricular cartilage were CD3-positive (T cells) (Figure 4) and the rest (30–40%) were CD79a-positive (B cells). Neither bacteria nor fungi were detected within the pinna by special staining (data not shown). Based on these findings, a diagnosis of bilateral auricular lymphoplasmacytic chondritis and perichondritis was made. The microscopic feature of the skin nodules was multifocal nodular hyperkeratotic and hyperplastic dermatitis, typical of bovine cutaneous papillomatosis (consistent with the gross pathology and clinical diagnosis). Other microscopic lesions included reactive lymphoid hyperplasia in multiple lymph nodes with mild depletion of medullary sinuses and protein casts within occasional medullary renal tubules with rare multifocal interstitial lymphocyte aggregates. No lesions were detected in other cartilaginous tissues.

3. Discussion

Auricular chondritis accompanied by marked loss, disorganization, and fibrosis of the cartilage plate of the pinna was presented in this heifer. The lesion would have compromised the physical strength of the pinna consistent with clinical presentation of droopy ears.

Auricular chondropathy is extremely rare in the bovine species, and, to the authors' knowledge, there is only a single case report describing a similar condition in cattle [12]. This earlier report was described in Swiss Braunvieh cattle [12]; this breed exhibits a predisposition to malformations of the pinnae, with involvement of the epiglottis and the arytenoid cartilage in some animals [13]. Other cartilaginous tissues were not affected in the current case nor in the previous case report in two heifers [12], a horse [11], and laboratory rats [5, 14]. In contrast, auricular chondritis induced experimentally by immunization with type II collagen is accompanied by arthritis in rats and mice [4, 15, 16]. Also, a recent report in a cat describes a polychondritis with involvement of the cartilage of the pinnae, costae, larynx, trachea, and limbs [10].

In the previous report of bovine auricular chondritis, a difference in the length of the long arms of the X chromosome was observed; however, the cause and pathogenesis were not determined [12]. The bilateral presentation deep within the cartilage and away from the skin makes extension from dermatitis associated with dermatophytosis or papillomatosis unlikely. Furthermore, the inflammation at the lateral edge where the ear tag was applied was minimal to absent, which makes trauma an unlikely cause. A mild trauma associated with insertion of ear tag likely happened at a very young age and there was no history of lesions of the ear/pinna before the recent presentation. These observations together with the multifocal and random T lymphocyte-dominated inflammation strongly suggest an immune-mediated etiopathogenesis. In this regard, the presence of widespread papillomatosis and previous history of dermatophytosis in this animal suggests an underlying systemic immunopathy. However, no abnormalities were detected in proportion of the different populations of lymphocytes. The mild lymphocytosis and neutrophilia were consistent with underlying fungal infection and papillomatosis. Furthermore, there were neither atrophic nor degenerative changes in the thymus and other lymphoid tissues to offer a morphological basis for immune suppression. Bovine viral diarrhea virus isolation to rule out persistent BVD infection was negative.

Auricular chondritis in human beings is part of a rare autoimmune disease complex known as relapsing polychondritis. This condition involves several cartilaginous structures including the pinnae, nose, trachea, joints, and eyes, resulting in clinical manifestations of cyclical and destructive auricular chondritis, polyarthritis, nasal chondritis, ocular inflammation, audiovestibular damage, and respiratory tract chondritis [1, 2]. A similar condition has been described in laboratory rodents, notably in rats, a species that has been proposed as a model for relapsing polychondritis in human beings. In rats, it has been reported as an idiopathic/spontaneous [5, 6] or as experimental type II collagen-induced condition [4]. Interestingly, development of bilateral auricular chondritis has

been reported secondary to unilateral application of metallic ear tags in rats [6] and mice [7]. In the later report, the auricular chondritis was characterized by the predominance of CD4-positive T lymphocytes, increased expression of Th1-type cytokines, and upregulation of metallothionein- (MT-) I and MT-II. This suggests an autoimmune disease triggered by the presence of metal ions released from metal ear tags [7]. The etiology of relapsing polychondritis in human beings is unknown; however, consistent with autoimmune etiopathogenesis, antibodies to cartilage proteins were identified in the sera of patients with this condition [15]. No tests for autoantibodies to cartilage proteins were done in our case; however, the pathological findings are consistent with an autoimmune pathogenesis.

To our knowledge, this is the first report of auricular chondritis in Jersey cattle and the second report in cattle as a whole. Further cases of auricular chondritis may be found if the pinna is routinely examined in cattle with a similar clinical presentation.

Conflict of Interests

The authors have no financial or personal relationships with other people or organizations that could inappropriately influence this work.

Acknowledgments

The authors thank Dr. Ian Barker for the gross pathology and initial histopathological interpretation of the case and the University of Guelph Animal Health Laboratory for histological and immunohistochemical service.

References

[1] A. P. Rozin, E. Gez, and R. Bergman, "Recurrent auricular chondritis and cartilage repair," *Annals of the Rheumatic Diseases*, vol. 64, no. 5, pp. 783–784, 2005.

[2] J. L. Lamoureux, J. H. Buckner, C. S. David, and D. S. Bradley, "Mice expressing HLA-DQ6a8β transgenes develop polychondritis spontaneously," *Arthritis Research and Therapy*, vol. 8, no. 4, article R134, 2006.

[3] T. Lahmer, M. Treiber, A. von Werder et al., "Relapsing polychondritis: an autoimmune disease with many faces," *Autoimmunity Reviews*, vol. 9, no. 8, pp. 540–546, 2010.

[4] W. J. McCune, A. L. Schiller, R. A. Dynesius-Trentham, and D. E. Trentham, "Type II collagen-induced auricular chondritis," *Arthritis and Rheumatism*, vol. 25, no. 3, pp. 266–273, 1982.

[5] D. J. Prieur, D. M. Young, and D. F. Counts, "Auricular chondritis in fawn-hooded rats. A spontaneous disorder resembling that induced by immunization with type II collagen," *The American Journal of Pathology*, vol. 116, no. 1, pp. 69–76, 1984.

[6] M. Kitagaki, T. Suwa, M. Yanagi, and K. Shiratori, "Auricular chondritis in young ear-tagged Crj:CD(SD)IGS rats," *Laboratory Animals*, vol. 37, no. 3, pp. 249–253, 2003.

[7] M. Kitagaki and M. Hirota, "Auricular chondritis caused by metal ear tagging in C57BL/6 mice," *Veterinary Pathology*, vol. 44, no. 4, pp. 458–466, 2007.

[8] D. A. Delmage and D. F. Kelly, "Auricular chondritis in a cat," *Journal of Small Animal Practice*, vol. 42, no. 10, pp. 499–501, 2001.

[9] B. Gerber, M. Crottaz, C. von Tscharner, and V. Schärer, "Feline relapsing polychondritis: two cases and a review of the literature," *Journal of Feline Medicine and Surgery*, vol. 4, no. 4, pp. 189–194, 2002.

[10] T. Baba, A. Shimizu, T. Ohmuro et al., "Auricular chondritis associated with systemic joint and cartilage inflammation in a cat," *Journal of Veterinary Medical Science*, vol. 71, no. 1, pp. 79–82, 2009.

[11] J. R. Bowers and R. F. Slocombe, "Auricular chondrosis in a horse," *Australian Veterinary Journal*, vol. 87, no. 6, pp. 219–221, 2009.

[12] U. Bleul, E. Ahrens, G. Stranzinger, T. Sydler, S. Ohlerth, and U. Braun, "Auricular chondropathy in two Swiss Braunvieh heifers," *Veterinary Record*, vol. 159, no. 26, pp. 890–892, 2006.

[13] U. Bleul, G. Stranzinger, and T. Sydler, "Polychondritis: a new disease in Swiss Braunvieh?" *Schweizer Archiv fur Tierheilkunde*, vol. 153, no. 11, pp. 526–529, 2011.

[14] B. J. McEwen and N. J. Barsoum, "Auricular chondritis in Wistar rats," *Laboratory Animals*, vol. 24, no. 3, pp. 280–283, 1990.

[15] T. Fujiyoshi, K. Cheng, M. S. Krug, and T. Yoo, "Molecular basis of type II collagen autoimmune disease: observations of arthritis, auricular chondritis and tympanitis in mice," *ORL*, vol. 59, no. 4, pp. 215–229, 1997.

[16] D. S. Bradley, P. Das, M. M. Griffiths, H. S. Luthra, and C. S. David, "HLA-DQ6/8 double transgenic mice develop auricular chondritis following type II collagen immunization: a model for human relapsing polychondritis," *The Journal of Immunology*, vol. 161, no. 9, pp. 5046–5053, 1998.

24

Nasal Adenocarcinoma in a Horse with Metastasis to Lung, Liver, and Bone and Review of Metastasis in Nine Horses with Sinonasal Tumors

Ashley Hanna,[1] Susanne M. Stieger-Vanegas,[1] Jerry R. Heidel,[2] Melissa Esser,[1] John Schlipf,[1] and Jacob Mecham[1]

[1]*Department of Clinical Sciences, College of Veterinary Medicine, Oregon State University, Magruder Hall, Corvallis, OR 97331, USA*
[2]*Department of Biomedical Sciences, College of Veterinary Medicine, Oregon State University, Magruder Hall, Corvallis, OR 97331, USA*

Correspondence should be addressed to Susanne M. Stieger-Vanegas; susanne.stieger@oregonstate.edu

Academic Editor: Franco Mutinelli

Sinonasal neoplasia metastasizing to distant organs is rare in horses. This case report describes the clinical and imaging findings of a horse with sinonasal neoplasia, which had metastasized to the lung, liver, and humerus. Additionally, the prevalence of sinonasal neoplasia and their incidence of distant metastasis among horses that presented to the Oregon State University Veterinary Teaching Hospital (OSU-VTH) were estimated. Of 5,558 equine patients who presented to the OSU-VTH in the last nine years, 1.4% were diagnosed with sinonasal disease and 10.3% of these cases had sinonasal neoplasia with only one having confirmed distant metastasis. This case was an eleven-year-old quarter horse which was evaluated due to a history of a right forelimb lameness of three weeks duration. Two and a half months later he presented again, this time for unilateral epistaxis and persistent right forelimb lameness. Radiography of the right elbow noted an increasingly irregular, periosteal response and osteolytic lesion of the right distal humeral condyle. At the time of the second presentation, nasosinal endoscopy identified a lobulated mass in the region of the ethmoid turbinates. Histopathology of this mass revealed an adenocarcinoma of nasal origin with metastasis to the lung, liver, and right humerus.

1. Introduction

Adenocarcinomas in the horse are uncommon but have been reported to occur in a variety of locations including lung, intestine, kidney, skin, lacrimal gland, testes, ovary, mammary tissue, sinuses, and nasal passages [1–7]. Adenocarcinomas of nasal and paranasal sinus origin are rare tumors affecting equids but can cause significant morbidity. More commonly the tumors originate in the maxillary area than in the nasal area [1]. They are often aggressive, locally invasive neoplasias that carry a poor prognosis [8]. These tumors have been reported to extend from the nasal cavity and paranasal sinuses through the cribriform plate into neural tissue and often tend to metastasize to regional lymph nodes [1, 9]. Distant metastases of nasal adenocarcinomas to the lung have been described in two horses; however, this appears

to be a rare occurrence. This is likely in part secondary to the low number of affected animals submitted for necropsy and in part due to the limitations of the current diagnostic techniques available evaluating the horses [1, 8]. Though there has been no evidence of equine nasal adenocarcinoma metastasis to bone, there are reports of intestinal and renal adenocarcinomas metastasizing to the axial and appendicular skeleton [2, 7, 10].

Neoplasia involving the appendicular skeleton in horses can cause severe lameness that is often attributed to bone pain, soft tissue pathology, or a nonpathologic fracture. Metastatic lesions as well as primary bone neoplasia can cause significant osseous destruction, which is caused by an increased osteoclastic activity secondary to a dysregulation of the normal bone homeostasis. The osseous destruction in combination with focal inflammation and increasing

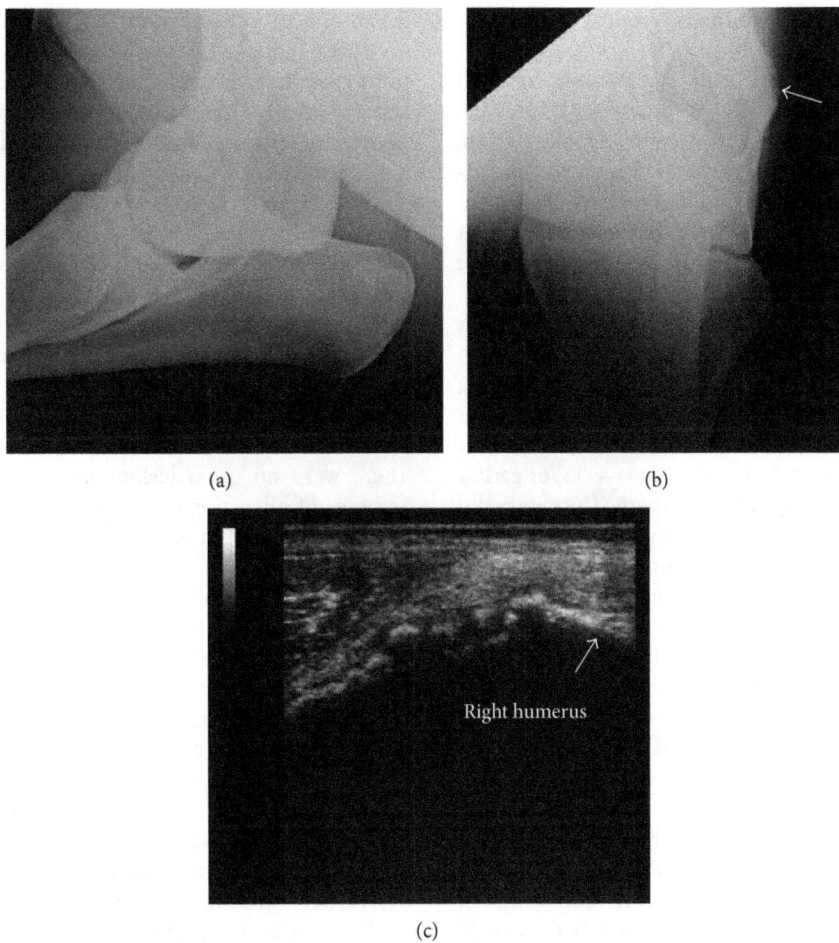

(a)

(b)

(c)

FIGURE 1: Radiographs of the right elbow at first presentation in (a) lateromedial and (b) craniocaudal views. A faint lucency is noted in the lateral aspect of the condyle of the right humerus. There is mild periosteal bone proliferation on the lateral aspect of the distal humerus metaphysis and condyle (marked by white arrow), which is best noted in the craniocaudal view. (c) Ultrasound image of the lateral aspect of the condyle of the right humerus. A marked irregularity of the bone surface just proximal of the origin of the lateral collateral ligament (marked by white arrow) of the right elbow joint is noted.

tissue acidity results in sensitized and partially destroyed peripheral nerve endings resulting in a high level of pain [11]. Osteosarcoma, fibrosarcoma, and chondrosarcoma involving bone have been documented infrequently in horses. In none of these horses metastatic lesions were present at necropsy, suggesting that the incidence of metastasis might also be low in these tumor types; however larger case series are needed to confirm this finding [12]. This case report describes a case of nasal adenocarcinoma with distant metastasis to multiple organs including liver, lung, and the distal right humerus. To the authors' knowledge this is the only report of nasal adenocarcinoma in the horse with metastasis to bone.

2. Case Presentation

An eleven-year-old quarter horse gelding used for pleasure riding first presented to the Oregon State University Veterinary Teaching Hospital (OSU-VTH) for a right forelimb lameness of three weeks' duration. He had been treated with oral flunixin meglumine (Banamine, Merck Animal Health, Whitehouse Station, NJ, USA) at a dose of 1.1 mg/kg once per

day by the owners with no improvement. At presentation, the horse displayed a grade 4/5 right forelimb lameness, was dragging his toe, and was reluctant to further flexion of the limb. On physical examination, the horse stood with his right forelimb in slight flexion and his toe pointed. He had a positive response to hoof testers on his right forelimb. Palpation of the right forelimb elicited a mild pain response at the origin of the lateral collateral ligament of the elbow.

Localized abaxial sesamoid perineural anesthesia of the right forelimb did not improve the lameness. Intra-articular anesthesia of the elbow joint resulted in mild improvement but did not resolve the lameness. Radiographs of the right elbow (Figures 1(a) and 1(b)) revealed a mild irregularity of the lateral cortex of the metaphysis of the humerus and the epicondyle of the humerus at the origin of the lateral collateral ligament (Figure 1(b)). Ultrasound of the origin of the lateral collateral ligament demonstrated irregular bony margins at the lateral cortex of the distal humerus metaphysis extending to the proximal aspect of the attachment of the lateral collateral ligament (Figure 1(c)), which at the time was thought to be consistent with trauma secondary to injury of the lateral collateral ligament.

The horse was sent home with instructions for stall rest, administration of 2.2 mg/kg of oral phenylbutazone (Butapaste, Butler Schein Animal Health, Dublin, Ohio, USA) twice per day, and application of a 5″ strip of topical 1% diclofenac sodium (Surpass, Boehringer Ingelheim Vetmedica, St. Joseph, MO, USA) over the right elbow joint twice per day. According to the owner the phenylbutazone was not providing adequate analgesia and was discontinued. Therefore oral gabapentin (Neurontin, Pfizer, New York, NY, USA) at a dose of 4.5 mg/kg twice per day and oral firocoxib (Equioxx, Merial, Duluth, GA, USA) at a dose of 0.1 mg/kg once per day were prescribed. While receiving gabapentin and firocoxib the horse became sound at the walk. It was recommended to reevaluate the horse in two weeks, or earlier if the horse was not improving with treatment. The owner did not schedule a visit and was contacted by phone two weeks following the initial examination and reported that the horse was still sound at walk. No other concerns about the horse were voiced at that time.

Two and a half months after his initial visit the horse presented again with a complaint of a mild intermittent left sided epistaxis over the last two months. The most recent episode of epistaxis was more severe and longer in duration than previously. At the time of presentation the horse was receiving gabapentin and firocoxib at the doses previously prescribed. On physical exam the horse had a constant drip of blood coming from his left nostril. Rectal temperature, heart rate, and respiratory rate were within normal limits. Blood work revealed a packed cell volume of 35% (reference range 32–53%) and total protein of 8 g/dL (reference range 5.7–7.9 g/dL).

The day following admittance, endoscopy revealed a lobulated mass in the region of the left ethmoid turbinates. A biopsy of the mass was obtained and submitted for histopathology.

Radiographs of the skull (Figures 2(a), 2(b), and 2(c)) and right elbow (Figures 3(a) and 3(b)) were subsequently performed. Radiographs of the skull revealed a poorly defined, irregularly outlined soft tissue opacity in the region of the left ethmoid turbinates (Figure 2(c)). Radiographs of the right elbow were compared to the previous radiographs and moderate, irregular periosteal proliferation at the distolateral aspect of the humerus in the location of the origin of the lateral collateral ligament of the elbow was noted (Figures 3(a) and 3(b)). The periosteal proliferation was more pronounced than on the previous radiographs (Figures 1(a) and 1(b)). In addition a heterogeneous lucency was present in the distomedial aspect of the humeral condyle that was not appreciated on the previous radiographs. Based on the most recent radiographs, a healing avulsion fracture was considered unlikely. At this time an underlying aggressive process was suspected with the most likely differential diagnosis being neoplasia, and less likely osteomyelitis.

Histologically, the ethmoidal mass consisted of neoplastic epithelial cells arranged in tubuloacinar, tubular, and solid patterns, all of which were transected by bands of fibrovascular tissue harboring large numbers of mixed mononuclear

inflammatory cells (Figure 4). The neoplastic cells featured moderate anisocytosis and anisokaryosis, with frequent mitotic figures. Mucous-filled spaces and foci of necrosis accompanied by neutrophilic inflammation interrupted the neoplastic cell populations. The findings were consistent with a diagnosis of nasal adenocarcinoma.

Due to multiple lesions with poor prognoses, the owner elected humane euthanasia. The horse underwent a complete necropsy. The mass in the region of the left ethmoid turbinates measured 9 × 5 × 3 cm. It was attached to the turbinates near their caudal extent but did not penetrate the cribriform plate (Figure 2(d)). Dissection of the condyle of the right humerus showed areas of variable malacia (Figure 3(c)). Gross pathology in the lungs included patchy atelectasis, pulmonary edema, and foci of pleural thickening. There were no gross lesions present in any other organs. Samples of all major organs as well as those having visible lesions were fixed in neutral buffered formalin for histologic examination.

Histologic features of the mass from the left ethmoid turbinates were similar to those found in the previous biopsy and remained consistent with nasal adenocarcinoma (Figure 4(a)). The liver and lung had intravascular accumulations of similar clustered neoplastic epithelial cells; in the lung these cells formed tubuloacinar patterns. There were similar accumulations of epithelial cells invading the bone of the right distal humerus (Figure 4(b)). Based upon these findings and the absence of other potential primary tumors, a final diagnosis of nasal adenocarcinoma with metastasis to liver, lung, and distal humerus was made.

To estimate the prevalence of sinonasal neoplasia, medical records of the Oregon State University Veterinary Teaching Hospital from July 2004 to April 2013 were reviewed for equids diagnosed with sinonasal disease. Of these equids diagnosed with sinonasal disease, all equids with confirmed sinonasal neoplasia were evaluated for presenting clinical signs, diagnostic tests performed, and imaging and histopathologic findings. Of 5,558 equine patients that presented to the Oregon State University Veterinary Teaching Hospital in the last nine years, 78 horses and one mule were diagnosed with sinonasal disease (1.4% of the total number of horses seen). Of these, seven horses and one mule were diagnosed with a neoplasia originating in the nasal or paranasal sinus (0.14% of the total number of horses seen). All of the cases with sinonasal neoplasia presented with nasal discharge. 75% had unilateral nasal discharge. One horse started with unilateral nasal discharge, which became later bilateral. Only two of the cases with sinonasal neoplasia had epistaxis. In these 8 cases the following other changes were noted: facial deformities ($n = 2$, 25%), external lymphadenopathy ($n = 2$, 25%), dyspnea ($n = 2$, 25%), fever ($n = 1$, 13%), ocular discharge ($n = 1$, 13%), exophthalmos ($n = 1$, 13%), and lameness ($n = 1$, 13%). The following diagnostic tests were performed in the 8 cases of sinonasal neoplasia: skull radiographs ($n = 6$, 75%), endoscopy ($n = 7$, 88%), sinusoscopy ($n = 2$, 25%), biopsies ($n = 6$, 75%), and necropsy ($n = 4$, 50%). Histologic diagnoses of these tumors were lymphoma ($n = 2$), adenocarcinoma ($n = 2$), and squamous cell carcinoma, osteoma, respiratory transitional

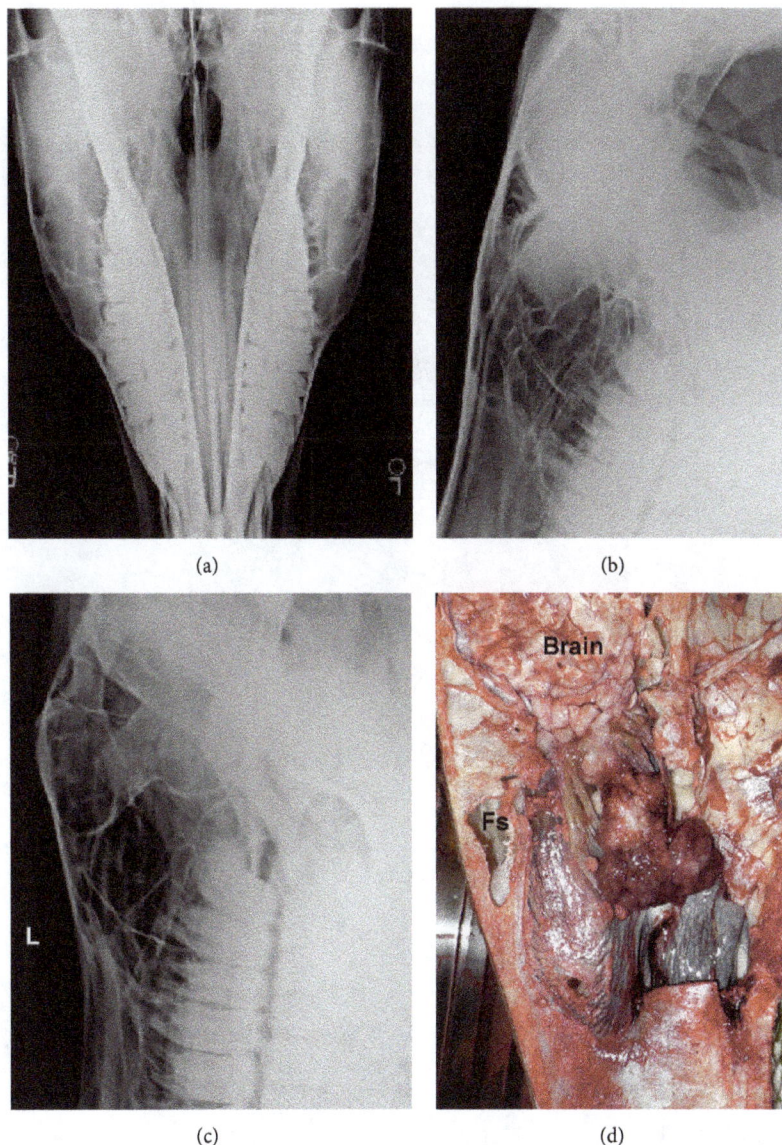

(a)

(b)

(c)

(d)

FIGURE 2: Radiographs of the skull at the time of second presentation in (a) dorsoventral and (b) lateral views. An indistinct soft tissue attenuating area is summating with the left turbinate region rostral to the rostral border of the choanae. (c) Oblique radiographic view of the left frontal and maxillary area. An indistinct soft tissue attenuating area is noted summating with the left lateral aspect of the ethmoid area. (d) Photographic image of the skull cut open in a left parasagittal plane. A dark red to tan mass is noted in the left ethmoid region attached to the caudal aspect of the turbinates. The mass does not extend through the cribriform plate. Fs: frontal sinus.

carcinoma, and undifferentiated carcinoma in one case each. Of the 7 horses, including the horse described in this case report, 2 had enlargement of local lymph nodes, one due to lymphoma and in the other there was no evidence of neoplastic cells. The horse described in this case report was the only one with confirmed distant metastasis of a sinonasal neoplasm.

3. Discussion

The incidence of sinonasal tumors in the population of equine patients seen at our facility is low and similar to that previously reported [1, 13, 14]. The horse diagnosed with nasal adenocarcinoma with metastasis to lung, liver, and distal

humerus was unique as the first presenting complaint was related to the metastatic lesion and not the primary disease. Epistaxis from the nasal adenocarcinoma occurred later in the disease process and was not confirmed to be associated with the ongoing lameness until necropsy.

Neoplasia of the paranasal sinuses and nasal cavity is a relatively rare cause of epistaxis in horses. More common causes include exercise induced pulmonary hemorrhage, guttural pouch mycosis, ethmoid hematoma, and trauma [15]. Often the first diagnostic step in horses with suspected sinonasal disease is endoscopy. If further information regarding the lesion is desired, radiography is traditionally used. Radiographs have proven useful for initial evaluation in horses with sinonasal neoplasia; however they are limited

(a)

(b)

(c)

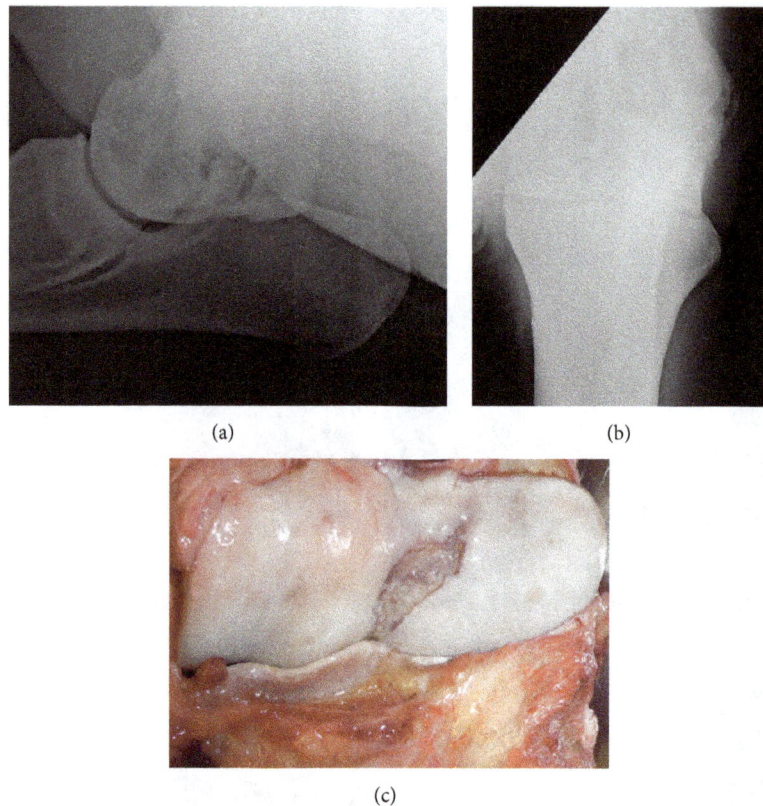

FIGURE 3: Radiographs of the right elbow at second presentation in (a) lateromedial and (b) craniocaudal view. Severe osteolysis of the right humeral condyle and marked irregularity and osteolysis of the lateral epicondyle of the right humerus are noted. (c) Photographic image of the right humeral condyle from the cranial aspect of the right humerus. A large defect secondary to osseous metastasis is noted in the centrolateral aspect of the condyle of the right humerus.

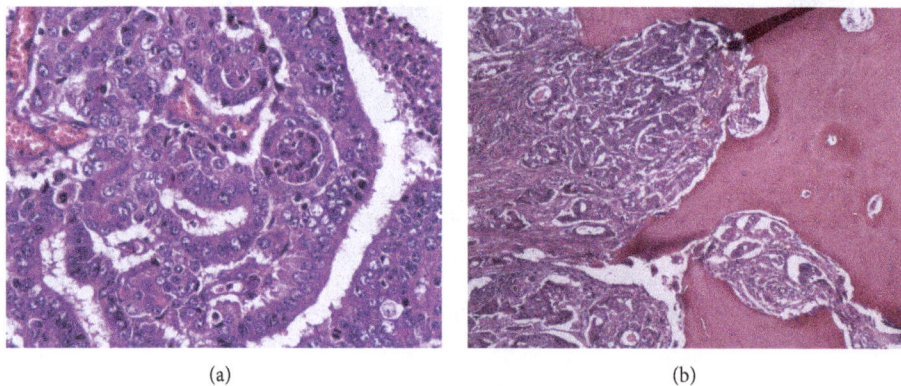

(a)

(b)

FIGURE 4: (a) Left ethmoid mass. The nasal adenocarcinoma effaces normal turbinates. The patterns of neoplastic cell distribution varied between tubular (shown) and solid. Hematoxylin and eosin, 400x. (b) Right humerus. Metastatic nasal adenocarcinoma, with tubular pattern, invading cortical bone. Hematoxylin and eosin, 100x.

in their ability to localize the lesion to the correct location. In this case radiography was the only imaging modality done, as treatment was not pursued. However, in cases of sinonasal neoplasia where surgery is warranted or further prognostic information is desired CT and MRI have shown to be beneficial [16, 17]. The advantages of CT include the ability to better evaluate disease extension, assess involvement of surrounding osseous structures, and more precisely localize

the disease [16]. MRI has been suggested to be more accurate than CT to determine the degree of brain involvement as well as damage to the soft tissues surrounding the orbit. A potential drawback of MRI is the intense sensitivity to inflammatory changes, which could lead to over diagnosis of a benign lesion [17].

Based on the presence of a nasal adenocarcinoma in this patient, the absence of other primary sites of adenocarcinoma in this horse, and metastatic epithelial cells invading the humerus, we present this as the first report of an adenocarcinoma of nasal or paranasal sinus origin metastasizing to bone in a horse. There have been reports in horses of adenocarcinomas originating from other sites that have metastasized to bone, causing significant lameness. This includes two cases of intestinal and one of renal adenocarcinoma with metastatic osseous involvement [2, 10, 18]. In all of the cases of metastatic adenocarcinoma to bone, the horses developed a significant lameness at some point in the disease process. This emphasizes the importance of evaluating the patient thoroughly as some clinical signs associated with the primary disease process may easily be overlooked.

This case report displays that sinonasal neoplasia in the horse can lead to distant metastatic disease. Clinical signs may be associated with the metastatic lesions and not necessarily be the result of the primary tumor. This case also serves as a reminder that osseous neoplasia is uncommon in horses but might be a significant source of lameness. Although metastatic disease associated with nasal adenocarcinoma in the horse is rare further evaluation for presence of metastatic disease should be performed prior to initiation of therapy.

Conflict of Interests

The authors declare that there is no conflict of interests regarding the publication of this paper.

References

[1] K. W. Head and P. M. Dixon, "Equine nasal and paranasal sinus tumours. Part 1: review of the literature and tumour classification," *Veterinary Journal*, vol. 157, no. 3, pp. 261–278, 1999.

[2] M. Oosterlinck, E. Raes, S. Verbraecken et al., "Severe lameness caused by metastatic renal adenocarcinoma of the third phalanx in a Warmblood mare," *Equine Veterinary Education*, vol. 23, no. 10, pp. 512–516, 2011.

[3] G. H. Edington and D. F. Cappell, "Adenocarcinoma of undescended testicle in the horse: (?) secondary growths in lung and mediastinum," *Proceedings of the Royal Society of Medicine*, vol. 24, pp. 1139–1140, 1931.

[4] F. L. Matheis, K. Birkmann, M. Ruetten, S. A. Pot, and B. M. Spiess, "Ocular manifestations of a metastatic adenocarcinoma in a horse," *Veterinary Ophthalmology*, vol. 16, no. 3, pp. 214–218, 2013.

[5] F. E. T. Pauwels, S. J. Wigley, J. S. Munday, and W. D. Roe, "Bilateral ovarian adenocarcinoma in a mare causing haemoperitoneum and colic," *New Zealand Veterinary Journal*, vol. 60, no. 3, pp. 198–202, 2012.

[6] G. P. Reppas, S. A. McClintock, P. J. Canfield, and G. F. Watson, "Papillary ductal adenocarcinoma in the mammary glands of two horses," *Veterinary Record*, vol. 138, pp. 518–519, 1996.

[7] J. A. Wright and G. B. Edwards, "Adenocarcinoma of the intestine in a horse: an unusual occurrence," *Equine Veterinary Journal*, vol. 16, no. 2, pp. 136–137, 1984.

[8] J. L. Davis, B. C. Gilger, K. Spaulding, I. D. Robertson, and S. L. Jones, "Nasal adenocarcinoma with diffuse metastases involving the orbit, cerebrum, and multiple cranial nerves in a horse,"

[9] J. F. Zaruby, M. A. Livesey, and D. H. Percy, "Ethmoid adenocarcinoma perforating the cribriform plate in the horse," *The Cornell Veterinarian*, vol. 83, no. 4, pp. 283–289, 1993.

[10] L. M. East, P. F. Steyn, C. E. Dickinson, and A. A. Frank, "Occult osseous metastasis of a colonic adenocarcinoma visualized with technetium tc 99m hydroxymethylene diphosphate scintigraphy in a horse," *Journal of the American Veterinary Medical Association*, vol. 213, pp. 1167–1170, 1998.

[11] C. M. Kane, P. Hoskin, and M. I. Bennett, "Cancer induced bone pain," *British Medical Journal*, vol. 350, article h315, 2015.

[12] J. M. Bush, R. L. Fredrickson, and E. J. Ehrhart, "Equine osteosarcoma: a series of 8 cases," *Veterinary Pathology*, vol. 44, no. 2, pp. 247–249, 2007.

[13] C. H. Boulton, "Equine nasal cavity and paranasal sinus disease: a review of 85 cases," *Journal of Equine Veterinary Science*, vol. 5, pp. 267–275, 1985.

[14] P. M. Dixon and K. W. Head, "Equine nasal and paranasal sinus tumours: part 2: a contribution of 28 case reports," *Veterinary Journal*, vol. 157, no. 3, pp. 279–294, 1999.

[15] B. P. Smith, *Large Animal Internal Medicine*, Elsevier Health Sciences, 4th edition, 2008.

[16] D. D. Cissell, E. R. Wisner, J. Textor, F. C. Mohr, P. V. Scrivani, and A. P. Théon, "Computed tomographic appearance of equine sinonasal neoplasia," *Veterinary Radiology and Ultrasound*, vol. 53, no. 3, pp. 245–251, 2012.

[17] C. Tessier, A. Brühschwein, J. Lang et al., "Magnetic resonance imaging features of sinonasal disorders in horses," *Veterinary Radiology and Ultrasound*, vol. 54, no. 1, pp. 54–60, 2013.

[18] H. W. Jann, M. A. Breshears, R. W. Allison et al., "Occult metastatic intestinal adenocarcinoma resulting in pathological fracture of the proximal humerus," *Equine Veterinary Journal*, vol. 41, no. 9, pp. 915–917, 2009.

25

Hypertrophic Osteodystrophy in Two Red Wolf (*Canis rufus*) Pups

Jenessa L. Gjeltema,[1,2,3] **Robert A. MacLean,**[3,4] **Eli B. Cohen,**[1] **and Ryan S. De Voe**[3,5]

[1]*Departments of Clinical and Molecular Biomedical Sciences, College of Veterinary Medicine, North Carolina State University, 1060 William Moore Drive, Raleigh, NC 27607, USA*
[2]*North Carolina Zoo, Asheboro, NC 27205, USA*
[3]*Environmental Medicine Consortium, College of Veterinary Medicine, North Carolina State University, Raleigh, NC 27207, USA*
[4]*Audubon Nature Institute, 6500 Magazine Street, New Orleans, LA 70118, USA*
[5]*Disney's Animal Kingdom, Orlando, FL 32830, USA*

Correspondence should be addressed to Jenessa L. Gjeltema; jenessa_gjeltema@ncsu.edu

Academic Editor: Sheila C. Rahal

A 6-month-old red wolf (*Canis rufus*) pup presented for evaluation of progressive thoracic and pelvic limb lameness, joint swelling, and decreased body condition. Radiographic evaluation revealed medullary sclerosis centered at the metaphyses of multiple long bones, well-defined irregular periosteal proliferation, and ill-defined lucent zones paralleling the physes, consistent with hypertrophic osteodystrophy (HOD). Biopsies of affected bone revealed medullary fibrosis and new bone formation. The pup improved following treatment with nonsteroidal anti-inflammatories, opioids, and supportive care over the course of 4 weeks. Metaphyseal periosteal bone proliferation persisted until the animal was humanely euthanized several years later for poor quality of life associated with bilateral cranial cruciate ligament rupture. A second red wolf pup of 4.5 months of age presented for evaluation of lethargy, kyphotic posture, and swollen carpal and tarsal joints. Radiographs revealed bilateral medullary sclerosis and smooth periosteal reaction affecting multiple long bones, suggestive of HOD. Further diagnostics were not pursued in this case to confirm the diagnosis, and the clinical signs persisted for 4 weeks. In light of these two case reports, HOD should be recognized as a developmental orthopedic disease in growing red wolves.

1. Introduction

Hypertrophic osteodystrophy (HOD), also referred to as metaphyseal osteopathy, is a developmental disease affecting the metaphyses of bones in young growing animals. Altered vascularity, necrosis, suppurative inflammation, and modeling of bone at the affected metaphyses have been described [1, 2]. Affected animals may exhibit signs of discomfort, lameness, and general malaise related to the condition. Nutritional, infectious, vaccine-associated, and congenital causes have been implicated in the development of this disease; however, the exact pathogenesis remains unknown [3–9]. The disease has been well documented in domestic canines (*Canis lupus familiaris*), and there have also been reports of the disease in domestic cats (*Felis domesticus*) and Iberian lynx (*Lynx pardinus*) [10–12].

The International Union for the Conservation of Nature (IUCN) currently lists the red wolf as critically endangered [13]. While once considered extinct in the wild in 1980, reintroduction programs have since established a small population in the Southeastern United States of America. This report describes the presentation, diagnosis, and management of HOD in one red wolf (*Canis rufus*) pup and the presentation and management of suspected HOD in a second pup.

2. Case 1

A captive bred male red wolf pup of 6 months of age presented for evaluation of progressive lameness of the thoracic and pelvic limbs, joint swelling, and decreased body condition over the course of nine days. The animal was housed with six other conspecifics including four littermates in a natural

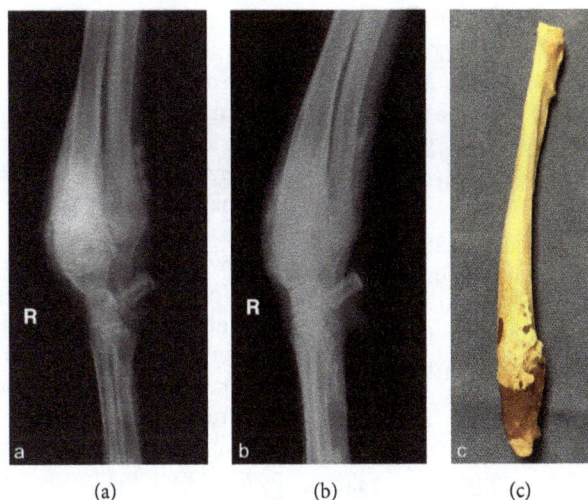

(a)   (b)   (c)

FIGURE 1: Radiographs and gross photograph obtained of the right distal limb from the red wolf pup of case 1 depicting characteristic bone lesions consistent with hypertrophic osteodystrophy. (a) Lateral radiograph day 9. The distal radial and ulnar metaphyses are distally flared with severe, well-defined, and irregular to palisading periosteal bone formation and medullary sclerosis. An irregular zone of lucency is present proximal to the distal radial physis. (b) Lateral radiograph day 62. There is reduction of the prior distal radial and ulnar periosteal bone formation and medullary sclerosis. The distal radial subphyseal linear lucency is no longer present. (c) Postmortem gross image of the right radius demonstrating well-defined, irregular periosteal bone formation at the metaphysis.

substrate outdoor enclosure with access to several den boxes. All wolves were fed Mazuri® exotic canine formulated diet #5MN2 (Mazuri®, PMI® Nutrition International, Inc., Brentwood, MO 63144, USA) ad libitum and were supplemented with a moist canned food temporarily at the time of weaning. There were no reported complications during parturition. The pup was treated for ascariasis but had been normal with an unremarkable medical history up to the time of presentation. It had received preventive care including periodic deworming and routine vaccinations, and none of its littermates demonstrated clinical signs.

The animal was immobilized to perform a full physical examination and diagnostics using midazolam (Akorn Inc., Lake Forest, IL 60045, USA; 0.17 mg/kg) intramuscularly followed by mask-induction with isoflurane gas. On physical examination, the pup had a thin body condition at a weight of 14 kg and was noticeably smaller than its littermates. Swelling with associated heat was present bilaterally at the carpi, tarsi, and stifle joints. All joints had normal range of motion with no crepitus palpated during flexion or extension.

A complete blood count and serum biochemistry were performed and compared to values listed for red wolves in the International Species Information System (ISIS) database [14]. There was marked eosinophilia ($4,765 \times 10^6$ cells/L; ISIS values 144–2,393) consistent with underlying endoparasitism, a decreased blood urea nitrogen (3.2 mmol/L; ISIS values 3.8–14.4) possibly related to the animal's young age or a decreased intake of dietary protein, and hyperphosphatemia (2.45 mmol/L; ISIS values 0.62–2.28) with elevated alkaline phosphatase (319 U/L; ISIS values 7–73) consistent with growth in a young animal. Fecal floatation analysis was performed with sodium nitrate solution, which revealed occasional ova consistent with Toxocara and Ancylostoma sp.

Differential diagnoses included hypertrophic osteodystrophy, septic arthritis, and osteomyelitis.

Orthogonal screen-film radiographs were obtained (Figure 1(a)). Centered at the metaphyses and extending into the diaphyses of multiple long bones bilaterally (proximal humeri, proximal and distal radii, distal ulnae, distal femur, and proximal and distal tibiae and fibulae) increased medullary opacity was present resulting in loss of visualization of trabeculation, consistent with sclerosis. At these sites, there was also varying degrees of well-defined, irregularly marginated periosteal bone formation resulting in flaring of the metaphyses, which was palisading in some regions. The periosteal change was most severe at the distal antebrachia as well as the proximal and distal aspects of the crura. Additionally, within the proximal humeri, distal radii and ulnae, and proximal and distal tibiae, ill-defined irregularly linear zones of lucency were present within the metaphyseal bone, which paralleled the physes. The adjacent physes were well defined. Within the proximal diaphysis of the left ulna, faint, ill-defined, and increased medullary opacity was present. Complete evaluation of soft tissues at all sites was hindered due to technique, but concurrent soft-tissue swelling at these sites was suspected. The primary differential for the polyostotic change centered at the metaphyses of multiple long bones was HOD. Concurrent osteomyelitis was also considered. The diaphyseal sclerosis within the left proximal ulna was most consistent with panosteitis or other causes of bone infarction.

The pup was treated supportively with buprenorphine (American Regent, Inc., Shirley, NY 11967, USA; 0.008 mg/kg) subcutaneously, meloxicam (Metacam®, Boehringer Ingelheim Vetmedica, Inc., St. Joseph, Mo 64506, USA; 0.2 mg/kg) intramuscularly, and a fentanyl transdermal patch (Dura-gesic®, ALZA corp., Vacaville, CA 95688, USA; 50 mcg/hr). Meloxicam was also prescribed (0.1 mg/kg) orally once daily for 10 days and a single dose of pyrantel pamoate (Strongid T®, Pfizer Inc., New York, NY 10017, USA; 32 mg/kg) orally. Over the next week, the pup maintained an appetite; however, its lameness and joint swelling persisted.

A follow-up procedure was performed on day 18 after the onset of clinical signs. The animal was anesthetized using midazolam (0.2 mg/kg) and buprenorphine (0.01 mg/kg) intramuscularly followed by mask induction with isoflurane gas. On physical examination there was progressive swelling of the previously affected joints. These joints were subjectively less warm to the touch than at the original evaluation of the animal. A complete blood count showed resolution of the previous eosinophilia (1,420 × 10^6 cells/L; ISIS values 144–2,393). A serum biochemistry revealed a decreased blood urea nitrogen (1.79 mmol/L; ISIS values 3.8–14.4), hyperphosphatemia (2.49 mmol/L; ISIS values 0.62–2.28), and elevated alkaline phosphatase activity (103 U/L; ISIS values 7–73). Orthogonal radiographs of the thorax, abdomen, and shoulders were performed, which showed a static appearance of the proximal humeral metaphyseal sclerosis and subphyseal lucency. No thoracic or abdominal abnormalities were identified radiographically.

Bone biopsies were performed at the metaphyses of the distal left radius and the right proximal tibia using aseptic technique. Two 15 ga core biopsies were obtained from each site and placed into 10% buffered formalin for histopathologic evaluation. Following the procedure, meloxicam (0.15 mg/kg) was administered intramuscularly. Recovery from anesthesia was uneventful. Three additional blood samples were collected under manual restraint for aerobic and anaerobic bacterial culture on days 20, 23, and 25 using aseptic technique.

Histopathology of the bone biopsies indicated diffuse moderate medullary fibrosis with new bone formation. No signs of active inflammation were present in the submitted samples. No bacterial growth was present after 14 days from the first two blood cultures; however, *Clostridium bifermentans* was cultured from the final sample. Due to this positive blood culture result, a complete blood count, serum biochemistry, and an additional follow-up blood culture sample were obtained on day 35. The complete blood count revealed a mild monocytosis (1,803 × 10^6 cells/L; ISIS values 87–1,214) indicative of chronic inflammation. A serum biochemistry revealed a decreased blood urea nitrogen (3.57 mmol/L; ISIS values 3.8–14.4), hyperphosphatemia (2.65 mmol/L; ISIS values 0.62–2.28), and elevated alkaline phosphatase activity (103 U/L; ISIS values 7–73) similar to the animal's previous results. Because *Clostridium bifermentans* is only rarely reported to cause osteomyelitis in children and elderly humans, it was presumed to be an environmental contaminant [15]. A follow-up fecal analysis revealed no evidence of parasites.

Caretakers reported marked improvement of the animal's gait and ability to move by day 28, with no additional episodes of lameness through day 60. A physical examination was performed on day 62 in preparation for transfer of the animal to another facility. Radiographs were repeated (Figure 1(b)). Metaphyseal and diaphyseal medullary scleroses as well as periosteal bone formation remained at the prior sites but were markedly reduced. An additional similar lesion to the other long bones was present within the second metatarsal bilaterally. This region was not imaged on prior dates and this may have been present previously as opposed to being a novel lesion. The prior palisading periosteal bone production and subphyseal lucent zones were no longer present. The prior left ulnar proximal diaphyseal sclerosis was also no longer present. The imaged physes remained open.

For the following two years, periodic physical examinations were performed, which demonstrated persistent bilateral carpal and stifle swelling. At 30 months of age, the animal developed severe right pelvic limb lameness. Based on physical examination and stifle radiography, cranial cruciate ligament rupture with associated stifle osteoarthrosis was diagnosed. The animal was treated with restricted activity, nonsteroidal anti-inflammatory medications, and supplementation with glucosamine and chondroitin. The lameness improved but did not completely resolve. At 34 months of age, the animal developed severe bilateral pelvic limb lameness. Physical examination and radiographic findings were suggestive of bilateral cranial cruciate ligament rupture and associated osteoarthrosis. These radiographs were not available for review by the authors of this case report. The animal was not responsive to medical management with restricted activity and administration of nonsteroidal anti-inflammatory medications. Due to a poor overall quality of life related to the lameness, humane euthanasia was elected.

Gross necropsy confirmed the diagnosis of bilateral cranial cruciate ligament rupture. There were defects of the articular cartilage on the lateral femoral condyle and osteophytosis of both stifles. Thickening of the lateral collateral ligaments and joint capsules of both stifles was also noted. Moderate medial and lateral flaring of the metaphyses with periosteal proliferation of bone was noted at the distal radii (Figure 1(c)). No other musculoskeletal abnormalities were found, and other than several missing teeth, the remainder of the necropsy findings were normal.

3. Case 2

A captive-bred male red wolf pup of 4.5 month of age presented as an emergency for a rectal prolapse that failed to resolve with medical management. The wolf was housed with 5 siblings, and their diet consisted of Science Diet Canine Adult Active formula (Hills Pet Nutrition Inc., Topeka, KS 66603, USA), carnivore diet (Bravo Packing, Inc., Penns Grove, NJ 08069, USA), and occasional rats or mice. It had received preventive care including periodic deworming and routine vaccinations, and none of its littermates demonstrated clinical signs. A cecal inversion was diagnosed by ultrasound, and an exploratory laparotomy was subsequently performed. An ileocolic intussusception with cecal inversion was discovered. A subtotal colectomy and distal ileectomy with ileocolic anastomosis was performed, and the animal recovered uneventfully. No other abnormalities were noted at this time.

Approximately 2 weeks later, the wolf presented for lethargy and a kyphotic posture, presumed to be related to abdominal pain. The animal was examined under sedation with medetomidine (Domitor®, Pfizer Inc.; 0.05 mg/kg) intramuscularly and was administered intravenous crystalloid fluids, ticarcillin disodium, and clavulanate potassium (Timentin®, GlaxoSmithKline, Inc., Philadelphia, PA 19112, USA; 30 mg/kg IV q6 h for 2 d) and meloxicam (0.1 mg/kg IM, q24 h for 2 d). His temperature was elevated (41.1°C) after manual restraint and sedation. Abdominal and thoracic radiographs as well as a complete blood count were considered unremarkable. The animal was discharged on oral antibiotics (amoxicillin clavulanate, Clavamox®, Pfizer Inc.; 250 mg PO q12 h for 14 d) and oral meloxicam daily, as needed.

The animal's kyphotic posture worsened 2 weeks after surgery and another examination under anesthesia was conducted at four weeks after surgery. All complete blood count and serum biochemistry results were within species values reported by ISIS, other than a mild monocytosis (1577 × 10^6 cells/L; species values 87–1,214). An abdominal ultrasound revealed a suspected gastrointestinal foreign body, and an exploratory laparotomy was performed, which was considered to be within normal limits. Carpal and tarsal joints were noted to be swollen bilaterally during the exam. Orthogonal view radiographs of the thorax, abdomen, hips, and distal limbs obtained during the procedure were submitted to a consulting radiology service (Insight Radiology, San Diego, CA 92111, USA). Centered at the diaphysis and metaphyses of the distal femurs, radii, and ulnae bilaterally, smooth, well-defined periosteal bone formation was present. Medullary sclerosis was also identified. Similar lesions were noted in the proximal humerus, bilaterally. The distal aspects of the left 8th and 10th ribs were flared and were more lucent than adjacent ribs. The radiographic appearance was suggestive, but not specific for a systemic disorder of cartilage formation or cartilage inflammation characteristic of HOD. These images were not available for further review by the authors of this case report.

The animal was managed successfully with oral meloxicam for the next 3 months. During this time, whenever anti-inflammatory therapy was discontinued, the animal would become anorexic. After 3 months, his treatment was then tapered and discontinued successfully. The animal's adult weight was 32.5 kg. He died acutely of unrelated causes at 20 months of age. Histopathology of the bones was not pursued at the time of necropsy.

4. Discussion

Hypertrophic osteodystrophy is an important developmental disease that affects the bones of growing animals. This report describes one confirmed and one suspected case of hypertrophic osteodystrophy in two red wolf pups, which to the author's knowledge has not been previously reported in this species. In the first case, a diagnosis of HOD in multiple long bones with concurrent panosteitis at the left ulna was made based on clinical history, radiographic findings, bone

biopsy, and negative blood cultures. Hypertrophic osteodystrophy was also suspected in the second wolf pup based on radiographic findings, although additional diagnostics were not performed to confirm the diagnosis. The onset of disease for the red wolf pups of this report occurred between 5 and 6 months of age. This is consistent with what is frequently seen in domestic dogs (Canis familiaris), with pups under 6 months of age considered to be at the highest risk of developing the disease [16]. Common clinical signs in domestic dogs include pyrexia, lethargy, anorexia, lameness, soft-tissue swelling at affected bones, and ostealgia [8]. The severity of disease varies, and some cases have episodic recurrence of clinical signs. The presentation of both red wolf pups was similar to that seen in domestic canines and included lameness and soft-tissue swelling. Although anorexia was not documented in the first case due to the presence of several other conspecifics within its shared enclosure, a degree of anorexia or decreased appetite was likely in considering the animal's thin body condition at presentation.

Long bones including the radius, ulna, and tibia are most commonly affected in dogs, and the disease is usually bilateral. Radiographs of the red wolves described in this report revealed involvement of many of the long bones, with the radii, ulnae, and tibias most severely affected. Early radiographic abnormalities of affected bones may include radiolucent zones within the metaphyses parallel to the physis as well as soft-tissue swelling. As the disease progresses, there may be increased metaphyseal medullary opacity along with periosteal or extraperiosteal new bone formation [1, 4]. In some cases, development of clinical signs may precede radiographic abnormalities. Increased metaphyseal medullary opacity with associated periosteal new bone formation was seen in both red wolf pups. These radiographic findings indicated chronicity, seen in later stages of HOD. The subphyseal lysis that was concurrently seen in the first case may represent incomplete resolution of the initial stages of disease or an acute on chronic occurrence. The earliest stages of the disease in the red wolf pups were not captured radiographically. This is likely due to delay between initial onset of clinical signs and acquisition of radiographs.

Treatment of this disease is symptomatic and supportive with specific therapies directed at alleviation of pain, inflammation, and pyrexia associated with the condition. Nonsteroidal anti-inflammatory medications or steroids are appropriate and effective for treatment of HOD [8], and crystalline fluid therapy, nutritional support, opioid pain medications, and other supportive care measures may also be clinically indicated in some cases. The wolf of the first case report responded favorably to treatment with nonsteroidal anti-inflammatory medications, opioids, and intermittent crystalline fluid therapy. The wolf in the second case responded well to nonsteroidal anti-inflammatory therapy alone.

Clinical signs can persist for days to weeks in domestic canines with relapses occurring in some individuals. In the first case, clinical improvement occurred 4 weeks following initial presentation, and no relapses occurred following recovery. Despite clinical improvement, the animal of the first case report had residual skeletal abnormalities at affected bones that persisted throughout its life. These abnormalities were evident on the preserved skeletal remains from this animal. Reports in the literature indicate that some animals with developmental orthopedic disease may also experience subsequent cranial cruciate ligament rupture [17]. While plausible, it is not known if the residual skeletal abnormalities seen in the first case contributed to the development of bilateral cranial cruciate ligament rupture several years later. This case was considered severe due to the extent of the lesions, number of affected bones, the lengthy clinical course, and the persistent proliferative bone lesions that did not resolve despite clinical improvement. Although these factors are suggestive of a severe case, clinical signs indicating pain were subtle and less apparent than expected. This may be due to behavioral differences between domestic dogs and red wolves. Clinical signs for the wolf in the second case appeared to resolve after 3 months of therapy and residual lesions were not clinically apparent; however, no histologic evidence was obtained postmortem.

Excessive dietary calcium, phosphorous, protein, and energy have been identified as factors leading to developmental orthopedic diseases in dogs and could play a role in the development of HOD [18, 19]. The specific nutritional requirements for red wolves are unknown and the current husbandry guidelines are based on recommendations for domestic dogs, including feeding a high quality commercial dry dog food with additional supplementation provided at and following whelping [20]. Use of a commercial growth formulation for red wolf pups is not currently recommended due to the feeding challenges related to managing red wolves in family groups that minimize habituation to humans. The average weight of adult male red wolves is 27.6 kg [21], which is comparable in size to many large breed domestic dogs that are prone to rapid growth and developmental bone disease [6]. The adult weights for the wolves of this case series were 25 kg for the first case and the 33 kg for the second case. The wolf of the first case was maintained on a diet consisting predominantly of Mazuri® exotic canine formula provided ad libitum. Ad libitum feeding of large breed dogs has been associated with an increased occurrence of skeletal abnormalities and developmental bone diseases. The diet fed to the wolf of the first case also contains 1.7% calcium and 0.96% phosphorous on a dry matter basis and exceeds the dietary calcium recommendations established by the National Research Council for large breed puppies at risk for developmental orthopedic disease [22]. The wolf of the second case was fed Science Diet Adult Active formula, which has 1.04% calcium and 0.8% phosphorous on a dry matter basis. This diet is within the recommended range, and the extent to which nutritional factors contributed to the development of hypertrophic osteodystrophy in either case is unknown.

Infection with Canine Distemper Virus (CDV) and vaccination have also been implicated as other potential etiologies for HOD. Viral RNA has been found in the metaphyses of CDV-infected dogs, and a strong correlation has been established between CDV infection and metaphyseal bone lesions from young dogs [7, 23, 24]. Additionally, several reports have described systemic clinical signs similar to those associated with CDV in cases of HOD [2, 3, 5]. Although these findings are suggestive of a link between CDV and HOD, clear evidence of a relationship between the two diseases has not been established [16]. Reports have also described its clinical onset occurring several weeks following multiple doses of polyvalent vaccines including modified live CDV, canine adenovirus type 2, and *Leptospira* bacterin [3, 5]. Both pups in this report did receive polyvalent vaccines at routine 2-3-week intervals from 2 to 4 months of age, but neither pup nor any littermates exhibited gastrointestinal signs, respiratory signs, hyperkeratotic footpads, or neurologic deficits consistent with what is seen with CDV. PCR analysis of bone biopsies for CDV RNA was not performed for either red wolf pup and viral or vaccination-related causes for the development of HOD in these cases cannot be completely ruled out.

It is believed that genetics may be a contributing factor in the development of HOD in some cases. Breed predispositions have been identified in domestic canines [6, 16], and familial trends also occur in breeds, such as the Weimaraner [2, 3, 5]. This indicates that heredity may play a large role in the disease for some cases. None of the littermates of the two pups described in this case report exhibited clinical signs of HOD, and familial trends were not identified in these cases. However, an underlying genetic cause of this disease in red wolves remains a possibility and may be of concern for future red wolf breeding recommendations.

Captive breeding programs continue to play a large role in conservation and management efforts for the red wolf. The captive red wolf population consists of about 180 wolves, which was founded from 12 individuals [17]. Understanding disease susceptibility and etiology in red wolves is important for making appropriate and well-informed management decisions that balance the goals of maintaining genetic diversity with the risk of perpetuating potentially genetic diseases within the population. Although the underlying pathogenesis of HOD remains poorly understood, the potential for genetic, nutritional, infectious, and vaccine-associated causes makes it a disease of particular concern and interest for the future management of this species.

Conflict of Interests

The authors declare that there is no conflict of interests regarding the publication of this paper.

Acknowledgments

The authors would like to sincerely thank Chris Lasher, Katy Harringer, Sherry Samuels, Kathy Long, the Virginia Living Museum, and the Museum of Life and Science for their cooperation and assistance with this case report.

References

[1] H. Meier, S. T. Clark, G. B. Schnelle, and D. H. Will, "Hypertrophic osteodystrophy associated with disturbance of vitamin C synthesis in dogs," *Journal of the American Veterinary Medical Association*, vol. 130, no. 11, pp. 483–491, 1957.

[2] J. C. Woodard, "Canine hypertrophic osteodystrophy, a study of the spontaneous disease in littermates," *Veterinary Pathology*, vol. 19, no. 4, pp. 337–354, 1982.

[3] V. Abeles, S. Harrus, J. M. Angles et al., "Hypertrophic osteodystrophy in six weimaraner puppies associated with systemic signs," *The Veterinary Record*, vol. 145, no. 5, pp. 130–134, 1999.

[4] J. Grondalen, "Metaphyseal osteopathy (hypertrophic osteodystrophy) in growing dogs: a clinical study," *Journal of Small Animal Practice*, vol. 17, no. 11, pp. 721–735, 1976.

[5] S. Harrus, T. Waner, I. Aizenberg et al., "Development of hypertrophic osteodystrophy and antibody response in a litter of vaccinated Weimaraner puppies," *Journal of Small Animal Practice*, vol. 43, no. 1, pp. 27–31, 2002.

[6] E. LaFond, G. J. Breur, and C. C. Austin, "Breed susceptibility for developmental orthopedic diseases in dogs," *Journal of the American Animal Hospital Association*, vol. 38, no. 5, pp. 467–477, 2002.

[7] A. P. Mee, M. T. Gordon, C. May, D. Bennett, D. C. Anderson, and P. T. Sharpe, "Canine distemper virus transcripts detected in the bone cells of dogs with metaphyseal osteopathy," *Bone*, vol. 14, no. 1, pp. 59–67, 1993.

[8] N. Safra, E. G. Johnson, L. Lit et al., "Clinical manifestations, response to treatment, and clinical outcome for Weimaraners with hypertrophic osteodystrophy: 53 cases (2009–2011)," *Journal of the American Veterinary Medical Association*, vol. 242, no. 9, pp. 1260–1266, 2013.

[9] K. S. Schulz, J. T. Payne, and E. Aronson, "*Escherichia coli* bacteremia associated with hypertrophic osteodystrophy in a dog," *Journal of the American Veterinary Medical Association*, vol. 199, no. 9, pp. 1170–1173, 1991.

[10] C. Adagra, D. Spielman, A. Adagra, and D. J. Foster, "Metaphyseal osteopathy in a British shorthair cat," *Journal of Feline Medicine and Surgery*, vol. 17, no. 4, pp. 367–370, 2015.

[11] F. Martínez, X. Manteca, and J. Pastor, "Retrospective study of morbidity and mortality of captive Iberian lynx (*Lynx pardinus*) in the ex situ conservation programme (2004–June 2010)," *Journal of Zoo and Wildlife Medicine*, vol. 44, no. 4, pp. 845–852, 2013.

[12] J. Queen, D. Bennett, S. Carmichael et al., "Femoral neck metaphyseal osteopathy in the cat," *The Veterinary Record*, vol. 142, no. 7, pp. 159–162, 1998.

[13] B. T. Kelly, A. Beyer, and M. K. Phillips, "*Canis rufus*," The IUCN Red List of Threatened Species Version 2014.2, 2014, http://www.iucnredlist.org.

[14] J. A. Teare, "*Rhinoceros unicornis*, conventional American units 2013," in *ISIS Physiological Reference Intervals for Captive Wildlife: A CD-ROM Resource*, International Species Information System, Bloomington, Minn, USA, 2013.

[15] D. R. Scanlan, M. A. Smith, H. D. Isenberg, S. Engrassia, and E. Hilton, "*Clostridium bifermentans* bacteremia with metastatic osteomyelitis," *Journal of Clinical Microbiology*, vol. 32, no. 11, pp. 2867–2868, 1994.

[16] T. A. Munjar, C. C. Austin, and G. J. Breur, "Comparison of risk factors for hypertrophic osteodystrophy," *Veterinary and Comparative Orthopaedics and Traumatology*, vol. 11, pp. 37–43, 1998.

[17] R. A. Read and G. M. Robins, "Deformity of the proximal tibia in dogs," *Veterinary Record*, vol. 111, no. 13, pp. 295–298, 1982.

[18] K. Dämmrich, "Relationship between nutrition and bone growth in large and giant dogs," *Journal of Nutrition*, vol. 121, pp. 114s–121s, 1991.

[19] A. Hedhammer, F. Wu, and L. Krook, "Overnutrition and skeletal disease," *Cornell Veterinarian*, vol. 64, supplement 1, pp. 128–135, 1974.

[20] W. Waddell, "Population analysis and breeding and transfer plan," Red Wolf (*Canis rufus gregoryi*) AZA Species Survival Plan Program, 2010.

[21] J. L. Paradiso and R. M. Nowak, "*Canis rufus*," *Mammalian Species*, no. 22, pp. 1–4, 1972.

[22] National Research Council ad hoc Committee on Dog and Cat Nutrition, *Nutrient Requirements of Dogs and Cats*, National Academies Press, Washington, DC, USA, 2006.

[23] W. Baumgärtner, R. W. Boyce, S. Alldinger et al., "Metaphyseal bone lesions in young dogs with systemic canine distemper virus infection," *Veterinary Microbiology*, vol. 44, no. 2–4, pp. 201–209, 1995.

[24] W. Baumgärtner, R. W. Boyce, S. E. Weisbrode, S. Aldinger, M. K. Axthelm, and S. Krakowka, "Histologic and immunocytochemical characterization of canine distemper-associated metaphyseal bone lesions in young dogs following experimental infection," *Veterinary Pathology*, vol. 32, no. 6, pp. 702–709, 1995.

26

Followup of a Dog with an Intraocular Silicone Prosthesis Combined with an Extraocular Glass Prosthesis

Gwendolyna Romkes and Johanna Corinna Eule

Small Animal Clinic, Faculty of Veterinary Medicine, Freie Universität Berlin, Oertzenweg 19b, 14163 Berlin, Germany

Correspondence should be addressed to Gwendolyna Romkes, gwendolyna.romkes@gmail.com

Academic Editors: S. Hecht and C.-T. Lin

Because of unpredictable corneal changes, evisceration and implantation of a silicone prosthesis does not always lead to a satisfying cosmetic result. This paper describes the use of an intraocular silicone prosthesis in combination with an extraocular glass prosthesis and shows a followup of two and a half years in a nonexperimental study. An intraocular silicone prosthesis was implanted after evisceration of the left eye in a five-month-old Bernese mountain dog. A glass prosthesis was fitted four weeks after evisceration. Two and a half years after the operation, the dog is in good health and free of medication. No short-term or long-term complications were seen. The owners do not have trouble with handling the glass prosthesis. The combination of both prostheses shows a perfect solution to retrieve a normal looking and moving eye after evisceration.

1. Introduction

In both human and veterinary ophthalmology several surgical options are described to treat an end-stage glaucomatous eye that does not respond to medical therapy.

The easiest and fastest procedure is enucleation of the eye. Evisceration and implantation of a silicone prosthesis is an alternative which gives a better cosmetic result [1–6].

A disadvantage of evisceration and silicone implantation in dogs is the neovascularization of the cornea immediately after evisceration. One to two months after the operation, the cornea will be completely vascularized [2, 4, 6, 7]. Parallel to this process, the cornea becomes fibrotic and sometimes also pigmented [6]. The extent of blood vessel regression and the degree of pigmentation and/or opacification varies between canine eyes. Opacification can lead to unsatisfying cosmetic results [4, 7]. In a questionnaire for dog owners of eviscerated patients, 62% of the owners were very content with the result. Less satisfaction was caused by dense fibrosis of the cornea [5]. Still, all owners were happy to have chosen evisceration instead of enucleation. To improve the cosmetic appearance, in human medicine evisceration is always combined with an extraocular prosthesis (scleral shell or "artificial eye") [8–10]. An extraocular prosthesis combined with an intraocular prosthesis shows a better motility than an extraocular prosthesis alone [9, 10]. Table 1 gives an overview of selected options to restore anatomical structure after exenteration, enucleation, or evisceration. Figure 1 shows the anatomic relationship of the two prostheses.

Transscleral cyclophotocoagulation with diode laser or cryotherapy in combination with an Ahmed gonioimplantation in dogs with primary glaucoma has a success rate of approximately 76%, and most of the patients still need long-term medication [12, 13]. Therefore, this method is reserved for acute glaucomatous eyes, which are still visible or are believed to have a change to regain vision.

Ciliary body ablation by intravitreal gentamicin injection for the treatment of end-stage glaucoma is thought to correlate with the development of malignant intraocular tumours [14].

This paper shows a followup of two and a half years of a dog with an intraocular silicone prosthesis combined with an extraocular glass prosthesis after evisceration.

TABLE 1: Overview of selected options to restore anatomical structure after exenteration, enucleation, or evisceration [8, 10, 11]. Depending on the procedure and the selected prosthesis, a second prosthesis or an "artificial eye" can be placed between the first prosthesis and the eyelids. Porous implants like hydroxyapatite can be combined with a coupling or peg system, to give the second implant better motility [8, 10].

Surgical procedure	Prosthesis material	Site of implantation	Coupling system	Second prosthesis	Eyelid movement	Globe movement
Exenteration	Silicone Hydroxyapetite	Intraorbital	No		—	—
Enucleation	Silicone	Intraorbital	No		—	
				Acrylic	+	—
				Glass	+	—
	Hydroxyapetite	Intraorbital	No		—	
				Acrylic	+	—
				Glass	+	—
			Yes	Acrylic	+	++
Evisceration	Silicone	Intraocular	No	—	+	++++
				Bandage lens	+	++++
				Acrylic	+	+++
				Glass	+	+++
	Hydroxyapetite	Intraocular	No	—	+	++++
				Bandage lens	+	++++
				Acrylic	+	+++
				Glass	+	+++
			Yes	Acrylic	+	++++

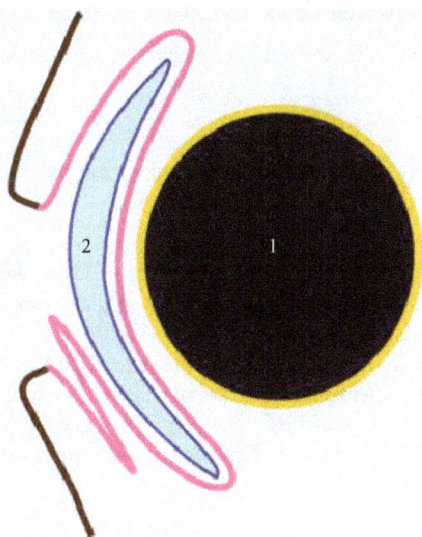

FIGURE 1: Anatomical position of different prostheses. 1: intraocular prosthesis introduced within the empty tunica fibrosa after evisceration. 2: second extraocular prosthesis or "artificial eye," lying between the conjunctiva (third eyelid in animals) and eyelids. Brown: eyelid skin, pink: conjunctiva, and yellow: tunica fibrosa.

2. Case Report

A three-month-old, male Bernese mountain dog was presented to a private veterinarian after a cat claw injury in his left eye. Ophthalmic examination, including fluorescein staining, Seidel Test, slit lamp biomicroscopy and B-mode ultrasound, led to the diagnosis of corneal perforation without injury of the lens. Under general anesthesia, the corneal wound was cleaned and afterwards closed with simple interrupted sutures (Vicryl 8/0, Ethicon, Johnson & Johnson, Norderstedt, Germany). An additional nictitating membrane flap was performed to protect the corneal wound. Postoperative treatment included topical treatment with neomycin, gramicidin, and polymyxin B eye drops TID (Polyspectran, Alcon, Freiburg, Germany) and atropine eye drops SID (Atropine-POS 1%, Ursapharm, Saarbrücken, Germany) and systemic treatment with amoxycillin-clavulanic acid 12.5 mg/kg BID (Clavaseptin, Vétoquinol, Ravensburg, Germany) for two weeks and carprofen 4 mg/kg SID (Rimadyl, Pfizer, Karlsruhe, Germany) for six weeks.

After six weeks, the eye became blind and the dog was referred. Ophthalmic examination of the blind eye revealed secondary glaucoma with an intraocular pressure of 29 mmHg measured by rebound tonometry (TonoVet, Acrivet-Veterinary Division, Hennigsdorf, Germany). Topical treatment including carbonic anhydrase-inhibitor and β-blocker eye drops QID (dorzolamide 2% and timolol 0.5%, Cosopt, Merck Sharp & Dohme-Chibret, Clermont-Ferrand, France) and prostaglandin-analog eye drops BID (Travoprost 40 μg/mL, Travatan, Alcon, Hemel Hempstead, United Kingdom) was initiated, but the intraocular pressure could not be controlled below 20 mmHg to prevent further damage. Seven weeks after the injury, the blind eye became buphthalmic (Figure 2). The owners elected to eviscerate the eye and chose an extraocular prosthesis to be installed.

2.1. Surgery Part I: Intraocular Prosthesis. The dog underwent general anesthesia. The left eye was cleaned in a routine

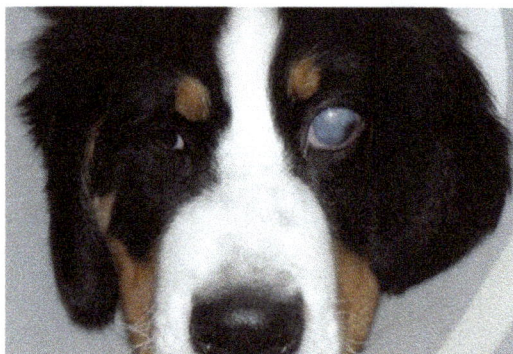

FIGURE 2: Four-and-a-half-month-old Bernese mountain dog with end-stage, glaucomatous left eye seven weeks after cat claw injury.

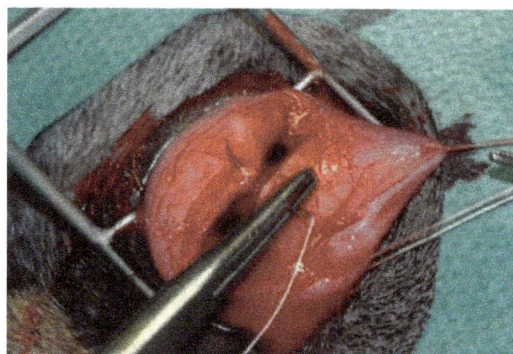

FIGURE 4: Closure of the sclera above the intraocular silicone prosthesis.

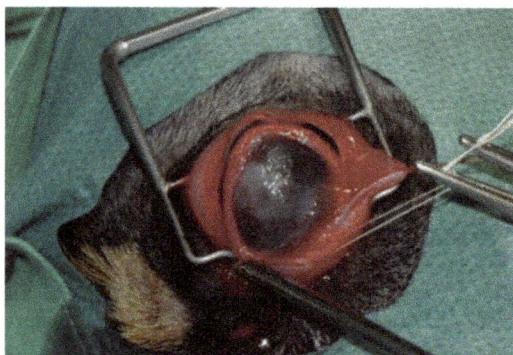

FIGURE 3: Perilimbal perforating scleral incision as preparation for implantation of intraocular silicone prosthesis.

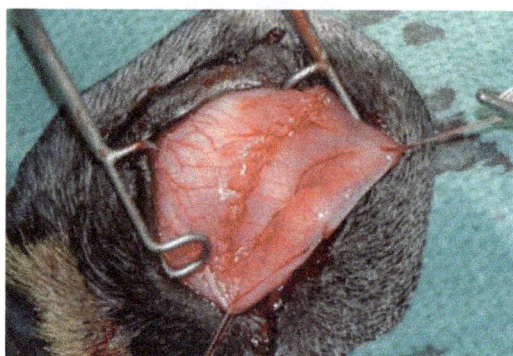

FIGURE 5: Closure of the conjunctiva above the sclera.

manner for eye surgery. A Barraquer eyelid speculum was placed to open the eyelids. The conjunctiva was prepared for a 360° flap by a complete perilimbal incision with a Stevenson's scissor. The cornea was excised by a 360° scleral incision with a Beaver blade nr. 65 and Stevenson's scissor 1 mm behind the limbus (Figure 3).

The content of the globe was removed with a lens loop, leaving an empty scleral shell. An 18 mm silicone prosthesis (Acrivet-Veterinary Division, Hennigsdorf, Germany) (size of the healthy eye, measured as the distance between the posterior surface of the cornea and the anterior surface of the sclerawith B-mode ultrasound) was placed into the scleral shell with a Carter sphere introducer (Acrivet-Veterinary Division, Hennigsdorf, Germany). The sclera was closed above the prosthesis with interrupted horizontal mattress sutures (Vicryl 6/0, Ethicon, Johnson & Johnson, Norderstedt, Germany) (Figure 4).

The 360° limbal-based conjunctival flap was closed above the sclera in a simple continuous pattern by the use of the Vicryl 6/0 (Figure 5).

A temporary tarsorrhaphy with the use of a monofilament suture material (Dafilon 4/0, Braun Aesculap, Tuttlingen, Germany) was performed to protect the empty fornix (Figure 6).

The sclera and conjunctiva healed within two weeks, and after which the tarsorrhaphy was released.

2.2. Surgery Part II: Extraocular Prosthesis. Three weeks after the surgery, an extraocular prosthesis of glass was prepared by an ocularist (Figure 7).

The prosthesis was placed into the fornix, above the conjunctiva, sclera, and intraocular prosthesis (Figure 1). The extraocular prosthesis was kept in place by its shape, the third eyelid and the eyelids resting over the border of the prosthesis.

2.3. Postoperative Care. Postoperative treatment included systemic treatment with amoxycillin-clavulanic acid 12.5 mg/kg BID (Clavaseptin, Vétoquinol, Ravensburg, Germany) and metamizol 20 mg/kg TID (Novaminsulfon, Ratiopharm, Ulm, Germany) for five days. No topical treatment was applied. The wound was examined one day, one week, and two weeks after surgery. No further systemic or local medication was indicated.

2.4. Prosthesis Handling. The glass prosthesis has to be taken out every evening. The prosthesis is placed overnight in a generally available lens cleaner (for example Boston Simplus all in one, Bausch & Lomb, Berlin, Germany). In the morning, the conjunctival sack is flushed with a generally

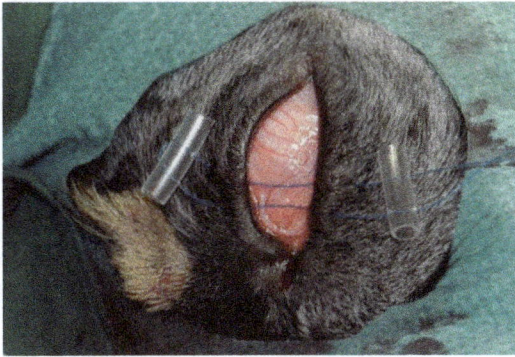

FIGURE 6: Temporary tarsorrhaphy to protect the empty fornix.

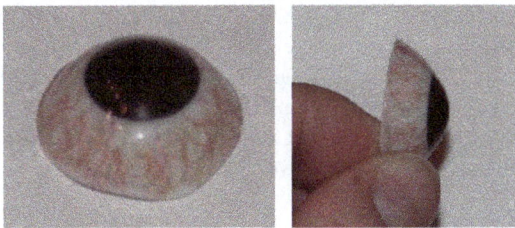

FIGURE 7: Artificial glass eye (extraocular prosthesis).

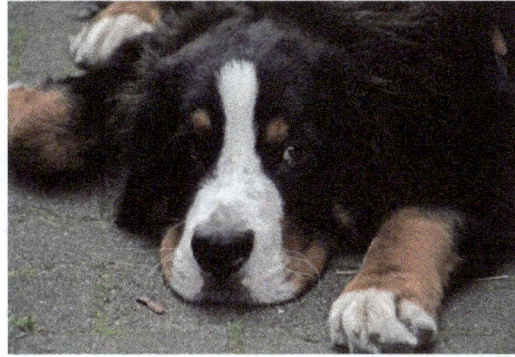

FIGURE 8: Six-and-a-half-month-old Bernese mountain dog with intraocular and extraocular prosthesis two months after surgery.

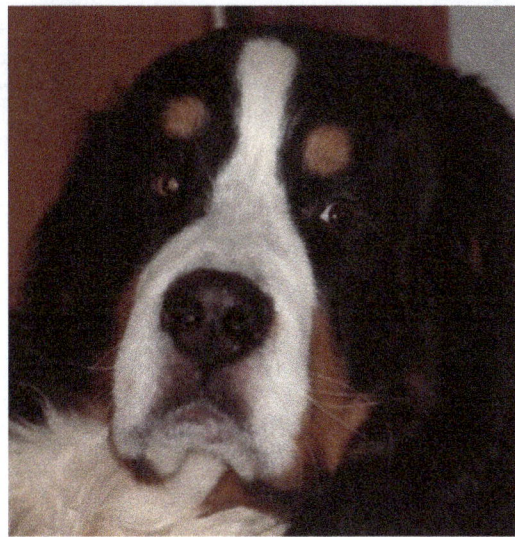

FIGURE 9: Two-year-old Bernese mountain dog one and a half year after surgery.

available eye cleaner (e.g., Albrecht, Aulendorf, Germany), and the prosthesis is placed back into the fornix.

2.5. Followup. Pictures were taken two months, one and a half year, and two and a half years after surgery (Figures 8, 9, and 10).

The extraocular prosthesis was replaced by the same ocularist for a new prosthesis after one year and after two and a half years. By experience, the ocularist was able to fit the last prosthesis in such a manner that less white of the prosthesis is seen. The only (long-term) complication is a little intermittent serous secretion. There is no history of a bacterial infection or insufficient tear production. Schirmer's tear test readings were always above 15 mm per minute. The dog is happy, does not need any medication and behaves and looks like a dog with two normal eyes. The dog does not show any discomfort with the intraocular and extraocular prosthesis.

The owners are very satisfied with the cosmetic result and do not feel inconvenienced by the handling of the extraocular prosthesis. Given the same circumstances, they would make the same decision again.

3. Discussion

3.1. Evisceration versus Enucleation. In human ophthalmology, the main advantage of evisceration over enucleation is that evisceration is described as the easier procedure with less orbital manipulation, hemorrhage, and reduced postoperative swelling, pain, and associated trauma [8]. In human ophthalmology eviscerations are also associated with fewer complications than enucleation due to less periocular

damage caused during evisceration [15, 16]. Postoperatively the globe still moves normally, because during evisceration extraocular muscles and their attachments are not disturbed [8]. Different studies in dogs have shown that evisceration and implantation of a silicone prosthesis is easy to learn, easy to practice and shows a very low complication rate in well-selected cases [5, 6]. In dogs, postoperative pain after evisceration is comparable with postoperative pain after enucleation [5]. Postoperative local therapy is needed for two to three weeks after evisceration, and therefore, the postoperative care is more intensive as after enucleation, but this was not inconvenient to owners and dogs [5].

3.2. Stimulating Appropriate Orbital Growth in Infants. Kennedy [17] describes that facial asymmetry and cosmetic deformity can occur following enucleation. Some studies in human ophthalmology describe that enucleation of one eye in infancy or childhood accompanied by insertion of an implant does not cause a cosmetically significant orbital variation [18, 19]. An experimental study in young cats

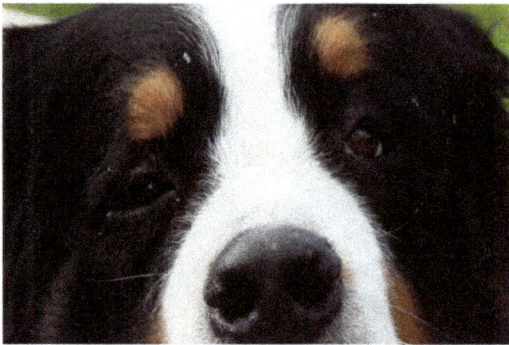

FIGURE 10: Three-year-old Bernese mountain dog two and a half years after surgery.

testing tissue expanders in the anophthalmic orbit after enucleation showed that insufficient tissue expanding led to asymmetric skull development [20]. In the presented case a tissue expander implant was not available at the time of surgery. The combination of an intraocular silicon prosthesis with an extraocular glass prosthesis did not lead to visible facial asymmetry. Additional radiographic studies to measure the volume of both orbitae are lacking due to clinical irrelevance in the presented patient.

3.3. Operation Technique. In this case the evisceration was combined with a full-thickness keratectomy, because the eye was so buphthalmic. Additionally, in human ophthalmology excision of the cornea is described for those patients who may still have corneal sensation or corneal pain. The removal of the cornea allows the sclera edges to be united, which provides a secure wound closure [8]. As the owners of the dog already decided preoperatively for a second extraorbital prosthesis, it was attempted to establish the best basis for this second prosthesis. Without the cornea, no cornea-related complications, such as a deep (nonhealing) ulcer, can develop.

Due to the preoperative buphthalmic eye, the silicone implant, which was the size of the other normal eye, could be introduced, and the sclera wound could be opposed without tension releasing incisions or posterior radial sclerotomies, which may be used in human ophthalmology [8, 9]. A buphthalmic globe contracts around the implant within one to two months to conform to the size of the implanted sphere [2].

3.4. Implant Material. In dogs, implantation of silicone prosthesis after evisceration has been used already for many years [1–6]. In more recent studies with well-selected cases, no extrusion of the prosthesis was seen and no secondary enucleation was needed [2, 5, 6].

The first extraocular prostheses for humans were made of glass, mainly produced in Germany. During World War II, an increased demand for glass eyes and limited export from Germany led to the development of acrylic prostheses [11]. Glass causes no allergic reactions [10]. The manufacturing of the prosthesis takes approximately one hour. The measurement and placement in the patient can be done during one consultation [10]. Disadvantages of glass are the gradual break down of the smooth surface over time and the need to renew the prosthesis every one or two years [21]. Furthermore, glass can become very cold in windy or cold weather. This can cause pain to the eyelids in contact with the prosthesis [10]. Acrylic prostheses have a very large mechanically resistance and therefore last five to ten years. After manufacturing, the prosthesis can be molded several times. The measurement and placement in the patient takes normally two to three visits. Theoretically, acrylics can cause allergic reactions. To maintain the surface smooth and clean, the prosthesis has to be polished once a year [21]. In Germany, ocularists prefer to use glass whereas, for example, in the Netherlands the ocularists prefer to use acrylic prostheses [22]. In the presented case, the ocularist preferred to use glass for the extraocular prosthesis.

In an eviscerated eye without keratectomy in which a fibrotic cornea develops a tinted bandage lens can be tried to camouflage the white appearance. Care must be taken with those eyes that develop a lower tear production.

3.5. Prosthesis Motility. The motility of an intraocular prosthesis together with the extraocular prosthesis can be further increased by addressing a motility coupling system, like a peg, between the two prostheses [10, 23]. This improvement is reported to be relatively small in effect and neutralized by the need of a second anesthesia or sedation and increased rate of complications like persistent discharge, pain, and peg extrusion [9, 10, 24, 25].

3.6. Postoperative Complications. Different studies show that 10% of the eviscerated canine eyes developed a keratoconjunctivitis sicca (KCS) [4, 5, 26], but within this presented case no signs of KCS were seen.

This paper shows that the combination of both prostheses offers a good treatment option with very good cosmetic results, with no discomfort for the dog and no need for additional medication.

References

[1] A. H. Brightman, W. G. Magrane, R. W. Huff, and L. C. Helper, "Intraocular prosthesis in the dog," *Journal of the American Animal Hospital Association*, vol. 13, no. 4, pp. 481–485, 1977.

[2] R. E. Hamor, R. D. Whitley, S. A. McLaughlin et al., "Intraocular silicone prostheses in dogs: a review of the literature and 50 new cases," in *Journal of the American Animal Hospital Association*, vol. 30, pp. 66–69, 1994.

[3] S. A. Koch, "Intraocular prosthesis in the dog and cat: the failures," *Journal of the American Veterinary Medical Association*, vol. 179, no. 9, pp. 883–885, 1981.

[4] C. T. Lin, C. K. Hu, C. H. Liu, and L. S. Yeh, "Surgical outcome and ocular complications of evisceration and intraocular prosthesis implantation in dogs with end stage glaucoma: a review of 20 cases," *Journal of Veterinary Medical Science*, vol. 69, no. 8, pp. 847–850, 2007.

[5] E. Ruoss, B. M. Spiess, M. B. Rühli et al., "Intascleral silicone prosthesis in the dog: a retrospective study of 22 cases," *Tierärztliche Praxis*, vol. 25, no. 2, pp. 164–169, 1997.

[6] D. A. Wilkie, B. C. Gilger, A. van der Woerdt et al., "Implantation of intraocular silicone protheses," *Der praktische Tierarzt*, vol. 12, pp. 1097–1100, 1994.

[7] K. N. Gelatt and R. D. Whitley, "Surgery of the orbit," in *Veterinary Ophthalmic Surgery*, K. N. Gelatt and J. Peterson Gelatt, Eds., pp. 63–86, Elsevier Saunders, Philadelphia, Pa, USA, 2011.

[8] W. P. Chen, "Evisceration," in *Oculoplastic Surgery, The Essentials*, W. P. Chen, Ed., pp. 347–353, Thieme, New York, NY, USA, 2001.

[9] D. R. Jordan and L. Mawn, "Enucleation, evisceration, and exenteration," in *Basic Techniques of Ophthalmic Surgery*, J. P. Dunn and P. D. Langer, Eds., pp. 305–319, American Academy of Ophthalmology, San Fransisco, Calif, USA, 2009.

[10] M. L. R. Rasmussen, "The eye amputated—consequences of eye amputation with emphasis on clinical aspects, phantom eye syndrome and quality of life," *Acta Ophthalmologica*, vol. 88, no. 2, pp. 1–26, 2010.

[11] D. Sami, S. Young, and R. Petersen, "Perspective on orbital enucleation implants," *Survey of Ophthalmology*, vol. 52, no. 3, pp. 244–265, 2007.

[12] E. Bentley, P. E. Miller, C. J. Murphy, and J. V. Schoster, "Combined cycloablation and gonioimplantation for treatment of glaucoma in dogs: 18 cases (1992–1998)," *Journal of the American Veterinary Medical Association*, vol. 215, no. 10, pp. 1469–1472, 1999.

[13] J. S. Sapienza and A. Van Der Woerdt, "Combined transscleral diode laser cyclophotocoagulation and Ahmed gonioimplantation in dogs with primary glaucoma: 51 Cases (1996–2004)," *Veterinary Ophthalmology*, vol. 8, no. 2, pp. 121–127, 2005.

[14] F. D. Duke, T. D. Strong, E. Bentley, and R. R. Dubielzig, "Canine ocular tumors following ciliary bodyablation with intravitreal gentamicin," *Veterinary Ophthalmology*. In press.

[15] R. K. Dortzbach and J. J. Woog, "Choice of procedure. Enucleation, evisceration, or prosthetic fitting over globes," *Ophthalmology*, vol. 92, no. 9, pp. 1249–1255, 1985.

[16] T. Nakra, G. J. B. Simon, R. S. Douglas, R. M. Schwarcz, J. D. McCann, and R. A. Goldberg, "Comparing outcomes of enucleation and evisceration," *Ophthalmology*, vol. 113, no. 12, pp. 2270–2275, 2006.

[17] R. E. Kennedy, "The effect of early enucleation on the orbit in animals and humans," *Advances in Ophthalmic Plastic and Reconstructive Surgery*, vol. 9, pp. 1–39, 1992.

[18] C. Hintschich, F. Zonneveld, L. Baldeschi, C. Bunce, and L. Koornneef, "Bony orbital development after early enucleation in humans," *British Journal of Ophthalmology*, vol. 85, no. 2, pp. 205–208, 2001.

[19] G. M. Howard, R. S. Kinder, and A. S. MacMillan Jr., "Orbital growth after unilateral enucleation in childhood," *Archives of ophthalmology*, vol. 73, no. 1, pp. 80–83, 1965.

[20] M. A. Cepela, W. R. Nunery, and R. T. Martin, "Stimulation of orbital growth by the use of expandable implants in the anophthalmic cat orbit," *Ophthalmic Plastic and Reconstructive Surgery*, vol. 8, no. 3, pp. 157–169, 1992.

[21] T. Lyberg and M. Grip, "Ocular prosthesis production in Norway," *Tidsskrift for den Norske laegeforening*, vol. 110, no. 20, pp. 2663–2664, 1990.

[22] C. Hintschich and L. Baldeschi, "Rehabilitation of anophthalmic patients. Results of a survey," *Ophthalmologe*, vol. 98, no. 1, pp. 74–80, 2001.

[23] N. Y. Yi, S. A. Park, M. B. Jeong et al., "Comparison of orbital prosthesis motility following enucleation or evisceration with sclerotomy with or without a motility coupling post in dogs," *Veterinary Ophthalmology*, vol. 12, no. 3, pp. 139–151, 2009.

[24] D. R. Jordan, S. S. Chan, L. Mawn et al., "Complications associated with pegging hydroxyapatite orbital implants," *Ophthalmology*, vol. 106, no. 3, pp. 505–512, 1999.

[25] A. Shoamanesh, N. K. Pang, and J. H. Oestreicher, "Complications of orbital implants: a review of 542 patients who have undergone orbital implantation and 275 subsequent peg placements," *Orbit*, vol. 26, no. 3, pp. 173–182, 2007.

[26] T. Blocker, A. Hoffman, D. J. Schaeffer, and J. A. Wallin, "Corneal sensitivity and aqueous tear production in dogs undergoing evisceration with intraocular prosthesis placement," *Veterinary Ophthalmology*, vol. 10, no. 3, pp. 147–154, 2007.

27

Vacuum-Assisted Closure Combined with a Myocutaneous Flap in the Management of Osteomyelitis in a Dog

Jeremy L. Shomper,[1,2] Julia V. Coutin,[1] and Otto I. Lanz[1]

[1] Department of Small Animal Clinical Sciences, Virginia-Maryland Regional College of Veterinary Medicine,
  Blacksburg, VA 24061, USA
[2] University of Missouri, College of Veterinary Medicine, Columbia, MO 65211, USA

Correspondence should be addressed to Jeremy L. Shomper; shomperj@missouri.edu

Academic Editors: L. Espino López, N. D. Giadinis, C. M. Loiacono, F. Martinho, L. G. Papazoglou, and D. M. Wong

Case Description. A 2.5-year-old female spayed mixed breed dog presented to the Teaching Hospital for draining tracts on the left medial aspect of the tibia. Two years prior to presentation, the patient sustained a left tibial fracture, which was repaired with an intramedullary (IM) pin and two cerclage wires. Multiple antimicrobials were utilized during this time. *Clinical Findings.* Radiographs were consistent with left tibial osteomyelitis. The implant was removed and the wound was debrided. *Treatment and Outcome.* A bone window on the medial aspect of the tibia was created in order to facilitate implant removal. The wound and associated bone window were treated with vacuum assisted closure (VAC) in preparation for reconstructive surgery. Adjunctive VAC therapy was utilized following the caudal sartorius myocutaneous flap. Complications following this surgery included distal flap necrosis and donor site dehiscence. *Clinical Relevance.* This presents a difficult case of canine osteomyelitis with subsequent wound care in which VAC and a myocutaneous flap were useful adjunctive treatments for osteomyelitis. This is the first report of VAC in the management of canine osteomyelitis and management with a myocutaneous flap.

1. Introduction

Muscle is the most versatile tissue for reconstructive surgery and is used in a variety of reconstructive surgical procedures ranging from soft tissue to orthopedics. Muscle flaps, for the most part, are easily dissected and are harvested with little donor site morbidity [1]. Donor muscle selection is based on the dimensions of the defect and function or purpose of the reconstructive procedure and can be harvested alone or as a composite flap (skin and muscle) [2–4]. Muscle flaps augment vascular supply of compromised wounds by inducing angiogenesis, which is used for the management of chronic osteomyelitis, shearing wounds to the distal extremities, decubital ulcers, and ablative oncological procedures [3–5]. The increased blood supply through transferred muscle enhances the host defense mechanism to a compromised wound by increasing local concentrations of immunoglobulins, complement, neutrophils, and oxygen tension [2, 6]. The use of vacuum assisted closure (VAC) therapy is well described as an alternative strategy in the management of a variety of wounds encountered in human medicine and surgery [7–11]. The uses of VAC therapy in human surgery include decubital ulcers, degloving injuries, distal extremity wounds, as a means to secure split thickness skin grafts in anatomically challenging areas, poststernotomy dehiscence following cardiac surgery, open peritonitis, abdominal wound dehiscence and perineal wounds [7–11]. VAC therapy is the controlled application of subatmospheric pressure to a wound using a therapy unit to intermittently or continuously convey negative pressure to a specialized wound dressing to help promote wound healing. The case described below illustrates the simultaneous use of a muscle flap and VAC therapy for the treatment of osteomyelitis in a dog.

2. Case Report

A 2.5-year-old female spayed mixed breed dog presented to the Veterinary Teaching Hospital for chronic draining

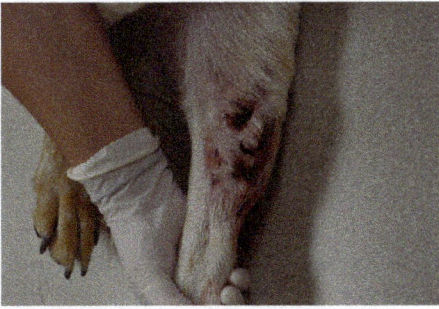

FIGURE 1: Medial aspect of the left hind limb on presentation. The nonhealing draining tracts revealed deep subcutaneous pocketing with purulent discharge.

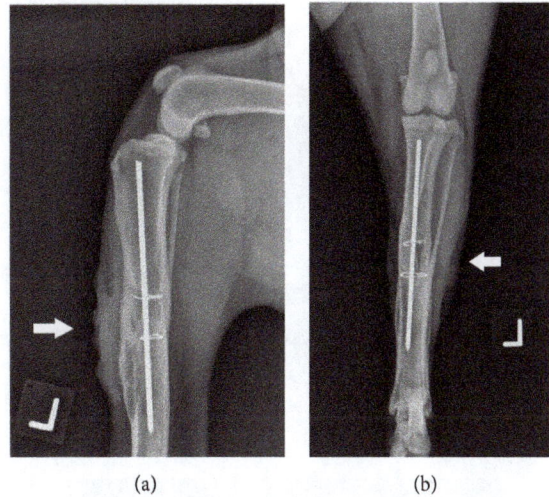

(a)   (b)

FIGURE 2: Lateral (a) and craniocaudal (b) radiographs of the left tibia. Note that the cerclage wires within the bone are broken with appreciable lucency surrounding the proximal wire. There does not seem to be lucency associated with the intramedullary pin. A large area of remodeled bone is also present on the cranial cortex of the tibia. On the craniocaudal image, between the two cerclage wires, there is an area of lucent bone surrounding a more radiopaque bone suggestive of a sequestrum. The arrows indicate soft tissue swelling and subcutaneous edema surrounding the mid-diaphyseal area. The radiographic interpretation was consistent with osteomyelitis and associated cellulitis.

tracts located on the left medial aspect of the tibia. Pertinent medical history included a tibial fracture that was repaired with an intramedullary (IM) pin and cerclage wires two years prior to presentation, which was just prior to the time of adoption at an unknown veterinary clinic. Multiple antimicrobials were utilized over the course of 2 years with only temporary resolution of clinical signs with recurrence after cessation of antimicrobials. Upon presentation, the medial aspect of the left hind limb was warm, swollen, and painful upon palpation, and a serosanguinous discharge was noted focally at the area of the midtibial diaphysis. The affected area was clearly demarcated with a dark purple discoloration noted around the periphery (Figure 1). No other abnormalities were noted on physical examination. Initial diagnostics included a complete blood count (CBC), serum biochemistry profile, and radiographs of the left tibia. Both the CBC and biochemistry profile were within normal limits. Radiographs revealed an intramedullary Steinman pin with 2 broken cerclage wires circling the mid-diaphysis of the tibia. Exuberant periosteal reaction was noted with much of the cerclage wires being overgrown with bone. A zone of lucency was noted around the proximal wire as were soft tissue swelling, gas, and bony lysis (Figures 2(a) and 2(b)). The radiographic interpretation was consistent with osteomyelitis and surrounding cellulitis.

The patient was taken to surgery for implant removal. A medial approach to the left tibia was utilized and the draining tracts were excised and underlying necrotic tissue was debrided. An approximately 10 cm × 5 cm section of devitalized tissue was removed. A round burr and Surgairtome (Surgairtome Two, Hall Power Instruments, ConMed Linvatec, Largo, FL) were used to make a 1.5 cm × 4 cm bone window in order to remove excess periosteum, the broken cerclage wires, and the Steinman pin. It was noted that the Steinman pin was freely moveable both proximally and distally within the medullary canal. Cultures were obtained from the Steinman pin surface prior to removal as well as the deep tissue. Culture samples were submitted for aerobic, anaerobic, and fungal cultures. A sample of exuberant periosteum was also submitted for histopathologic analysis. During surgery a suspected sequestrum was identified and removed (Figure 3). The wound was lavaged and debrided following implant removal, leaving an open bone window. Hemostasis

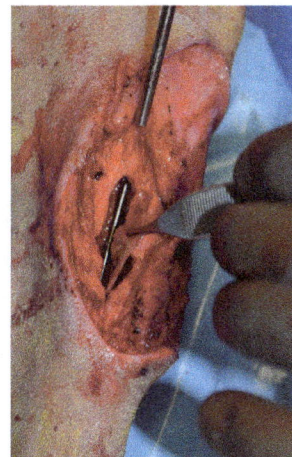

FIGURE 3: Intraoperative image of the medial wound after debridement of the necrotic tissues and creation of a bone window. The suction tip is placed over the proximal aspect of the tibia. Within the bone window, the intramedullary pin is still present and the thumb forceps are removing a necrotic bone segment suspected to be a sequestrum.

was assessed as adequate. A vacuum assisted closure (VAC) system (V.A.C. Freedom Wound System, Kinetic Concepts Inc., San Antonio, TX) was placed over the tibial window and associated wound. The polyurethane foam dressing (V.A.C., GranuFoam, Kinetic Concepts Inc., San Antonio, TX) was cut to the size of the wound and placed over the bone

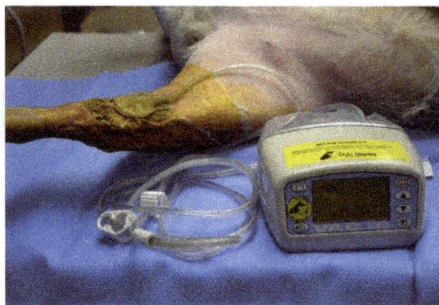

FIGURE 4: The VAC system was applied to wound and set at a negative pressure of 125 mmHg.

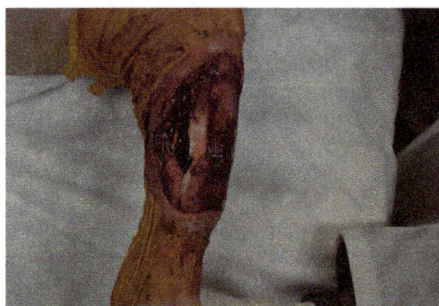

FIGURE 5: The wound and exposed bone after five days of negative pressure wound therapy.

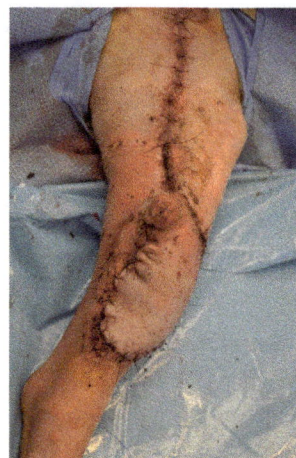

FIGURE 6: The medial aspect of the left hind limb taken intraoperatively after the completion of the caudal sartorius myocutaneous flap.

window and wound directly. The self-adhesive drape was then placed and the evacuation tubing (V.A.C., T.R.A.C. Pad, Kinetic Concepts Inc., San Antonio, TX) was placed over the foam-dressing interface (Figure 4). A modified Robert Jones bandage with a lateral splint was placed over the VAC system, which was set to maintain negative pressure of 125 mmHg.

Culture results of the IM pin revealed *Corynebacterium* spp. as well as an unidentified gram + organism. Treatment was initiated with sulfamethoxazole/trimethoprim (15 mg/kg (6.8 mg/lb), PO, q 12 h for 4 weeks) based upon susceptibility results. Histopathology of the submitted periosteal tissue revealed necrotic tissue infiltrated with lymphocytes, plasma cells, and neutrophils, consistent with chronic connective tissue inflammation. Postoperative medication included tramadol (3 mg/kg (1.3 mg/lb), PO, q 8 h) and carprofen (2.2 mg/kg (1 mg/lb), PO, q 12 h). Bandage changes were performed at 2-3-day intervals to assess granulation tissue formation (Figure 5). All bandage changes were performed under sedation with dexmedetomidine (5 mcg/kg (2.3 mcg/lb), IV) and butorphanol (0.2 mg/kg (0.9 mg/lb), IV). Sedation was reversed with atipamezole (0.05 mg/kg (0.02 mg/lb), IM). At the time of bandage changes, the wound was lavaged with sterile saline and the VAC was replaced at 125 mmHg. During the recovery period, packed cell volume and total solids were measured and were within normal limits. Postoperative radiographs were not performed due to monetary constraints.

Two weeks following implant removal adequate granulation tissue was noted covering the bone window and a caudal sartorius myocutaneous flap was performed (Figure 6). Packed cell volume (PCV) and total solids (TS) remained within normal limits and were 46% and 7 g/dL prior to reconstructive surgery. Following reconstructive surgery the VAC system was replaced but the negative pressure setting of 50 mmHg was applied over the recipient flap. Additionally, the foam dressing was placed over a petrolatum impregnated gauze (Adaptic, Johnson & Johnson, New Brunswick, NJ) used as an interface dressing. The proximal donor site was closed using subcutaneous and intradermal sutures. The VAC system was supported by a lateral splint and a modified Robert Jones bandage. Bandage changes under sedation were performed every 2 days. Serosanguinous discharge was noted beginning from the day after surgery from the donor site incision. Dehiscence occurred at the proximal donor site four days after surgery at which time, approximately 30% of the skin over the distal aspect of the myocutaneous flap was also noted to be necrotic (Figure 7). This wound, as well as the donor site wound, was then debrided and dressed with the negative pressure treatment. The VAC system was applied over the open wound, the surviving portion of the myocutaneous flap, and the donor site at a negative pressure setting of 50 mmHg. Bandage change was performed 3 days later. After healthy granulation tissue was noted 5 days after debridement, a full thickness mesh skin graft was placed over the distal aspect of the myocutaneous flap. The VAC system was replaced over the graft and myocutaneous flap donor site at 50 mmHg with a lateral splint and modified Robert Jones bandage. Bandage changes were performed every 3 days. After 9 days, the negative pressure therapy was discontinued. Outpatient bandage changes and wound care were continued until the skin graft had healed. The skin graft and donor site healed without further complication and the myocutaneous flap donor site healed by second intention. At 6-month and 1-year follow up conversation by phone, the patient was reported to be using the limb without appreciable

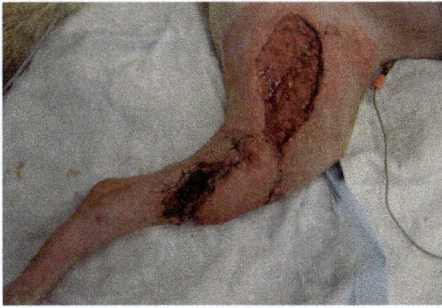

FIGURE 7: The medial aspect of the left hind limb at bandage change 4 days after reconstructive surgery. The portion of the necrotic skin over the flap was later debrided and treated with a mesh skin graft. The proximal donor wound was treated and healed by second intention.

lameness. The wounds had healed and fur coat had returned over the surgery sites.

3. Discussion

This case describes the use of VAC in the management of chronic osteomyelitis and subsequent myocutaneous flap wound reconstruction. Over ten years ago, Fleischmann and Morykwas introduced the concept of applying negative pressure to wounds in order to promote rapid wound healing [7, 8]. The VAC was quickly accepted as an efficacious treatment modality for wound management in human medicine and is recently being used with more frequency in veterinary medicine [12–14]. Indications for VAC therapy include acute, subacute, and chronic wounds, degloving injuries, reconstructive procedures, decubital ulcers, and burn wounds [7–9, 12, 15]. Clinical reports revealed that VAC was beneficial for treating osteomyelitis, promoting granulation tissue, and reducing the need for reconstructive tissue transfer [11, 16, 17]. VAC was initially utilized in the dog reported here to facilitate granulation tissue formation in an open wound with established osteomyelitis in preparation for reconstructive surgery. It was determined that all nonviable bone was debrided prior to the dressing placement. VAC was subsequently utilized to support additional reconstructive procedures. To our knowledge, this is the first case of VAC in the management of tibial osteomyelitis and subsequent myocutaneous flap in a dog.

The effect of VAC therapy on bacterial clearance and subsequent infection is debatable [13, 18]. In regards to using VAC for osteomyelitis treatment, studies have compared VAC use to conventional wound dressing in open tibial fractures [19]. Results showed that VAC reduced the risk of deep infection by almost 80% when compared to conventional dressing [19]. In agreement with this study, studies and case reports of osteomyelitis treated with negative pressure increased granulation tissue formation, decreased number of reconstructive procedures and have variably affected bacterial burden [5, 11, 20]. With this in mind, the VAC system was chosen to treat the patient in this report. In the case presented here,

bacterial culture confirmed preexisting bacterial osteomyelitis with multiple Gram positive organisms. Implant removal, surgical debridement, and VAC therapy in conjunction with appropriate antimicrobial selection and a myocutaneous flap were successful in managing this case, allowing decreased frequency of bandage changes, rapid creation of granulation tissue within the wound, and resolution of clinical signs.

In veterinary medicine, continuous negative pressure of 125 mmHg is commonly used as it provides marked benefit to wound healing while minimizing patient discomfort [12, 13]. In this patient, these standard settings were used initially to facilitate granulation tissue formation. Following reconstructive surgery with a caudal sartorius myocutaneous flap, VAC therapy was applied at 50 mmHg. Although some authors make recommendations that subatmospheric pressure settings of only 50 mmHg are needed to reduce edema over closed incisions or skin grafts, clinical cases report a 95% success rate with split thickness skin grafting and adjunctive negative pressures between 75 and 125 mmHg [7, 21–23]. The negative pressure setting of 50 mmHg was chosen based on clinical experience with skin grafts treated adjunctively with VAC therapy at our institute.

Although granulation tissue was witnessed within the wound and bone window, a caudal sartorius myocutaneous flap was chosen in the place of a skin graft for the additional protection the muscle flap would offer over the tibial bone window. The authors also chose to use a myocutaneous flap in this case because of its superior vascularity and beneficial properties pertaining to refractory osteomyelitis. Mycocutaneous flaps are well defined in the literature for adjunctive treatment of osteomyelitis [2, 6]. The caudal sartorius myocutaneous flap, despite being a type IV muscle, was reported to be an extremely reliable flap due to its blood supply from the saphenous artery and vein and reverse saphenous blood flow as described for the reverse saphenous conduit flap [3, 4]. Possible explanations for the distal myocutaneous flap necrosis seen in this case include lack of proximal muscle excision as was recommended during the original study by Weinstein et al., excessive flap shear in lieu of lateral splint stabilization, or hindered blood flow due to the nature of segmental blood supply to the muscle [3]. The authors initially had concern that the VAC system may have impaired the local blood supply to the flap with excessive negative pressure and subsequent areas of hypoxia, but this is considered unlikely as a decrease in local ischemia and reperfusion injury to free muscle flaps in humans treated with adjunctive negative pressure treatment of 125 mmHg was reported [24]. Although this beneficial effect was not elicited in dogs, we believe that the pressure applied to the wound was potentially subtherapeutic because of the lower negative pressure setting in addition to an interface dressing, which also decreased the pressure delivered over the wound. That being said, the distal aspect of the flap healed without complication following appropriate wound care and surgical placement of a full thickness mesh skin graft. Dehiscence of the donor site was likely due to excessive tension, and therefore the wound was treated and allowed to heal by second intention without further complication. Interestingly, VAC has recently been reported to successfully maintain viability of a tissue flap following partial dehiscence [25]. Moreover, VAC has been associated with increased skin graft acceptance rates and less graft necrosis [26].

Complications considered during the management of this case included ongoing blood loss and hypoproteinemia resulting from application of negative pressure over the medullary cavity. Repeated laboratory values were used to monitor these parameters which remained stable throughout the case. Hemorrhage as a result of VAC is reported sparsely in the literature [27–29]. Furthermore, tibial artery erosion secondary to treatment with VAC was described recently in a traumatic open fibular wound report [27]. In that report, the arterial erosion and subsequent hemorrhage were multifactorial due to concurrent anticoagulant therapy, fungal infection with *Aspergillus*, and the concurrent placement of the VAC system over the exposed artery [27]. In the case reported here, at the time of surgery, there was adequate hemostasis with no appreciable vessels that would be exposed to the VAC foam dressing. Additionally, no adverse effects were noted as a result of transient loss of negative pressure in this case.

In conclusion, the indications for VAC in both human and veterinary medicine are expanding. Originally VAC was examined for use in chronic nonhealing wounds, and the therapeutic benefits in veterinary medicine seen with VAC are starting to be appreciated in its diverse applications which are largely derived from human medicine. Regardless of the type of wound, it is imperative to thoroughly debride the wound before applying the VAC device [10]. Chronic osteomyelitis was once considered a contraindication of VAC therapy [10, 30]. In more recent years VAC has been proven effective in cases of osteomyelitis and traumatic wounds with exposed bone [10, 31, 32]. This case report illustrates VAC as an effective wound healing technique in a canine patient with an open tibial medullary cavity with chronic multiorganism osteomyelitis. This case also lends support to the use of VAC in patients with myocutaneous flap reconstructive surgeries as well as skin grafts.

Conflict of Interests

The authors of this paper have no financial or personal relationship with other people or organizations that could inappropriately influence or bias the content of this paper.

References

[1] J. M. Miller, O. I. Lanz, and D. A. Degner, "Rectus abdominis free muscle flap for reconstruction in nine dogs," *Veterinary Surgery*, vol. 36, no. 3, pp. 259–265, 2007.

[2] S.-L. Chen, T.-M. Chen, T.-D. Chou, S.-C. Chang, and H.-J. Wang, "Distally based sural fasciomusculocutaneous flap for chronic calcaneal osteomyelitis in diabetic patients," *Annals of Plastic Surgery*, vol. 54, no. 1, pp. 44–48, 2005.

[3] M. J. Weinstein, M. M. Pavletic, and R. J. Boudrieau, "Caudal sartorius muscle flap in the dog," *Veterinary Surgery*, vol. 17, no. 4, pp. 203–210, 1988.

[4] D. A. Degner and R. Walshaw, "Medial saphenous fasciocutaneous and myocutaneous free flap transfer in eight dogs," *Veterinary Surgery*, vol. 26, no. 1, pp. 20–25, 1997.

[5] Z. Eyileten, A. R. Akar, S. Eryilmaz et al., "Vacuum-assisted closure and bilateral pectoralis muscle flaps for different stages of mediastinitis after cardiac surgery," *Surgery Today*, vol. 39, no. 11, pp. 947–954, 2009.

[6] D. P. Lew and F. A. Waldvogel, "Current concepts: osteomyelitis," *The New England Journal of Medicine*, vol. 336, no. 14, pp. 999–1007, 1997.

[7] L. C. Argenta and M. J. Morykwas, "Vacuum-assisted closure: a new method for wound control and treatment: Clinical experience," *Annals of Plastic Surgery*, vol. 38, no. 6, pp. 563–576, 1997.

[8] M. J. Morykwas, L. C. Argenta, E. I. Shelton-Brown, and W. McGuirt, "Vacuum-assisted closure: a new method for wound control and treatment: animal studies and basic foundation," *Annals of Plastic Surgery*, vol. 38, no. 6, pp. 553–562, 1997.

[9] C. M. Sciortino, G. S. Mundinger, D. P. Kuwayama, and S. C. Yang MS Sussman, "Case report: treatment of severe subcutaneous emphysema with a negative pressure wound therapy dressing," *Eplasty*, vol. 9, article e1, 2009.

[10] A. J. DeFranzo, L. C. Argenta, M. W. Marks et al., "The use of vacuum-assisted closure therapy for the treatment of lower-extremity wounds with exposed bone," *Plastic and Reconstructive Surgery*, vol. 108, no. 5, pp. 1184–1191, 2001.

[11] Y. Tan, X. Wang, H. Li et al., "The clinical efficacy of the vacuum-assisted closure therapy in the management of adult osteomyelitis," *Archives of Orthopaedic and Trauma Surgery*, vol. 131, no. 2, pp. 255–259, 2011.

[12] R. Ben-Amotz, O. I. Lanz, J. M. Miller, D. E. Filipowicz, and M. D. King, "The use of vacuum-assisted closure therapy for the treatment of distal extremity wounds in 15 dogs," *Veterinary Surgery*, vol. 36, no. 7, pp. 684–690, 2007.

[13] M. Demaria, B. J. Stanley, J. G. Hauptman et al., "Effects of negative pressure wound therapy on healing of open wounds in dogs," *Veterinary Surgery*, vol. 40, no. 6, pp. 658–669, 2011.

[14] A. E. Guille, L. W. Tseng, and R. J. Orsher, "Use of vacuum-assisted closure for management of a large skin wound in a cat," *Journal of the American Veterinary Medical Association*, vol. 230, no. 11, pp. 1669–1673, 2007.

[15] C. Mullally, K. Carey, and R. Seshadri, "Use of a nanocrystalline silver dressing and vacuum-assisted closure in a severely burned dog," *Journal of Veterinary Emergency and Critical Care*, vol. 20, no. 4, pp. 456–463, 2010.

[16] S. J. Ford, S. Rathinam, J. E. King, and R. Vaughan, "Tuberculous osteomyelitis of the sternum: successful management with debridement and vacuum assisted closure," *European Journal of Cardio-thoracic Surgery*, vol. 28, no. 4, pp. 645–647, 2005.

[17] R. E. Hersh, A. K. Kaza, S. M. Long, S. M. Fiser, D. B. Drake, and C. G. Tribble, "A technique for the treatment of sternal infections using the Vacuum Assisted Closure device," *Heart Surgery Forum*, vol. 4, no. 3, pp. 211–215, 2001.

[18] T. Weed, C. Ratliff, D. B. Drake et al., "Quantifying bacterial bioburden during negative pressure wound therapy: does the wound VAC enhance bacterial clearance?" *Annals of Plastic Surgery*, vol. 52, no. 3, pp. 276–280, 2004.

[19] M. L. Blum, M. Esser, M. Richardson et al., "Negative pressure wound therapy reduces deep infection rate in open tibial fractures," *Journal of Orthopaedic Trauma*, vol. 26, no. 9, pp. 499–505, 2012.

[20] S. J. Lalliss, D. J. Stinner, S. M. Waterman, J. G. Branstetter, B. D. Masini, and J. C. Wenke, "Negative pressure wound therapy reduces pseudomonas wound contamination more than

staphylococcus aureus," *Journal of Orthopaedic Trauma*, vol. 24, no. 9, pp. 598–602, 2010.

[21] E. A. Azzopardi, D. E. Boyce, W. A. Dickson et al., "Application of topical negative pressure (vacuum-assisted closure) to split-thickness skin grafts: a structured evidence-based review," *Annals of Plastic Surgery*, vol. 70, pp. 23–29, 2013.

[22] L. A. Dainty, J. J. Bosco, J. W. McBroom, W. E. Winter III, G. S. Rose, and J. C. Elkas, "Novel techniques to improve split-thickness skin graft viability during vulvo-vaginal reconstruction," *Gynecologic Oncology*, vol. 97, no. 3, pp. 949–952, 2005.

[23] L. X. Webb, "New techniques in wound management: vacuum-assisted wound closure," *Journal of the American Academy of Orthopaedic Surgeons*, vol. 10, no. 5, pp. 303–311, 2002.

[24] S. U. Eisenhardt, Y. Schmidt, J. R. Thiele et al., "Negative pressure wound therapy reduces the ischaemia/reperfusion-associated inflammatory response in free muscle flaps," *Journal of Plastic, Reconstructive and Aesthetic Surgery*, vol. 65, no. 5, pp. 640–649, 2012.

[25] P. C. Bristow, K. L. Perry, Z. J. Halfacree, and V. J. Lipscomb, "Use of vacuum-assisted closure to maintain viability of a skin flap in a dog," *Journal of the American Veterinary Medical Association*, vol. 243, pp. 863–868, 2013.

[26] J. S. Bryden, K. A. Pitt, C. D. Weder et al., "Effects of negative pressure wound therapy on healing of free full-thickness grafts in dogs," *Veterinary Surgery*, vol. 42, pp. 511–552, 2013.

[27] R. A. White, R. A. Miki, P. Kazmier, and J. O. Anglen, "Vacuum-assisted closure complicated by erosion and hemorrhage of the anterior tibial artery," *Journal of Orthopaedic Trauma*, vol. 19, no. 1, pp. 56–59, 2005.

[28] G. A. Jones, J. Butler, I. Lieberman, and R. Schlenk, "Negative-pressure wound therapy in the treatment of complex postoperative spinal wound infections: complications and lessons learned using vacuum-assisted closure," *Journal of Neurosurgery*, vol. 6, no. 5, pp. 407–411, 2007.

[29] U. Sartipy, U. Lockowandt, J. Gäbel, L. Jidéus, and G. Dellgren, "Cardiac rupture during vacuum-assisted closure therapy," *Annals of Thoracic Surgery*, vol. 82, no. 3, pp. 1110–1111, 2006.

[30] W. Fleischmann, U. Becker, M. Mischoff et al., "Vacuum sealing: indication, technique, and results," *European Journal of Orthopaedic Surgery and Traumatology*, vol. 5, pp. 37–40, 1995.

[31] M. J. Adkesson, E. K. Travis, M. A. Weber, J. P. Kirby, and R. E. Junge, "Vacuum-assisted closure for treatment of a deep shell abscess and osteomyelitis in a tortoise," *Journal of the American Veterinary Medical Association*, vol. 231, no. 8, pp. 1249–1254, 2007.

[32] P. E. Banwell and M. Musgrave, "Topical negative pressure therapy: mechanisms and indications," *International wound journal*, vol. 1, no. 2, pp. 95–106, 2004.

28

Cutaneous Disease as Sole Clinical Manifestation of Protothecosis in a Boxer Dog

Emmanouil I. Papadogiannakis,[1,2] Emmanouil N. Velonakis,[3] Gregory K. Spanakos,[4] and Alexander F. Koutinas[5]

[1]*Department of Veterinary Public Health, National School of Public Health, 115 21 Athens, Greece*
[2]*Small Animal Dermatology Clinic, Alimos, 174 55 Athens, Greece*
[3]*Department of Applied Microbiology and Immunology, National School of Public Health, 115 21 Athens, Greece*
[4]*Department of Parasitology, Entomology and Tropical Diseases, National School of Public Health, 115 21 Athens, Greece*
[5]*Quality Veterinary Practice, 383 33 Volos, Greece*

Correspondence should be addressed to Emmanouil I. Papadogiannakis; dermpap1@otenet.gr

Academic Editor: Paola Roccabianca

Prototheca wickerhamii is ubiquitous, saprophytic achlorophyllous algae that cause opportunistic infections in the dog and cat and disseminated disease usually in immunocompromised animals. In this report an uncommon case of canine cutaneous protot/hecosis is presented. A 6-year-old female boxer was brought in with skin lesions that consisted of nodules and generalized footpad hyperkeratosis, depigmentation, and erosion. Cytology and histopathology showed pyogranulomatous inflammation along with organisms containing round sporangia with spherical sporangiospores. PCR and sequencing identified the causal organism as *Prototheca wickerhamii*. Therapy applied in this patient with either fluconazole alone or combination of amphotericin B and itraconazole proved effective only for footpad lesions but not for skin nodules. Systemic therapy seems to be ineffective for skin nodules, at least in chronic cases of canine cutaneous protothecosis. Although canine protothecosis usually presents with the disseminated form, cutaneous disease as sole clinical manifestation of the infection may also be witnessed.

1. Introduction

Prototheca spp. are ubiquitous, saprophytic achlorophyllous algae that cause opportunistic infections in both small animals and disseminated disease actually in the immunocompromised ones [1]. In the dog, protothecosis is usually manifested as a disseminated disease [1, 2]. Three species are currently recognized within the genus *Prototheca*: *P. stagnosa*, *P. zopfii*, and *P. wickerhamii*, with the latter two being the most commonly isolated species from dogs [2, 3].

Although ulcerative colitis [4], ocular disease that may lead to sudden blindness [5, 6], and granulomatous encephalomyelitis [7] may occur as single clinical entities or in various combinations [8, 9], the disseminated form of the disease is by far the most common in the dog [3, 10, 11].

This report describes a case of cutaneous protothecosis in a dog the breed of which tends to develop granulomatous skin diseases either infectious (e.g. leishmaniosis, leproid granulomas) or sterile [12].

2. Case Description

A six-year-old female boxer dog presented with a 13-month history of progressive and mildly pruritic skin lesions. The dog was current on vaccinations and deworming and was being fed on dry commercial food of high quality. Previous treatments included amoxicillin plus clavulanic acid (20 mg/Kg/12 h), cefalexin (25 mg/Kg/12 h) alone or in combination with prednisolone (0.5 mg/Kg/24 h for 1 week and then every other day) for a period of approximately 3 to 4 weeks each, but of no avail. The owner also reported that the dog had intermittently been experiencing nonambulatory lameness on the right front leg.

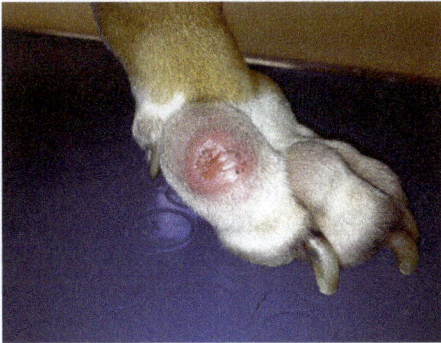

FIGURE 1: Nodules (one ulcerated) on the distal extremity and digits.

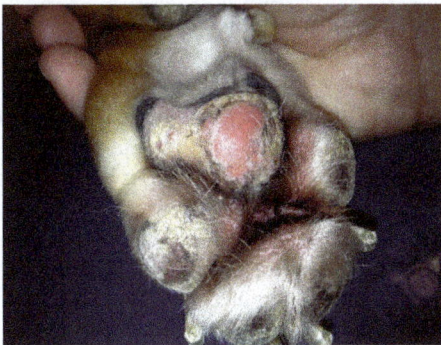

FIGURE 2: Hyperkeratosis, depigmentation, and erosions of footpads.

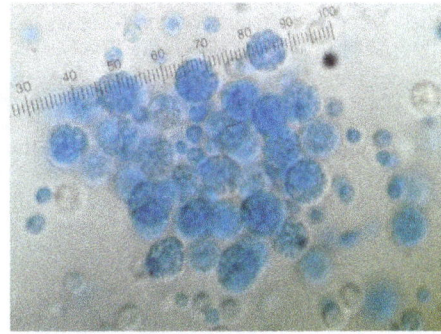

FIGURE 3: Light microscopy of lactophenol cotton blue slide preparations made of culture colonies revealed round sporangia containing spherical sporangiospores similar to those of *P. wickerhamii*.

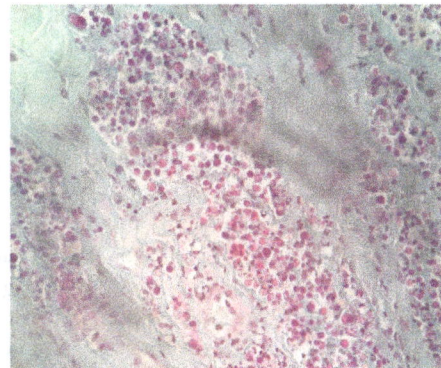

FIGURE 4: Nodular-to-diffuse, pyogranulomatous panniculitis with numerous *Prototheca*-like elements stained vividly purple with PAS stain.

Physical examination of the dog upon admission revealed no abnormality. On dermatological examination, 9 ulcerated and nonulcerated skin nodules were observed, ranged from 1 to 7 cm in diameter, and distributed mainly over bony prominences of distal extremities and digits of the front legs (Figure 1), left elbow, and right hock. Other skin lesions included footpad hyperkeratosis, crusting, depigmentation, and erosions (Figure 2).

At that time the main differentials included infectious or sterile nodules and neoplasia.

Fine needle aspiration (FNA) cytology made from material obtained from nonulcerated skin nodules revealed pyogranulomatous inflammation and numerous mainly extracellular round-shaped organisms, ranging from 20 to 30 μm in diameter, most containing 2 spores of approximately 10 μm in diameter. A tentative diagnosis of systemic mycosis was made. Culture of FNA material in dermatophyte test medium (DTM) was performed at room temperature. Furthermore, skin biopsies were obtained from intact nodules (the owner refused footpad lesions biopsy) along with blood and urine samples for further laboratory workup and serology. Survey thoracic and abdominal radiographs were also taken but were unremarkable.

Hematology, serum biochemistry, and urinalysis did not display any abnormalities and serology (snap ELISA, IDEXX®) for all of *Leishmania infantum*, *Ehrlichia canis*, and *Anaplasma phagocytophilum* antibodies and *Dirofilaria immitis* antigen was negative. After 4 days of incubation, smooth,

creamy, yeastlike colonies were grown on DTM. Light microscopy of lactophenol cotton blue slide preparations made of these colonies revealed round sporangia containing spherical sporangiospores similar to those of *P. wickerhamii* (Figure 3). *P. zopfii* cells are oval or cylindrical in shape, producing sporangia of larger diameter (15–25 μm) containing up to 20 sporangiospores. In contrast, *P. wickerhamii* cells tend to be round, forming sporangia (7–13 μm) containing up to 50 spherical sporangiospores [2].

Histopathology revealed nodular-to-diffuse, pyogranulomatous dermatitis and panniculitis (with lymphocytes, plasma cells, macrophages, and neutrophils) with numerous elements exhibiting *Prototheca* spp. morphology; their cell wall stained vividly purple with periodic acid Schiff (PAS) stain (Figure 4) and most of microorganisms were extracellular, either single or more often in groups, with only a few seen to be phagocytosed.

Approximately 1 mm³ of culture material was used for DNA isolation, by employing the QIAamp Mini Kit (QIAGEN, Hilden, Germany), and following the manufacturer's instructions. A portion of the 28S rRNA gene was amplified by using already published primers [13]. The band was excised from the gel and DNA was isolated using the DNA Isolation Spin-Kit Agarose (AppliChem, Darmstadt, Germany). The isolated DNA was subsequently sequenced with the PCR

Case: AATCCCAACGCCTGGCTCATGCTCTTCTTGAGAGACCGA³⁹
AB183198: AATCCCAACGCCTGGCTCATGCTCTTCTTGAGAGACCGA

Case: GGAACTTTCAGTACGGTGCCCCAGAAGAACCAATTCAC⁷⁷
AB183198: GGAACTTTCAGTACGGTGCCCCAGAAAAACCAACTCTT

Figure 5: Alignment of the sequence obtained in this case to the corresponding fragment of the GenBank number AB183198 sequence. Highlighted letters indicate the differences. The image was edited with Krita 2.8.5 (https://krita.org).

primers; PCR produced a ~350 bp band. As sequencing of the complete length of PCR product was not possible, a 77 bp sequence was obtained by employing the U2 primer. Beyond that fragment the double peaks were indicative of the presence of more than 1 strain. Similar sequences were searched in the GenBank with the aid of the Web interface of Blast software which returned 9 of these sequences that belonged to *Prototheca wickerhamii* strains; the higher similarity applied to GenBank number AB183198 sequence (Figure 5). This result confirmed the diagnosis of cutaneous protothecosis due to *Prototheca wickerhamii*.

As no treatment guidelines are available, the patient was treated with oral fluconazole (10 mg/Kg twice a day), based on reported agents likely to be most useful against *Prototheca* species such as amphotericin B (AMB), fluconazole, itraconazole, and possibly terbinafine [2]. Although significant clinical improvement was witnessed in footpad lesions after one month on fluconazole, this treatment regimen did little to slow the progression of skin nodules, because *Prototheca* organisms were found on cytology. At that time fluconazole administration was withdrawn and AMB was administered twice weekly as a subcutaneous infusion using a protocol developed to treat canine cryptococcosis [14]. Specifically, 0.5 mg AMB/Kg/sc per dose was administered twice weekly in 500 mL of 0.45% NaCl/2.5% dextrose fluids. The dog was given concurrently itraconazole (5 mg/Kg/per os, once daily). Due to nephrotoxicity, AMB was withdrawn after 7 infusions and the patient is still being treated with itraconazole alone for about six months. However, although skin nodules have not been improved with this treatment regimen, footpads remain close to normal.

3. Discussion

Protothecosis is a very uncommon disease that has been reported in humans [15], cattle [16], cats [17], and dogs [1–11]. In Greece this is the second reported case of canine protothecosis, the other one having been associated with colonic and rectal insult [4].

A striking similarity between this case report and the largest case series of canine protothecosis ever published [2] is the overrepresentation of boxer dogs suggesting a genetic predisposition to develop the infection [18]. The increased risk to this breed of developing infectious diseases in which cellular immunosuppression plays a crucial role [2] has been witnessed in cryptococcosis [19] and leishmaniosis [12]. Due to the fact that cutaneous nodules, either ulcerated or not, and generalized footpad hyperkeratosis accompanied by depigmentation and erosion were the main constituents of the

cutaneous disease in this dog and its many clinical similarities to canine leishmaniosis (*Leishmania infantum/chagasi*) [12, 20], made its exclusion with the aid of serology and cytology a diagnostic priority. Leproid granuloma (*Mycobacterium avium* complex), a top differential due to the many clinical similarities and the breed of the dog [21], was also ruled out with both cytology and histopathology.

The fact that the affected boxer was female complies with what has already been reported on several occasions [2]. Gender predisposition remains an unclarified issue and its association with female hormonal level has been argued [2].

Cutaneous protothecosis in dogs without other organ involvement is uncommon [22]. Colonic and rectal injury is the most consistent feature of *Prototheca* infection, even in the absence of overt colitis [2, 18]. Subclinical colitis would not be ruled out without colonoscopy and histopathology which were denied by the owner; his main concern was the skin lesions of his dog.

Footpad erosion and ulceration have been reported to occur in canine protothecosis [22], but not hyperkeratosis and depigmentation, although footpad biopsies should have been obtained in this case to confirm the presence of *Prototheca* organisms in those lesions. Portal of entry of *Prototheca* organism is thought to be skin wounds or colonic mucosa in disseminated disease in dogs with access to contaminated water or environmental sources [22, 23]. The patient described in this case had no obvious evidence of systemic disease and lived primarily indoors. Infection source for these reasons was uncertain. Footpad hyperkeratosis and depigmentation in this case could be explained by the chronicity of the disease that may worsen the already existing ones due to inflammation and keratinization abnormalities. Footpad erosion and/or ulceration albeit rarely reported [20, 23] was present in all four limbs and obviously was the cause of the intermittent lameness witnessed.

Therapy applied in this patient with either fluconazole alone or combination of AMB and itraconazole proved effective only for footpad lesions but not for skin nodules. Surgical excision of the nodules was not initially attempted because of their multifocal distribution mainly on the distal extremities. It was estimated that systemic therapy would probably reduce both the size and the number of nodules, thus facilitating their surgical removal later on. However, the systemic therapy administered seems to be ineffective for skin nodules, at least in chronic cases of canine cutaneous protothecosis.

4. Concluding Remarks

Although canine protothecosis usually presents with the disseminated form, cutaneous disease as sole clinical manifestation of the infection may also be witnessed.

Systemic therapy seems to be ineffective for skin nodules, at least in chronic cases of canine cutaneous protothecosis.

Conflict of Interests

None of the authors of this paper has a financial or personal relationship with other people or organizations that could inappropriately influence or bias the content of the paper.

Acknowledgments

The authors would like to thank Miss Bimba and Mrs. Vassalou for technical assistance.

References

[1] B. M. Pressler, "Prototothecosis and chlorellosis," in *Infectious Diseases of the Dog and Cat*, pp. 696–701, W. B. Saunders, Philadelphia, Pa, USA, 4th edition, 2013.

[2] V. J. Stenner, B. MacKay, T. King et al., "Prototothecosis in 17 Australian dogs and a review of the canine literature," *Medical Mycology*, vol. 45, no. 3, pp. 249–266, 2007.

[3] J. B. Thomas and N. Preston, "Generalised prototothecosis in a collie dog," *Australian veterinary journal*, vol. 67, no. 1, pp. 25–27, 1990.

[4] T. S. Rallis, D. Tontis, K. K. Adamama-Moraitou, M. E. Mylonakis, and L. G. Papazoglou, "Prototothecal colitis in a German Shepherd Dog," *Australian Veterinary Journal*, vol. 80, no. 7, pp. 406–408, 2002.

[5] A. E. Schultze, R. D. Ring, R. V. Morgan, and C. S. Patton, "Clinical, cytologic and histopathologic manifestations of prototothecosis in two dogs," *Veterinary Ophthalmology*, vol. 1, no. 4, pp. 239–243, 1998.

[6] J. R. Blogg and J. E. Sykes, "Sudden blindness associated with prototothecosis in a dog," *Australian Veterinary Journal*, vol. 72, no. 4, pp. 147–149, 1995.

[7] C. Font, J. Mascort, M. Márquez et al., "Paraparesis as initial manifestation of a *Prototheca zopfii* infection in a dog," *Journal of Small Animal Practice*, vol. 55, no. 5, pp. 283–286, 2014.

[8] M. Young, W. Bush, M. Sanchez, P. Gavin, and M. Williams, "Serial MRI and CSF analysis in a dog treated with intrathecal Amphotericin B for prototothecosis," *Journal of the American Animal Hospital Association*, vol. 48, no. 2, pp. 125–131, 2012.

[9] C. Salvadori, G. Gandini, A. Ballarini, and C. Cantile, "Prototothecal granulomatous meningoencephalitis in a dog," *Journal of Small Animal Practice*, vol. 49, no. 10, pp. 531–535, 2008.

[10] L. V. Lane, J. H. Meinkoth, J. Brunker et al., "Disseminated prototothecosis diagnosed by evaluation of CSF in a dog," *Veterinary Clinical Pathology*, vol. 41, no. 1, pp. 147–152, 2012.

[11] B. M. Pressler, J. L. Gookin, J. E. Sykes, A. M. Wolf, and S. L. Vaden, "Urinary tract manifestations of prototothecosis in dogs," *Journal of Veterinary Internal Medicine*, vol. 19, no. 1, pp. 115–119, 2005.

[12] M. N. Saridomichelakis and A. F. Koutinas, "Cutaneous involvement in canine leishmaniosis due to *Leishmania infantum* (syn. L. chagasi)," *Veterinary Dermatology*, vol. 25, no. 2, pp. 61–e22, 2014.

[13] G. S. Sandhu, B. C. Kline, L. Stockman, and G. D. Roberts, "Molecular probes for diagnosis of fungal infections," *Journal of Clinical Microbiology*, vol. 33, no. 11, pp. 2913–2919, 1995.

[14] R. Malik, A. J. Craig, I. Wigney, P. Martin, and D. N. Love, "Combination chemotherapy of canine and feline cryptococcosis using subcutaneously administered amphotericin B," *Australian Veterinary Journal*, vol. 73, no. 4, pp. 124–128, 1996.

[15] D. Thiele and A. Bergmann, "Prototothecosis in human medicine," *International Journal of Hygiene and Environmental Health*, vol. 204, no. 5-6, pp. 297–302, 2002.

[16] L. G. Corbellini, D. Driemeier, C. Cruz, M. M. Dias, and L. Ferreiro, "Bovine mastitis due to *Prototheca zopfii*: clinical, epidemiological and pathological aspects in a Brazilian dairy herd," *Tropical Animal Health and Production*, vol. 33, no. 6, pp. 463–470, 2001.

[17] J. E. Dillberger, B. Homer, D. Daubert, and N. H. Altman, "Prototothecosis in two cats," *Journal of the American Veterinary Medical Association*, vol. 192, no. 11, pp. 1557–1559, 1988.

[18] E. Bottero, E. Mercuriali, F. Abramo, B. Dedola, V. Martella, and E. Zini, "Fatal prototothecosis in four dogs with large bowel disease in Italy," *Veterinary Medicine Austria*, vol. 103, pp. 1–53, 2016.

[19] C. R. O'Brien, M. B. Krockenberger, D. I. Wigney, P. Martin, and R. Malik, "Retrospective study of feline and canine cryptococcosis in Australia from 1981 to 2001: 195 cases," *Medical Mycology*, vol. 42, no. 5, pp. 449–460, 2004.

[20] A. F. Koutinas, D. W. Scott, V. Kontos, and S. Lekkas, "Skin lesions in canine leishmaniasis (Kala-Azar): a clinical and histopathological study on 22 spontaneous cases in Greece," *Veterinary Dermatology*, vol. 3, no. 3, pp. 121–130, 1992.

[21] D. Santoro, M. Prisco, and P. Ciaramella, "Cutaneous sterile granulomas/pyogranulomas, leishmaniasis and mycobacterial infections," *Journal of Small Animal Practice*, vol. 49, no. 11, pp. 552–561, 2008.

[22] W. H. Miller, C. G. Griffin, and K. L. Campbell, "Prototothecosis," in *Small Animal Dermatology*, pp. 272–273, W. B. Saunders, Philadelphia, Pa, USA, 7th edition, 2013.

[23] A. Diesel, D. Liska, K. Russel, H. Minard, S. Lawhon, and A. Rodrigues-Hoffman, "Chronic cutaneous prototothecosis in a dog," in *Proceedings of the North American Veterinary Dermatology Forum*, vol. 25, p. 151, Phoenix, Ariz, USA, April 2014.

29

Cyclooxygenase Inhibitor Associated with Carboplatin in Treatment of Metastatic Nasal Carcinoma in Dog

Carlos Eduardo Fonseca-Alves,[1] **Aline Gonçalves Corrêa,**[1]
Fabiana Elias,[2] **and Sabryna Gouveia Calazans**[3]

[1] Department of Veterinary Clinic, School of Veterinary Medicine and Animal Science, Universidade Estadual Paulista, Botucatu, SP, Brazil
[2] Department of Veterinary Medicine, Federal University of Southern Border, Realeza, PR, Brazil
[3] Department of Veterinary Medicine, University of Franca, Franca, SP, Brazil

Correspondence should be addressed to Carlos Eduardo Fonseca-Alves; carloseduardofa@hotmail.com

Academic Editors: C. Hyun, C. M. Loiacono, and M. T. Mandara

A 10-year-old, intact male, pinscher was presented with unilateral bloodstained nasal discharge, sneezing, dyspnea, zygomatic arch deformity, submandibular lymph node increase, blindness in right eye, and exophthalmia. After clinical examination, it was found that the animal presented with upper respiratory tract dyspnea origin, possibly caused by an obstructive process. Complete blood count (CBC), ocular ultrasonography, thoracic radiographs, mandibular lymph node, and nasal sinus fine needle aspiration were performed. The right mandibular lymph node excisional biopsy was conducted and a tumor sample was obtained through the nasal fistula at hard palate. The material was processed, paraffin embedded, sectioned, and stained with hematoxylin and eosin. Immunohistochemical staining for cytokeratin (AE1/AE3), vimentin, and COX-2 was performed. After histopathological evaluation nasal carcinoma diagnosis was obtained. Chemotherapy was established with carboplatin 300 mg/m^2 intravenously— four cycles with intervals of 21 days—and firocoxib 5 mg/kg orally every 24 hours for 7 months. After 7 months the treatment started, the animal presented with ataxia, vocalization, hyperesthesia, and anorexia. Due the clinical condition presented, the animal owner opted for performing euthanasia. The chemotherapy protocol was effective causing the disease stagnation, minimizing the clinical signs, and extending patient survival and quality of life.

1. Introduction

Nasal tumors are uncommon and represent approximately 2% of all tumors in dogs [1]. Distant metastasis are rarely observed and when occur, prognosis is poor [2]. Older dogs have increased risk for nasal tumors, but it has been observed in dogs younger than six months to greater than 16 years old [3]. Nasal tumors are usually malignant and local invasion is common, with secondary extension to paranasal sinuses [4]. Clinical signs include unilateral or bilateral bloodstained discharge, dyspnea, facial deformity, and exophthalmos. In cases of cranial involvement, tumor can also cause neurological signs, especially seizures, but it only occurs in 20% of cases [5]. In these cases, the animal may present with pain, head pressing against the obstacles, and behavioral changes such as aggressiveness [6, 7]. Nasal tumor histopathological

evaluation is essential to establish the definitive diagnosis and computerized tomography is important for tumors extension evaluation in the nasal cavity [6]. The clinical stage is based on the tumor's size (T), in the World Health Organization (WHO) and TNM (tumor, node, and metastasis) classification system. Tumor staging can be based on skull radiographs or computerized tomography, thoracic radiographs, fine-needle aspiration, and cytological examination of enlarged palpably lymph nodes. The in vitro studies have demonstrated the possible role of cyclooxygenase (COX) inhibitor as a single agent to prevent the occurrence of tumors. Recent studies in spontaneous canine tumors and experimentally induced mouse tumors have shown that COX-2 inhibitors have antitumor and chemopreventive effects in several different types of cancer. However, no prospective studies evaluating the efficacy of COX-2 inhibitors drugs in cases of nasal carcinomas were conducted. The mechanisms by which COX inhibitors exert their antitumor effects are not completely understood, but studies have shown that COX-2-derived prostaglandins contribute to tumor cell resistance to apoptosis, new blood vessel formation, and tumor cell proliferation [8]. This paper reports clinical approach and describes a chemotherapy protocol in a dog with a primary nasal carcinoma presenting pulmonary and regional lymph node metastasis.

2. Case Report

A 10-year-old, intact male dog, pinscher was presented with unilateral nasal bloodstained discharge, sneezing, dyspnea, zygomatic arch deformity, submandibular lymph node increased, loss of vision in right eye, and exophthalmos. Physical examination revealed hard palate and oronasal fistula commitment. The animal has been presenting these clinical signs for three months and it was previously treated with amoxicillin 20 mg/kg, PO, BID, and prednisone 1 mg/kg, PO, BID. After clinical examination it was found that dyspnea origin was from the upper respiratory tract, possibly caused by an obstructive process. Submandibular lymph node cytological evaluation showed polyhedral shaped cells with oval to elongated nucleus with evident nucleoli; the cytoplasm was basophilic and well defined. There were intense anisocytosis, anisokaryosis, multinucleated giant cells, macrophages, and few lymphocytes, suggesting an epithelial tumor metastasis. Ocular ultrasound revealed a hypoechoic structure with uniform texture and irregular contours in retrobulbar space. The chest thoracic radiographs showed nodular interstitial pattern, suggestive of pulmonary metastasis. The skull radiographic evaluation revealed widespread loss of the shells details and small radiolucent areas on increased radiopacity areas. Excisional biopsy was performed on the right mandibular lymph node and the tumor sample was obtained through the nasal fistula at hard palate. Due to the limitation to surgically access of the chest, lung nodules biopsies were not performed. Material was processed, paraffin embedded, sectioned, and stained with hematoxylin and eosin. Histological evaluation of the nasal tumor revealed proliferation of round cells with oval and round nucleus, dispersed chromatin, prominent nucleoli, and bounded eosinophilic cytoplasm. These cells were arranged in palisades forming islands or robes. The tumor histopathology was compatible with the basal cell carcinoma (Figure 1), and metastasis with the same histological pattern of the primary tumor was detected in the submandibular lymph node. Immunohistochemical staining for cytokeratin antibody to confirm the diagnosis of carcinoma and COX-2 antibody to assess the expression of the primary tumor and lymph node metastasis was performed. Immunohistochemical staining was performed using peroxidase method and DAB. Slides were dewaxed in xylol and rehydrated in graded ethanol. For antigen retrieval, the slides were incubated in citrate buffer (pH 6.0) for 30 s in a pressure cooker (Pascal; Dako, Carpinteria, CA, USA). The sections were treated with freshly prepared 3% hydrogen peroxide in absolute methanol for 20 min to inhibit endogenous peroxidase activity and washed in Tris-buffer saline. Three primary antibodies were used: AE1/AE3 (monoclonal mouse,

Neomarkers, Fremont, CA, USA), vimentin (polyclonal mouse, Abcam, Cambridge, UK), and COX-2 (monoclonal mouse, Dako, Carpenteria, CA, USA), applied at dilutions of 1:50, 1:50, and 1:50, respectively, at 4°C temperature overnight. A signal amplification system with enzyme labeled polymer conjugated to a dual secondary antibody (Dako Envision System, Dako, Carpenteria, CA, USA) was used for AE1/AE3 and vimentin antibodies. For COX-2 antibody a similar signal amplification system (Advance, Dako, Carpenteria, CA, USA) was used. After each step in the process the slides were rinsed with Tris-buffered saline. The slides were developed with 3'-diaminobenzidine tetrahydrochloride (DAB, Dako, Carpenteria, CA, USA) for 5 min and counterstained with Harris haematoxylin. Positive and negative controls were performed for all antibodies by omitting the primary antibody and substituting with Tris-buffered saline. Positive stain for cytokeratin antibody in primary nasal tumor (Figure 2) and lymph node metastasis (Figure 3) and negative stain for vimentin antibody and strong expression of COX-2 protein in primary nasal tumor (Figure 4) and lymph node metastasis were found. Due to high expression of COX-2 in the primary tumor, it was decided to introduce the COX-2 inhibitors in the treatment protocol. Clinical staging of patient was conducted before start the chemotherapy protocol. The patient presented clinical stage T3N1M1 in accordance with WHO and stage T3 in accordance with Owen [7]. Chemotherapy with carboplatin 300 mg/m^2 intravenously—four cycles with intervals of 21 days—and firocoxib 5 mg/kg orally every 24 hours for 7 consecutive months were established. To evaluate the chemotherapy and COX-2 inhibitor treatment side effects, clinical and laboratory examinations (serum biochemistry and CBC) were carried out every 21 days. The patient presented no adverse effects. After the second chemotherapy cycle, the patient presented no more dyspnea, however, still presented unilateral bloody nasal discharge. After 7 months, the animal started with ataxia, vocalization, hyperesthesia, and anorexia. Due to the clinical condition presented, the animal owner requested euthanasia. Necropsy was performed and presence of a tumor in the nasal cavity was found, affecting palate, paranasal sinus, and retrobulbar space with optic nerve involvement, causing compression of the central nervous system. The lung parenchyma presented some nodules suggestive of metastasis. Fragments of lung nodules, sinus, and retrobulbar space were collected for histopathology. The histopathological analysis of specimens collected at necropsy confirmed the diagnosis obtained with biopsies performed previously and confirmed the presence of pulmonary metastases of nasal carcinoma. We performed immunohistochemical staining for COX-2 antibody of primary nasal tumor after treatment with carboplatin and COX-2 inhibitor. Immunohistochemistry showed low expression for the protein COX-2 (Figure 5).

3. Discussion

Some papers in the literature evaluated COX-2 expression in canine tumors, but few papers evaluated the expression of this specific protein associated with treatment using

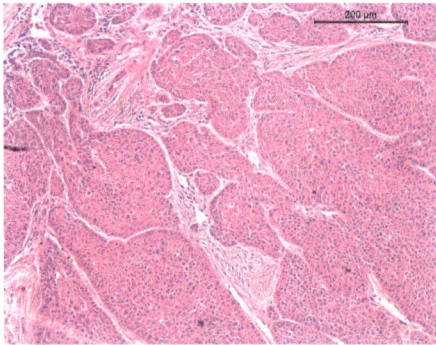

FIGURE 1: Histopathological appearance of of the canine nasal carcinoma. Note the proliferation of epithelial cells. Note moderate cellular pleomorphism. Hematoxylin and eosin (HE). Bar = 200 μm.

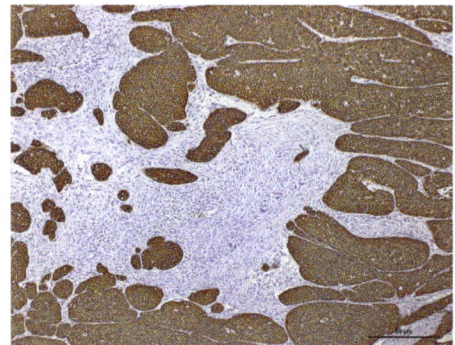

FIGURE 3: Immunolocalization of AE1/AE3 in lymph node metastasis of nasal carcinoma. Positive signal can be observed as the brown color in the cytoplasm of the cells or in the cytoplasm with hematoxylin counterstain. Bar = 50 μm.

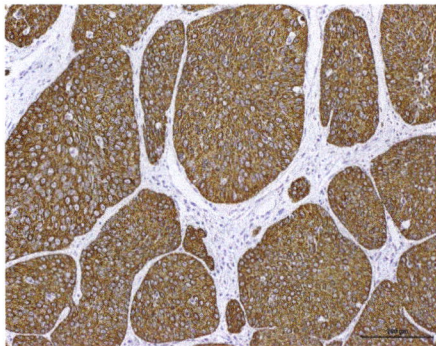

FIGURE 2: Immunolocalization of AE1/AE3 in nasal carcinoma. Positive signal can be observed as the brown color in the cytoplasm of the cells or in the cytoplasm with hematoxylin counterstain. Bar = 200 μm.

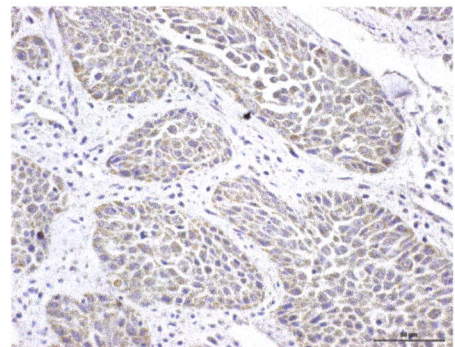

FIGURE 4: Immunolocalization of COX-2 in nasal carcinoma before treatment. Positive signal can be observed as the brown color in the cytoplasm of the cells or in the cytoplasm with hematoxylin counterstain. Bar = 50 μm.

COX-2 inhibitor. The immunohistochemistry found that the primary tumor and lymph node metastasis showed high expression of COX-2. Overexpression of COX-2 has been demonstrated in various canine neoplasms. Rassnick et al. [9] and Borzacchiello et al. [10] provided evidence of similar overexpression in canine nasal carcinomas. Recent studies in rodents, dogs, and humans indicated that COX-2 inhibitors may have chemopreventive and antitumor activity [10]. There is also evidence that COX-2 may increase tumor invasiveness and metastasis and this is important in angiogenic factors production [4].

The prognosis for dogs with nasal carcinomas that did not receive treatment other than palliative medications is poor [2]. Nasal carcinoma is uncommon in dogs and treatment is both difficult and controversial. The median survival time is 3.1 months, and the probability of surviving up to 1 and 2 years after diagnosis was only 12% and 2%, respectively [9]. Vanherberghen et al. [2] considered epistaxis as a poor prognosis; once the dogs had epistaxis at the time of diagnosis, the survival time was 88 days. Radiotherapy is the treatment that provides longer survival for these patients. Median survival times for dogs treated with radiation therapy range from 7.4 to 47.7 months. In this case the association between firocoxib

and carboplatin presented a survival rate closer to that one found in dogs treated with radiotherapy [11].

Based on studies that many different carcinomas express COX-2 and present increased PGE2 levels, COX-2 blockade has become an important component in antineoplastic therapy [12]. It is known that COX-2 may contribute to tumor aggressiveness by suppressing apoptosis, promoting angiogenesis and tumor invasion, and by tumor cell proliferation stimulation. Based on progression of epithelial tumor in humans, COX-2 showed a potentially powerful impact factor; therefore, COX-2 inhibition in canine tumors can be considered a strategy to improve outcome disease. The use of selective COX-2 inhibitors, could improve a variety of canine tumors response. However, tumors primarily treated with radiation therapy, as selective COX-2 inhibitors have been shown to improve the irradiation effect [13].

Despite the negative prognostic factors, after chemotherapy antineoplastic associated with nonsteroidal anti-inflammatory therapy the animal presented remission of clinical signs. In another study cisplatin combined with COX-2 inhibitors has been examined in many tumors. In transitional cell carcinoma, this combination increased the apoptotic index and demonstrated a positive effect on survival [14].

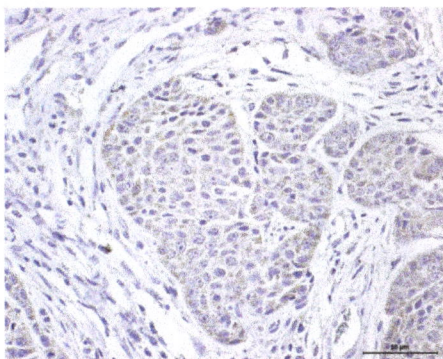

FIGURE 5: Immunolocalization of COX-2 in nasal carcinoma after treatment. Positive signal can be observed as the brown color in the cytoplasm of the cells or in the cytoplasm with hematoxylin counterstain. Bar = 50 μm.

Sorenmo et al. [12] evaluated the effect of carprofen or piroxicam administration in dogs with prostatic carcinoma. The authors found that COX-2 inhibitors associated with carboplatine use can offer positive effects on median survival times. Untreated dogs had a median survival time of 0.7 months with poor prognosis and treated dogs had a median survival time of 6.9 months, demonstrating the efficacy of COX-2 inhibitors.

4. Conclusion

The chemotherapy protocol used was effective providing the disease stagnation, minimizing the clinical signs, and increasing patient survival and quality of life.

Conflict of Interests

The authors report no conflict of interests. The authors alone are responsible for the content and writing of the paper.

References

[1] F. Millanta, S. Citi, D. Della Santa, M. Porciani, and A. Poli, "COX-2 expression in canine and feline invasive mammary carcinomas: correlation with clinicopathological features and prognostic fmolecular markers," Breast Cancer Research and Treatment, vol. 98, no. 1, pp. 115–120, 2006.

[2] M. Vanherberghen, M. J. Day, F. Delvaux, A. Gabriel, C. Clercx, and D. Peeters, "An immunohistochemical study of the inflammatory infiltrate associated with nasal carcinoma in dogs and cats," Journal of Comparative Pathology, vol. 141, no. 1, pp. 17–26, 2009.

[3] D. W. Wilson and D. L. Dungworth, "Tumors of the respiratory tract," in Tumors of Domestic Animals, D. J. Meuten, Ed., pp. 365–377, Iowa State Press, Ames, Iowa, USA, 2002.

[4] J. C. Woodard, "The respiratory system," in Veterinary Pathology, T. C. Jones, R. D. Hunt, and N. W. King, Eds., pp. 947–973, Williams & Wilkins, Baltimore, Md, USA, 6th edition, 1996.

[5] L. W. C. Chow, W. T. Y. Loo, and M. Toi, "Current directions for COX-2 inhibition in breast cancer," Biomedicine & Pharmacotherapy, vol. 59, supplement 2, pp. S281–S284, 2005.

[6] F. Ninomiya, S. Suzuki, H. Tanaka, S. Hayashi, K. Ozaki, and I. Narama, "Nasal and paranasal adenocarcinomas with neuroendocrine differentiation in dogs," Veterinary Pathology, vol. 45, no. 2, pp. 181–187, 2008.

[7] L. N. Owen, TNM Classification of Tumors in Domestic Animals, vol. 149, World Health Organization, Geneva, Switzerland edition, 1980.

[8] S. I. Mohammed, P. F. Bennett, B. A. Craig et al., "Effects of the cyclooxygenase inhibitor, piroxicam, on tumor response, apoptosis, and angiogenesis in a canine model of human invasive urinary bladder cancer," Cancer Research, vol. 62, no. 2, pp. 356–358, 2002.

[9] K. M. Rassnick, C. E. Goldkamp, H. N. Erb et al., "Evaluation of factors associated with survival in dogs with untreated nasal carcinomas: 139 cases (1993–2003)," Journal of the American Veterinary Medical Association, vol. 229, no. 3, pp. 401–406, 2006.

[10] G. Borzacchiello, O. Paciello, and S. Papparella, "Expression of cyclooxygenase-1 and -2 in canine nasal carcinomas," Journal of Comparative Pathology, vol. 131, no. 1, pp. 70–76, 2004.

[11] C. J. Henry, W. G. Brewer Jr., J. W. Tyler et al., "Survival in dogs with nasal adenocarcinoma: 64 cases (1981–1995)," Journal of Veterinary Internal Medicine, vol. 12, no. 6, pp. 436–439, 1998.

[12] K. U. Sorenmo, M. H. Goldschmidt, F. S. Shofer, C. Goldcamp, and J. Ferracone, "Evaluation of cyclooxygenase-1 and cyclooxygenase-2 expression and the effect of cyclooxygenase inhibitors in canine prostatic carcinoma," Veterinary and Comparative Oncology, vol. 2, no. 1, pp. 13–23, 2004.

[13] C. Petersen, S. Petersen, L. Milas, F. F. Lang, and P. J. Tofilon, "Enhancement of intrinsic tumor cell radiosensitivity induced by a selective cyclooxygenase-2 inhibitor," Clinical Cancer Research, vol. 6, no. 6, pp. 2513–2520, 2000.

[14] S. I. Mohammed, B. A. Craig, A. J. Mutsaers et al., "Effects of the cyclooxygenase inhibitor, piroxicam, in combination with chemotherapy on tumor response, apoptosis, and angiogenesis in a canine model of human invasive urinary bladder cancer," Molecular Cancer Therapeutics, vol. 2, no. 2, pp. 183–188, 2003.

30

Perivascular Wall Tumor in the Brain of a Dog

Margaret Cohn-Urbach,[1] **Annie Chen,**[1] **Gary Haldorson,**[2] **and Stephanie Thomovsky**[3]

[1]*Department of Veterinary Clinical Sciences, College of Veterinary Medicine, Washington State University, P.O. Box 647010, Pullman, WA 99164-7010, USA*

[2]*Department of Veterinary Microbiology and Pathology, College of Veterinary Medicine, Washington State University, P.O. Box 647040, Pullman, WA 99164-7040, USA*

[3]*Department of Veterinary Clinical Sciences, College of Veterinary Medicine, Purdue University, 625 Harrison Street, West Lafayette, IN 47907-2026, USA*

Correspondence should be addressed to Annie Chen; avchen@vetmed.wsu.edu

Academic Editor: Changbaig Hyun

A 9-year-old spayed female German shepherd mixed-breed dog presented for seizures. Magnetic resonance imaging revealed an irregularly marginated intraparenchymal cerebral mass. Microscopic examination of brain tissue collected postmortem demonstrated perivascular whorling and interwoven bundles of spindle-shaped cells. On immunohistochemistry, the tumor cells tested positive for vimentin and negative for factor VIII-related antigen, CD18, CD45, CD3, CD20, GFAP, S-100, and desmin. Immunohistochemistry results, in combination with histopathologic morphology, were suggestive of a perivascular wall tumor. To the authors' knowledge, this is the first case report to utilize both histopathology and immunohistochemistry to describe a perivascular wall tumor in the brain of a dog.

1. Introduction

Canine perivascular wall tumors are a group of soft tissue sarcomas that arise from structural and supportive cells of the vascular wall [1]. Prior to a report in 2007, the term hemangiopericytoma was widely used to describe all canine perivascular wall tumors [2]. As these tumors may have a range of histologic origins other than the pericyte, the broader term of "perivascular wall tumor" has been suggested [2]. The group encompasses tumors derived from various types of vascular mural cells excluding endothelial cells [2]. The cell of origin of the tumor includes the pericyte, myopericyte, myofibroblast, smooth muscle cell, and fibroblast [2]. Specific types of canine perivascular wall tumors include hemangiopericytoma, myopericytoma, angiomyofibroblastoma, angioleiomyoma, and angiofibroma [2]. When citing references on canine hemangiopericytomas in the following report, the authors infer that this information is also applicable to perivascular wall tumors. Since these tumors are described as a morphologic continuum, they can be difficult to subtype [1]. Utilization of an extensive panel

of immunohistochemical markers has been described, in an attempt to subtype canine perivascular wall tumors based on human subclassification schemes [2].

Canine hemangiopericytomas have traditionally been recognized histologically by the presence of whorls of spindle-shaped cells arranged in concentric layers around blood vessels [3]. However, canine perivascular wall tumors can show other histologic patterns such as bundles [2]. Hemangiopericytomas and other perivascular wall tumors most commonly occur in the skin and subcutis of dogs [4, 5]. However, there have been reports of primary hemangiopericytomas and perivascular wall tumors in the lung [6], orbit [7], spleen [8], pelvic cavity [9], mesentery [10], nasal cavity [11], frontal sinus [12], and nasopharynx of dogs [13].

To the authors' knowledge, this is the first case report written in the English language describing a perivascular wall tumor in the brain of a dog or any other nonhuman species. The diagnosis was made utilizing histological appearance combined with immunohistochemistry. A previous case report, written in Polish, describes a hemangiopericytoma in the brain of a dog [14]. However, in that paper the diagnosis was based solely on histopathological characteristics; immunohistochemistry was not performed [14].

2. Case Presentation

A 9-year-old spayed female German shepherd mixed-breed dog presented to Washington State University (WSU) Veterinary Teaching Hospital for an acute onset of seizures. Three generalized seizures had occurred 2.5 weeks prior to referral to the veterinary teaching hospital. A complete blood count and chemistry profile showed no significant findings. The patient was prescribed phenobarbital (2.3 mg/kg orally every 12 hours). Upon presentation to WSU, physical and neurologic examinations were normal; no abnormalities were detected on urinalysis or thoracic radiographs.

Magnetic resonance (MR) imaging by use of a 1.0 Tesla magnet (Philips Gyroscan, Philips Medical Systems, Andover, Massachusetts, USA) revealed an irregularly marginated intraparenchymal mass located within the right piriform lobe. The mass measured 1.5 × 1.3 cm in diameter. On T1-weighted images obtained following the intravenous administration of gadolinium DTPA-dimeglumine (Magnevist, Bayer Healthcare Pharmaceuticals, Wayne, New Jersey, USA), the lesion had heterogeneous contrast enhancement (Figure 1). There was significant parenchymal hyperintensity involving both the white and the gray matter on both T2-weighted and Fluid Attenuated Inversion Recovery (FLAIR) imaging, suggestive of perilesional edema (Figure 2). A mass effect was also observed at the level of the interthalamic adhesion resulting in compression of the right lateral ventricle, in addition to the right rostral and caudal colliculi. The major differentials for this lesion included neoplasia versus an inflammatory lesion.

Analysis of cerebrospinal fluid (CSF) collected at the atlantooccipital site revealed an elevated microprotein level of 104.5 mg/dL (reference range < 30 mg/dL) with a normal cell count of 1 nucleated cell/μL (reference range < 5 cells/μL). CSF cytology results were normal with very rare lymphocytes and erythrocytes observed. Prednisone (0.5 mg/kg orally every 12 hours), fluconazole (4 mg/kg orally every 12 hours), trimethoprim sulfamethoxazole (10 mg/kg orally every 12 hours), and clindamycin (11 mg/kg orally every 12 hours) were commenced while awaiting the results of infectious disease testing. Negative results were obtained on bacterial and fungal cultures of CSF and urine and fungal and protozoal blood and CSF titers. This included the failure to detect *Coccidioides*, *Histoplasma*, *Blastomyces*, and *Aspergillus* antibodies in serum by immunodiffusion, *Cryptococcus neoformans* antigen in serum by latex *Cryptococcus* agglutination, *Toxoplasma gondii* antibody in serum and CSF by enzyme-linked immunosorbent assay (ELISA), and *Neospora caninum* antibody in serum and CSF by immunofluorescence assay (IFA).

A brain biopsy was performed using a modified Brainsight stereotactic system as previously described [15]. Microscopic examination was suggestive of a perivascular wall tumor with prominent perivascular whorling of spindle-shaped cells. Due to the whorling pattern of the cells,

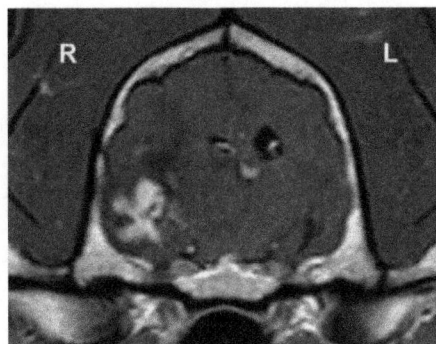

FIGURE 1: T1-weighted postcontrast transverse MR image of the brain at the level of the thalamus demonstrates a heterogeneous contrast-enhancing lesion in the right piriform lobe.

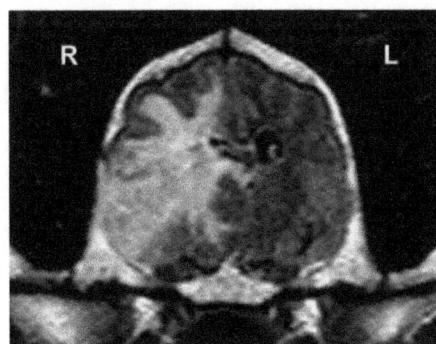

FIGURE 2: FLAIR transverse MR image of the brain at the level of the thalamus shows hyperintensity throughout the right cerebral hemisphere, most consistent with marked perilesional edema. A midline shift to the left results in compression of the right lateral ventricle and thalamus.

the diagnosis of an unusual and infiltrative meningioma was also considered.

Abdominal ultrasound performed during the initial screening process prior to MR imaging had revealed an enlarged left medial iliac lymph node. Histologic evaluation of an ultrasound guided Tru-Cut biopsy of the lymph node was consistent with a neuroendocrine carcinoma. At a later date, thoracic and abdominal computed tomography (CT) were performed with images obtained before and after contrast, in order to attempt to identify the location of the primary neuroendocrine tumor. However, no primary neuroendocrine tumor was identified via CT. CT also did not reveal any evidence of metastatic lesions arising from the primary brain tumor.

Two months following diagnostics and prior to the initiation of any specific oncologic treatment, the dog was euthanized due to acute necrotizing enteritis of unknown etiology and disseminated intravascular coagulation (DIC). Decisions regarding surgery, radiation therapy, and/or chemotherapy to address the brain tumor had been delayed pending immunohistochemical results.

A complete postmortem examination was performed. Brain tissue samples were collected and fixed in 10% neutral

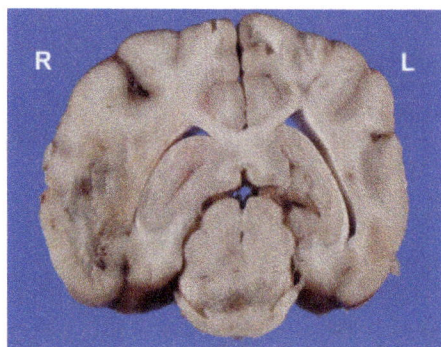

FIGURE 3: Macroscopic appearance of the cut surface of the brain at the level of the midbrain on postmortem examination. A focus of malacia is identified in the right piriform lobe.

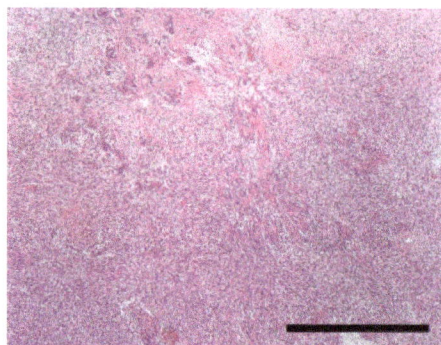

FIGURE 4: Perivascular wall tumor; right piriform lobe. The majority of the mass is comprised of spindle cells arranged in haphazardly oriented bundles. H&E ×40. Bar = 1 mm.

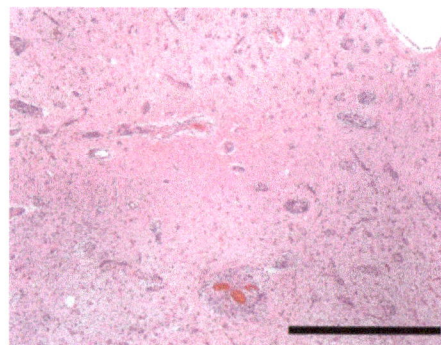

FIGURE 5: Perivascular wall tumor; right piriform lobe. The margins of the mass frequently have spindle cells predominantly arranged in whorls surrounding blood vessels infiltrating beyond the primary mass. H&E ×40. Bar = 1 mm.

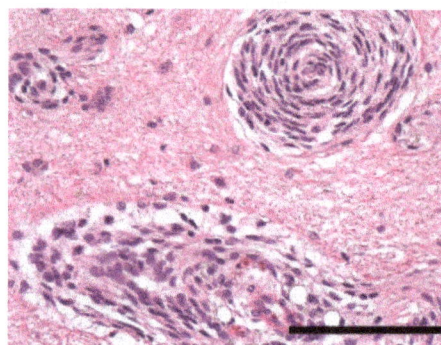

FIGURE 6: Perivascular wall tumor; right piriform lobe. Higher magnification demonstrating perivascular whorling of proliferative cells. H&E ×600. Bar = 200 μm.

buffered formalin for histopathologic examination. After fixation, an approximately $2.5 \times 2.0 \times 1.0$ cm focus of malacia involving the right piriform lobe was identified on the cut surface of the brain (Figure 3). Multifocal hemorrhages were observed within the gastric serosa, gastric and jejunal mucosa, pancreas, and mesentery. These hemorrhages were considered consistent with changes associated with DIC. The underlying cause for DIC was undetermined. In the region of the left medial iliac lymph node, there was a $5.0 \times 3.5 \times 3.0$ cm irregular, mottled tan to gray mass.

Tissue specimens were processed routinely and stained with hematoxylin and eosin for histopathologic examination. The focus of malacia in the brain was characterized microscopically by a broad area of cavitating necrosis within the neuropil in the region of the right piriform lobe. Within this focus there were severe rarefaction, mild gliosis, and infiltration of large numbers of large macrophages with foamy cytoplasm. Near the dorsal margin of this focus there was a densely cellular, poorly defined mass infiltrating the adjacent neuropil. In some regions the mass was composed primarily of interwoven bundles of spindle-shaped cells (Figure 4), while in other areas the predominant pattern was perivascular whorling of the proliferative cells (Figures 5-6). The perivascular whorls varied from three to ten cells in thickness. Nuclei of the proliferative cells varied from

round to oval in shape and from medium to large in size and had finely stippled chromatin and small nucleoli. Mitoses averaged one per five 400x fields. The malacia and proliferative tissue did not extend to the meningeal surface of the brain, and no communication of the mass with the superficial leptomeninges was evident grossly or microscopically. These microscopic findings were similar to the antemortem biopsy samples with the exception of very limited necrosis in the antemortem sample.

Microscopic examination of the left medial iliac lymph node confirmed the biopsy diagnosis of a neuroendocrine tumor. Although the tumor was suspected to be a metastatic lesion, no primary neuroendocrine tumor was identified on complete postmortem examination, which included histologic evaluation of the thyroid glands, adrenal glands, and pancreas. Additionally, no evidence of metastatic disease arising from the primary brain tumor was identified on postmortem examination.

Immunohistochemical staining was performed both on brain tissue samples collected antemortem via brain biopsy and also on postmortem tissue. Staining procedures were performed at Washington State University (Washington Animal Disease Diagnostic Laboratory) and Michigan State University (Diagnostic Center for Population and Animal

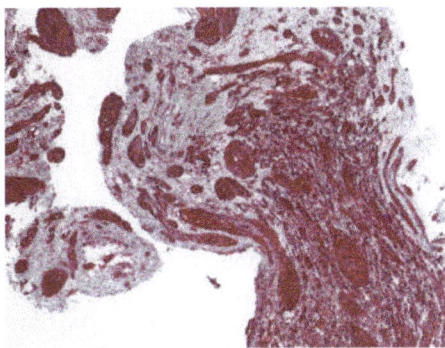

FIGURE 7: Perivascular wall tumor; right piriform lobe. The proliferative tumor cells displayed a positive reaction for vimentin.

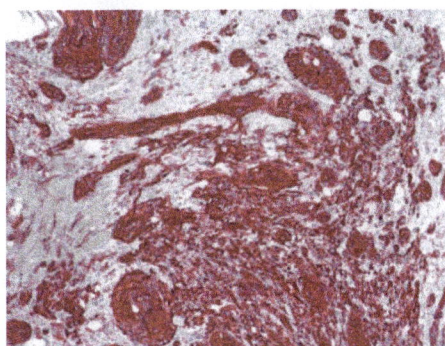

FIGURE 8: Perivascular wall tumor; right piriform lobe. The proliferative tumor cells displayed a positive reaction for vimentin.

Health). All immunohistochemistry procedures were run concurrently with positive control tissues; the test and control samples were run with positive and irrelevant negative primary antibodies.

Sections were tested with antibodies to vimentin, factor VIII-related antigen, CD3, glial fibrillary acidic protein (GFAP), S-100, desmin, synaptophysin, chromogranin A (Dako, Carpinteria, California, USA), CD18, CD45 (Leukocyte Antigen Biology Laboratory, Davis, California, USA), and CD20 (Thermo Scientific, Fremont, California, USA). The proliferative tumor cells tested positive for vimentin (Figures 7-8) and negative for factor VIII-related antigen, CD18, CD45, CD3, CD20, GFAP, S-100, synaptophysin, chromogranin A, and desmin. These immunohistochemistry results indicated that this tumor had a mesenchymal cell of origin. In combination with the histopathologic morphology, this suggested that the tumor was of perivascular wall origin.

3. Discussion

Immunohistochemistry was utilized in this case to confirm a diagnosis of perivascular wall tumor and rule out other major differentials. Positive vimentin staining demonstrated that the proliferative cells were of a mesenchymal or round cell origin [16]. Negative staining for factor VIII-related antigen and GFAP ruled out an endothelial cell of origin

(hemangiosarcoma) and astrocytic cell of origin (astrocytoma), respectively [16]. Negative staining for CD18, CD45, CD3 (T-cell), and CD20 (B-cell) ruled out a leukocytic cell of origin (histiocytic sarcoma and lymphoma) [16].

Negative staining for GFAP and S-100 made a peripheral nerve sheath tumor less likely [2]. While being rare, intracranial intraparenchymal peripheral nerve sheath tumors have been reported in dogs, without any association with cranial nerves [17]. However, the observation of spindle cells whorling around blood vessels and the prominence of the whorling pattern also were less supportive of a peripheral nerve sheath tumor [3]. Negative S-100 staining was also more suggestive of a perivascular wall tumor than a meningioma [18]. In a retrospective study of 30 canine intracranial meningiomas, 97% of the tumors were positive for S-100 [18]. In contrast, in a study of 31 canine hemangiopericytomas, all tumors stained negative for S-100 [4]. Additionally, while whorling of spindle-shaped cells around capillaries is recognized in a subset of transitional meningiomas [19], the abundance of whorling of spindle-shaped cells around larger blood vessels would be unusual for a meningioma. Combining the negative S-100 staining, prominent perivascular whorling, and lack of extension to the superficial leptomeninges, a meningioma was considered unlikely [18].

Desmin has been proposed to help in the subtyping of canine cutaneous perivascular wall tumors [2]. However, the negative result for desmin was not specific for any one type of perivascular wall tumor [2]. Synaptophysin and chromogranin A staining were also performed to investigate whether the brain tumor was related to the neuroendocrine tumor of the left medial iliac lymph node. Negative synaptophysin and chromogranin A staining confirmed that this was not a neuroendocrine tumor of the brain and that the two tumors found in the patient were unrelated.

Although canine perivascular wall tumors have only rarely been reported outside the skin and subcutis, the histopathologic appearance and immunohistochemical results of this intracranial tumor are consistent with those of canine cutaneous perivascular wall tumors [2, 4, 20]. In a study of 20 canine cutaneous perivascular wall tumors, all tumors were intensely vimentin positive and negative for CD18, factor VIII-related antigen, GFAP, and S-100 [2]. Case reports of canine hemangiopericytomas occurring outside the skin and subcutis have also stained positive for vimentin and negative for S-100 [6, 9]. As there are no specific immunohistochemical markers for perivascular wall tumors, a diagnosis is based on histopathologic appearance in combination with immunohistochemistry findings [2].

Intracranial perivascular wall tumors have been reported in humans, though they are rare [21]. Hemangiopericytomas account for less than 1% of all central nervous system tumors in humans [22]. Case reports also describe human intracranial myopericytomas and angioleiomyomas [23, 24]. However, these intracranial tumors are seen even less commonly than intracranial hemangiopericytomas in humans [23, 24]. Human myopericytomas and angioleiomyomas are most commonly seen in the subcutaneous tissues of the extremities [23, 25], a distribution similar to that of dogs. Whereas human hemangiopericytomas are also frequently seen in the extremities, the retroperitoneal region is the most common site [26]. Middle-aged adults are most frequently affected by these three types of tumors [25–27], which is comparable to the age of the canine patient in this present case report. On MRI, these intracranial tumors are most commonly extra-axial; however intra-axial locations have been reported [21, 23, 25, 28].

Surgical excision and radiation therapy have been employed as the fundamental treatment modalities for intracranial hemangiopericytomas, myopericytomas, and angioleiomyomas in humans [23, 25, 29]. Intracranial myopericytomas and angioleiomyomas show a benign clinical behavior and have a good prognosis with complete surgical resection [23, 25]. In contrast, recurrence and metastasis are commonly seen in intracranial hemangiopericytomas despite complete surgical resection and adjuvant radiation therapy [29].

Canine cutaneous perivascular wall tumors are locally invasive and occasionally recur [30] but are slow-growing and have very low metastatic potential [31]. When tumors do locally recur they are often following a long period of latency [5]. While canine cutaneous hemangiopericytomas and perivascular wall tumors are described as having low metastatic potential, reports have suggested that the presence of necrosis in hemangiopericytomas may indicate an increased potential for malignant behavior [3]. A large tumor size (>5 cm) has also been proposed as a significant prognostic indicator in canine cutaneous perivascular wall tumors [5]. Other than extensive necrosis and local invasion, this intracranial perivascular wall tumor did not demonstrate any additional features suggestive of increased malignancy. Specific subclassification of canine cutaneous perivascular wall tumors has been described by use of a large panel of immunohistochemical muscle markers [2]. However, no studies have investigated the significance of subclassification in determining prognosis in canine cutaneous perivascular wall tumors. Additionally, treatment of perivascular wall tumors is currently based on generalized recommendations for the group of soft tissue sarcomas.

In dogs, radical surgical excision has traditionally been recommended for treatment of cutaneous hemangiopericytomas [32]. Recent studies have similarly highlighted the importance of complete surgical excision in treatment of canine cutaneous perivascular wall tumors [33]. One study found that in all cases in which surgical margins for cutaneous perivascular wall tumors were complete, no recurrence was observed [33]. There has been reported success with the use of radiation therapy in cases of nonresectable soft tissue sarcomas [34]; however unfortunately no data is currently available regarding the effectiveness of radiation therapy specifically for canine perivascular wall tumors. Additionally, no veterinary studies have investigated effectiveness of surgical versus radiation treatment in dogs with perivascular wall tumors external to the skin and subcutis. In the case of intracranial tumors in dogs, wide surgical resection is often not feasible. Palliative radiotherapy and combination therapy of marginal surgical resection with radiotherapy would, therefore, be potential treatment options for perivascular wall tumors of the canine brain.

This report additionally presents a case of metastatic cancer of unknown primary, confirmed via abdominal and thoracic CT, and postmortem examination. Despite postmortem histopathologic evaluation confirming the medial iliac lymph node to be a neuroendocrine carcinoma, the primary tumor was never discovered. A retrospective study of 21 dogs with metastatic cancer of unknown primary identified carcinoma to be the most common histological type [35]. Additionally, amongst dogs in this study with carcinoma as the histological type, 67% of dogs had only a single metastatic site [35]. The median survival time for dogs with metastatic cancer of unknown primary was reported to be 30 days [35]. Survival time for the dog in this current report was 56 days following diagnosis of the left medial iliac neuroendocrine carcinoma. However, the reason for euthanasia was necrotizing enteritis, which appeared to be unrelated to the neuroendocrine carcinoma.

4. Conclusion

This case report describes a perivascular wall tumor in the brain of a dog, a tumor type that has been rarely identified in the brain of humans. While being an uncommon neoplasm, perivascular wall tumor should be considered as a differential diagnosis for an intraparenchymal cerebral mass in a dog.

Conflict of Interests

The authors declare that there is no conflict of interests regarding the publication of this paper.

References

[1] C. Palmieri, G. Avallone, M. Cimini, P. Roccabianca, D. Stefanello, and L. D. Salda, "Use of electron microscopy to classify canine perivascular wall tumors," *Veterinary Pathology*, vol. 50, no. 2, pp. 226–233, 2013.

[2] G. Avallone, P. Helmbold, M. Caniatti, D. Stefanello, R. C. Nayak, and P. Roccabianca, "The spectrum of canine cutaneous perivascular wall tumors: morphologic, phenotypic and clinical characterization," *Veterinary Pathology*, vol. 44, no. 5, pp. 607–620, 2007.

[3] M. J. Hendrick, A. E. Mahaffey, F. M. Moore, J. H. Vos, and E. J. Walder, *Histological Classification of Mesenchymal Tumors of Skin and Soft Tissues of Domestic Animals*, Armed Forces Institute of Pathology, Washington, DC, USA, 1998.

[4] M. Mazzei, F. Millanta, S. Citi, D. Lorenzi, and A. Poli, "Haemangiopericytoma: histological spectrum, immunohistochemical characterization and prognosis," *Veterinary Dermatology*, vol. 13, no. 1, pp. 15–21, 2002.

[5] D. Stefanello, G. Avallone, R. Ferrari, P. Roccabianca, and P. Boracchi, "Canine cutaneous perivascular wall tumors at first presentation: clinical behavior and prognostic factors in 55 cases," *Journal of Veterinary Internal Medicine*, vol. 25, no. 6, pp. 1398–1405, 2011.

[6] M. Vignoli, J. Buchholz, F. Morandi et al., "Primary pulmonary spindle cell tumour (haemangiopericytoma) in a dog," *Journal of Small Animal Practice*, vol. 49, no. 10, pp. 540–543, 2008.

[7] W. A. Beltran, M. A. Colle, L. Boulouha, A. Daude-Lagrave, P. Moissonnier, and B. Clerc, "A case of orbital hemangiopericytoma in a dog," *Veterinary Ophthalmology*, vol. 4, no. 4, pp. 255–259, 2001.

[8] M. J. Obwolo, "Primary splenic haemangiopericytoma in a German shepherd dog," *Journal of Comparative Pathology*, vol. 96, no. 3, pp. 285–288, 1986.

[9] H. S. Cho and N. Y. Park, "Primary haemangiopericytoma in the pelvic cavity of a dog," *Journal of Veterinary Medicine, Series A: Physiology Pathology Clinical Medicine*, vol. 53, no. 4, pp. 198–201, 2006.

[10] O. Katsuta, T. Doi, M. Yokoyama, Y. Okazaki, M. Tsuchitani, and F. Kidachi, "Vascular leiomyoma of the mesentery in a dog," *Journal of Comparative Pathology*, vol. 118, no. 2, pp. 155–161, 1998.

[11] K. E. Burgess, E. M. Green, R. D. Wood, and R. R. Dubielzig, "Angiofibroma of the nasal cavity in 13 dogs," *Veterinary and Comparative Oncology*, vol. 9, no. 4, pp. 304–309, 2011.

[12] R. M. Miller, "Angiofibroma in the frontal sinus of a dog," *Veterinary Medicine, Small Animal Clinician*, vol. 63, no. 8, pp. 772–773, 1968.

[13] J. L. Carpenter and T. A. Hamilton, "Angioleiomyoma of the nasopharynx in a dog," *Veterinary Pathology*, vol. 32, no. 6, pp. 721–723, 1995.

[14] Z. Soltysiak, S. Dzimira, and M. Nowak, "Two rare cases of brain tumors in dogs," *Medycyna Weterynaryjna*, vol. 59, pp. 221–223, 2003.

[15] A. V. Chen, F. A. Wininger, S. Frey et al., "Description and validation of a magnetic resonance imaging-guided stereotactic brain biopsy device in the dog," *Veterinary Radiology and Ultrasound*, vol. 53, no. 2, pp. 150–156, 2012.

[16] E. J. Ehrhart, D. A. Kamstock, and B. E. Powers, "The pathology of Neoplasia," in *Withrow and MacEwen's Small Animal Clinical Oncology*, S. J. Withrow, D. M. Vail, and R. L. Page, Eds., pp. 51–67, Elsevier Saunders, St. Louis, Mo, USA, 5th edition, 2013.

[17] N. Shihab, B. A. Summers, L. Benigni, A. W. McEvoy, and H. A. Volk, "Imaging diagnosis-malignant peripheral nerve sheath tumor presenting as an intra-axial brain mass in a young dog," *Veterinary Radiology and Ultrasound*, vol. 54, no. 3, pp. 278–282, 2013.

[18] P. Montoliu, S. Añor, E. Vidal, and M. Pumarola, "Histological and immunohistochemical study of 30 cases of canine meningioma," *Journal of Comparative Pathology*, vol. 135, no. 4, pp. 200–207, 2006.

[19] A. K. Patnaik, W. J. Kay, and A. I. Hurvitz, "Intracranial meningioma: a comparative pathologic study of 28 dogs," *Veterinary pathology*, vol. 23, no. 4, pp. 369–373, 1986.

[20] J. Pérez, M. J. Bautista, E. Rollón, F. C.-M. de Lara, L. Carrasco, and J. Martín De Las Mulas, "Immunohistochemical characterization of hemangiopericytomas and other spindle cell tumors in the dog," *Veterinary Pathology*, vol. 33, no. 4, pp. 391–397, 1996.

[21] P. M. Shetty, A. V. Moiyadi, and E. Sridhar, "Primary CNS hemangiopericytoma presenting as an intraparenchymal mass-case report and review of literature," *Clinical Neurology and Neurosurgery*, vol. 112, no. 3, pp. 261–264, 2010.

[22] B. L. Guthrie, M. J. Ebersold, B. W. Scheithauer, and E. G. Shaw, "Meningeal hemangiopericytoma: histopathological features, treatment, and long-term follow-up of 44 cases," *Neurosurgery*, vol. 25, no. 4, pp. 514–522, 1989.

[23] A. Rousseau, M. Kujas, R. van Effenterre et al., "Primary intracranial myopericytoma: report of three cases and review of the literature," *Neuropathology and Applied Neurobiology*, vol. 31, no. 6, pp. 641–648, 2005.

[24] S. V. Shinde, A. B. Shah, R. B. Baviskar, and J. R. Deshpande, "Primary intracranial multicentric angioleiomyomas," *Neurology India*, vol. 60, no. 1, pp. 115–117, 2012.

[25] L. Sun, Y. Zhu, and H. Wang, "Angioleiomyoma, a rare intracranial tumor: 3 case report and a literature review," *World Journal of Surgical Oncology*, vol. 12, article 216, 2014.

[26] F. R. Spitz, M. Bouvet, P. W. T. Pisters, R. E. Pollock, and B. W. Feig, "Hemangiopericytoma: a 20-year single-institution experience," *Annals of Surgical Oncology*, vol. 5, no. 4, pp. 350–355, 1998.

[27] T. Mentzel, A. P. Dei Tos, Z. Sapi, and H. Kutzner, "Myopericytoma of skin and soft tissues: clinicopathologic and immunohistochemical study of 54 cases," *The American Journal of Surgical Pathology*, vol. 30, no. 1, pp. 104–113, 2006.

[28] E. Spence, R. Chelvarajah, and C. Shieff, "Haemangiopericytoma with no dural attachment," *BMJ Case Reports*, vol. 2012, 2012.

[29] L. Chen, Y. Yang, X.-G. Yu, Q.-P. Gui, B.-N. Xu, and D.-B. Zhou, "Multimodal treatment and management strategies for intracranial hemangiopericytoma," *Journal of Clinical Neuroscience*, vol. 22, no. 4, pp. 718–725, 2015.

[30] E. Handharyani, K. Ochiai, T. Kadosawa, T. Kimura, and T. Umemura, "Canine hemangiopericytoma: an evaluation of metastatic potential," *Journal of Veterinary Diagnostic Investigation*, vol. 11, no. 5, pp. 474–478, 1999.

[31] N. A. Connery and C. R. Bellenger, "Surgical management of haemangiopericytoma involving the biceps femoris muscle in four dogs," *Journal of Small Animal Practice*, vol. 43, no. 11, pp. 497–500, 2002.

[32] J. A. McKnight, G. N. Mauldin, M. C. McEntee, K. A. Meleo, and A. K. Patnaik, "Radiation treatment for incompletely resected soft-tissue sarcomas in dogs," *Journal of the American Veterinary Medical Association*, vol. 217, no. 2, pp. 205–210, 2000.

[33] G. Avallone, P. Boracchi, D. Stefanello, R. Ferrari, A. Rebughini, and P. Roccabianca, "Canine perivascular wall tumors: high prognostic impact of site, depth, and completeness of margins," *Veterinary Pathology*, vol. 51, no. 4, pp. 713–721, 2014.

[34] T. Plavec, M. Kessler, B. Kandel, A. Schwietzer, and S. Roleff, "Palliative radiotherapy as treatment for non-resectable soft tissue sarcomas in the dog—a report of 15 cases," *Veterinary and Comparative Oncology*, vol. 4, no. 2, pp. 98–103, 2006.

[35] F. Rossi, L. Aresu, M. Vignoli et al., "Metastatic cancer of unknown primary in 21 dogs," *Veterinary and Comparative Oncology*, vol. 13, no. 1, pp. 11–19, 2015.

31

Atlantoaxial Synovial Cyst Associated with Instability in a Chihuahua

Franck Forterre,[1, 2] Núria Vizcaino Reves,[1, 3] Christina Stahl,[1, 4] Stephan Rupp,[5] and Karine Gendron[1, 4]

[1] Small Animal Clinic, Department of Clinical Veterinary Medicine, Vetsuisse Faculty, University of Berne, 3012 Berne, Switzerland
[2] Department of Neurosurgery, Vetsuisse Faculty, University of Berne, Länggassstrasse 128, 3012 Berne, Switzerland
[3] Department of Surgery, Vetsuisse Faculty, University of Berne, Länggassstrasse 128, 3012 Berne, Switzerland
[4] Department of Radiology, Vetsuisse Faculty, University of Berne, Länggassstrasse 128, 3012 Berne, Switzerland
[5] Tierklinik Hofheim, Im Langgewann 9, am Taunus, 65719 Hofheim, Germany

Correspondence should be addressed to Franck Forterre, franck.forterre@vetsuisse.unibe.ch

Academic Editors: J. Lakritz and F. Mutinelli

Objective. To describe an atlantoaxial degenerative cyst associated with instability. *Animal.* Chihuahua, male, 5 years old. *Methods.* Ever since colliding with a large dog two years prior to presentation, the dog suffered recurrent episodes of intractable cervical pain. Over time, the pain attacks increased in frequency and intensity. On presentation, pain was clinically localized to the high cervical region. No neurological deficits were observed. CT and MRI revealed an atlantoaxial degenerative articular cyst associated with instability, causing cervicomedullary compressive myelopathy. On MRI the cyst appeared hypointense in T1W and hyperintense in T2-weighted sequences, with rim enhancement. The dog was treated surgically by cyst fenestration and ventral stabilization using a 1.5 mm Butterfly Locking plate and cancellous bone graft placed within the atlantoaxial joint after cartilage removal. Histological examination of a sample of the cyst wall confirmed a degenerative articular cyst. The dog recovered uneventfully after surgery and remained pain free throughout the 2-year followup. *Conclusion.* Atlantoaxial degenerative articular cyst associated with instability is a rare finding in dogs. *Clinical Relevance.* The presence of an atlantoaxial degenerative articular cyst appears not to worsen the prognosis of instability treatment. Atlantoaxial fusion and cyst fenestration may provide good long-term results.

1. Introduction

Extradural spinal cysts occurring in dogs are relatively uncommon [1–5]. Canine spinal synovial cysts have been described in the cervical spine of large breed dogs, and at the thoracolumbar and lumbosacral junctions [1, 2, 4, 6].

Cysts associated with the atlantoaxial joint are an infrequent cause of cervicomedullary compression in humans [7] and, to the authors' knowledge, have not previously been described in dogs. The goal of the present short communication is to present a case of atlantoaxial cyst associated with instability in a dog.

2. Case History

2.1. History. A 5-year-old male Chihuahua was referred to our clinic with a suspicion of atlantoaxial instability because of recurrent cervical pain. Clinical signs had developed two years prior following a collision with a large dog. Episodes of pain had become more frequent and severe in the few months preceding the dog's presentation. No improvement was observed after an oral steroid therapy instituted by the private veterinarian.

2.2. Clinical Examination. The dog presented with a low head carriage. Physical examination, including a complete neurological examination, was otherwise normal. Pain could only be demonstrated upon gentle palpation of the high cervical region. Because of the suspected diagnosis, excessive manipulation of the neck was avoided. Based on the clinical findings, the lesion was localized in the upper cervical region. Differential diagnoses included atlantoaxial instability, cervical fracture/luxation, intervertebral disc disease, neoplasia,

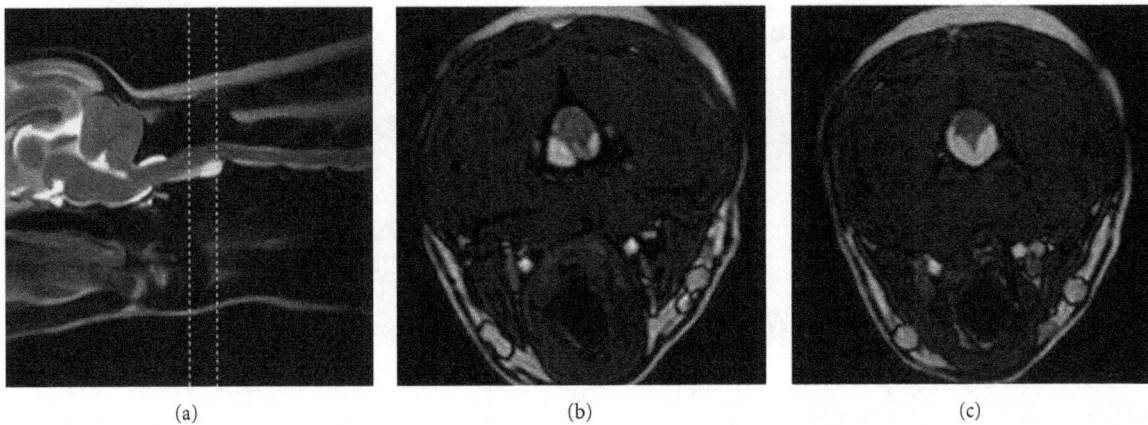

(a)   (b)   (c)

FIGURE 1: (a) Sagittal T2-weighted MR image showing a hyperintense cyst compressing the spinal cord. The vertical dotted lines indicate the level of the transverse images: middle image (cranial line) and right image (caudal line). (b) Transverse BASG at the level of the atlantoaxial joint demonstrating the cyst's origin from the right side of the atlantoaxial joint. (c) Transverse BASG at the caudal aspect of C2 showing the biconvex outline and ventral bilateral location of the cyst eliciting severe compression of the spinal cord.

inflammatory conditions (meningitis), or other conditions affecting soft tissues of the high cervical region.

Results of a blood and urine analysis were within normal limits.

Anesthesia and diagnostic imaging were performed as previously described in a prior study [8].

MRI revealed a well-circumscribed extradural space-occupying lesion extending from the area of the right atlantoaxial joint to the floor of the vertebral canal of the C2 body. The mass had a bilobed appearance and biconvex form at the C2 level, with rounded cranial and caudal borders, and compressed the spinal cord ventrally from both sides. The lesion was hypointense on T1-weighted images and markedly hyperintense on T2-weighted images. This signal suppressed in the FLAIR sequence, and an incomplete rim of contrast enhancement was present (Figure 1).

On CT, the cyst could not be visualized. An increased distance between the dens axis and the atlas, as well as an increased distance between the lamina dorsalis of the atlas and the axis were noted. Cranially to the dens axis, a small mineral dense fragment was present (Figure 2). The MRI findings, characterized by a fluid-filled lesion (with contents hypointense in T1-weighted and hyperintense in T2-weighted images) with postcontrast rim enhancement, suggested an articular cyst.

Differential diagnoses for such cystic lesions include arachnoid cysts, discal cysts, and dermoid sinus cysts, although intra- or extradural tumors and abscesses may need to be ruled out.

2.3. Surgery. A ventral midline incision and a routine approach were made at the ventral aspects of C1 to C3 [8]. A self-maintaining Gelpi retractor distracting the occipital bone and C3 allowed realignment of C1-C2. After identification of the ventral part of the atlantoaxial joint, the capsule was excised with a number 11 scalpel blade. A relatively large amount of clear synovial fluid flowed out of the joint capsule, and the remainder was aspirated. Analysis of the

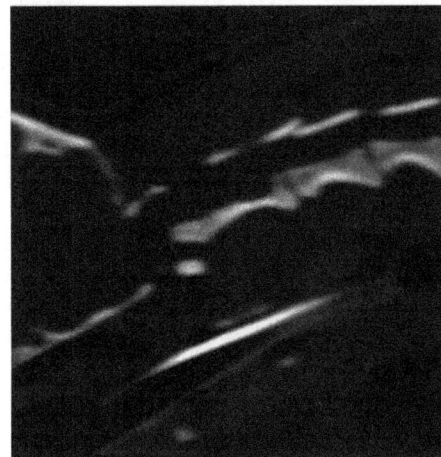

FIGURE 2: Sagittally reconstructed CT image showing the atlantoaxial subluxation and small mineral fragment cranial to the dens axis.

cyst fluid was not performed. Slight overdistraction exerted by the Gelpi retractor allowed good atlantoaxial opening and visualization of the dens, the articular cartilage and the dorsal cyst wall. The cyst wall was grasped with ophthalmic forceps and fenestration of the cyst was performed. The excised tissue sample was sent for histopathologic examination. The cartilage of the atlantoaxial joint was removed, cancellous bone was placed within the joint and the joint was stabilized with a 1.5 mm locking plate [8].

Postoperative care and followup have also been described in a previous study [8].

The dog was ambulatory tetraparetic the day after surgery. Physiotherapy, consisting in massages and coordination training, was begun on the first day after surgery. On the third day after surgery, locomotor deficits had disappeared, and the patient was discharged.

The dog was still clinically normal two years after surgery at which time a control CT was performed (Figure 3).

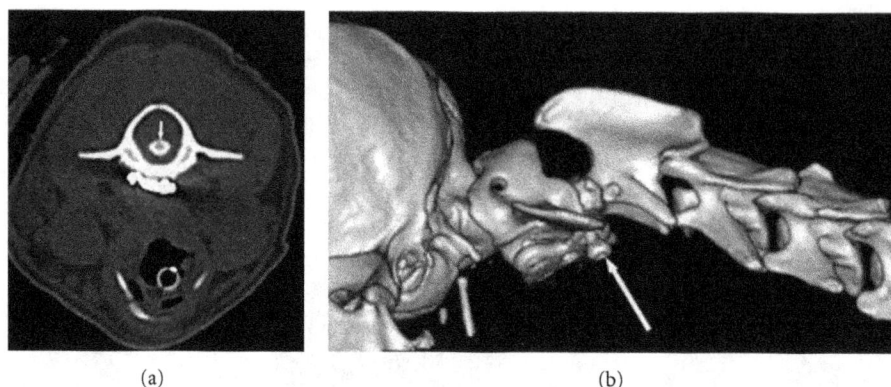

(a)   (b)

FIGURE 3: (a) Control CT scan after 2 years. The cyst appears not to have recurred; only a slight ventral cord compression elicited by the apex of the dens is visible (arrow). (b) Three-dimensional CT reconstruction showing the satisfactory positioning of the atlas and axis, and the loosening of the axial screws (arrow).

Despite loosening of the axial screws, atlantoaxial alignment had been preserved. It was not possible at this time to detect if synovial cyst had recurred, even after careful comparison between the control and the preoperative CT.

2.4. Histopathology. Tissue from the cyst wall was fixed in 10% buffered formalin, embedded in paraffin, sectioned at 5 μm, and stained with hematoxylin and eosin and Goldner's trichrome. The cyst wall was comprised of a thick layer of fibrous capsule with an inner layer of hypertrophic synoviocytes with apparent sloughing of cells into the cyst's lumen. Histopathological diagnosis was an intraspinal synovial cyst.

3. Discussion

Spinal articular cysts are a rare pathology in dogs and to the authors' knowledge have not been reported at the atlantoaxial joint until now. Approximately 30 cases have been described in the human literature [9, 10]. In people, cysts associated with the atlantoaxial joint are an infrequent cause of cervicomedullary compression [7].

The atlantoaxial articulation is a true synovial joint and is responsible for a large proportion of normal cervical mobility. The etiology of articular cysts is unclear, but they are assumed to be degenerative because minor chronic damage to articular surfaces produces a reactive proliferation of synovium or fibrocartilage that includes loculated collections of mucinous fluid [11]. Cysts may contain variable amounts of proteins, blood, or both. Pathological reports traditionally divide these cysts into two types: synovial cysts, which have an epithelial lining, and ganglion cysts, which do not. Synovial cysts are the result of synovial outpouchings through weakened capsular tissue [5]. Ganglion cysts arise from mucinous degeneration of the periarticular connective tissue [5]. Both are thought to develop secondary to degenerative joint disease. Degenerative osteoarthritic changes are frequently found at the level of the cyst, however the cyst and synovial space may be discontinuous [5]. There appears to be no significant clinical difference between these two cyst types. Although the term "juxtafacet cyst" has been used to include

both entities, the more general "spinal degenerative articular cyst" has been suggested because the atlantoaxial articulation is not a true facet [11].

In humans, synovial cysts are commonly located at the L4-L5 level of the lumbar spine. This segment experiences the greatest range of movement and is the most common site for degenerative disease. These findings may indicate that excessive stress to the facet joint is important in cyst generation [9]. We presume that a similar mechanism may be responsible for atlantoaxial cyst formation, namely, excessive stress to the atlantoaxial joint from repetitive chronic trauma associated with instability, which would lead to proliferation of synovium or fibrocartilage, and subsequent cyst formation. The same hypothesis has been formulated for atlantoaxial degenerative articular cysts in humans [9].

In the majority of cases, synovial cysts can be accurately differentiated from other lesions by their neuroanatomical location and specific MRI signal characteristics and contrast enhancement pattern. The classic appearance of a spinal synovial cyst is that of a well-defined, sharply marginated lesion adjacent to a degenerated facet joint, presenting signal intensities similar to cerebrospinal fluid (iso/hypointense on T1 and hyperintense on T2 weighted images) with peripheral rim enhancement after intravenous gadolinium administration [12]. Cysts may be isointense to CSF on T1W and T2W images if the contents are clear synovial fluid, or there may be high signal intensity on T1W images and T2W images if there is gelatinous or mucinous cyst material [5]. A communication between the synovial cyst and the facet joint can also be identified in some cases [2].

Nonetheless, a final diagnosis of atlantoaxial synovial cyst relies on histologic confirmation. Histopathologically, the cyst walls consist of fibrous or cartilaginous tissue and are usually lined with synovial epithelium, in part or along their entire surface, although this lining may be lacking in some cases [13]. Histological analysis suggests that inflammation does not play an important role in cyst formation.

In humans, various surgical approaches have proved to be equally effective in achieving adequate decompression, and in cases where cysts were incompletely removed, no ensuing complications or recurrences have been encountered [7, 11, 14]. Conservative treatment has also been described [13, 15, 16]. Furthermore, the possibility of a spontaneous regression of synovial cysts is a well-known but poorly understood phenomenon, at least in the lumbar spine [15]. One possible explanation would be a rupture of the cyst wall with leakage of the liquid content. A second and maybe more realistic possibility would be the reversal of the abnormal and prolonged microstresses applied to the joint that represent the primum movens of the cyst development [15]. In our case, the absence of clinical recurrence of the atlantoaxial degenerative articular cyst after ventral C1-C2 fusion may fit with this theory. In this paper it is surmised that the primary cause of progressive cystic degeneration was atlantoaxial instability, and stabilization of the joint may have allowed regression of the cyst. Although surgical management led to a good neurological outcome and no clinical cyst recurrence, the natural history of this atlantoaxial degenerative articular cyst remains unknown.

References

[1] C. S. H. Sale and K. C. Smith, "Extradural spinal juxtafacet (synovial) cysts in three dogs: case report," *Journal of Small Animal Practice*, vol. 48, no. 2, pp. 116–119, 2007.

[2] R. E. Levitski, A. E. Chauvet, and D. Lipsitz, "Cervical myelopathy associated with extradural synovial cysts in 4 dogs," *Journal of Veterinary Internal Medicine*, vol. 13, no. 3, pp. 181–186, 1999.

[3] B. Perez, E. Rollan, F. Ramiro, and M. Pumarola, "Intraspinal synovial cyst in a dog," *Journal of the American Animal Hospital Association*, vol. 36, no. 3, pp. 235–238, 2000.

[4] P. J. Dickinson, B. K. Sturges, W. L. Berry, K. M. Vernau, P. D. Koblik, and R. A. LeCouteur, "Extradural spinal synovial cysts in nine dogs," *Journal of Small Animal Practice*, vol. 42, no. 10, pp. 502–509, 2001.

[5] A. A. Webb, J. W. Pharr, L. J. Lew, and K. A. Tryon, "MR imaging findings in a dog with lumbar ganglion cysts," *Veterinary Radiology and Ultrasound*, vol. 42, no. 1, pp. 9–13, 2001.

[6] F. Forterre, S. Kaiser, M. Garner et al., "Synovial cysts associated with cauda equina syndrome in two dogs," *Veterinary Surgery*, vol. 35, no. 1, pp. 30–33, 2006.

[7] M. Zorzon, M. Skrap, S. Diodato, D. Nasuelli, and B. Lucci, "Cysts of the atlantoaxial joint: excellent long-term outcome after posterolateral surgical decompression. Report of two cases," *Journal of Neurosurgery*, vol. 95, supplement 1, pp. 111–114, 2001.

[8] M. Dickomeit, L. Alves, M. Pekarkova, D. Gorgas, and F. Forterre, "Use of a 1.5 mm butterfly locking plate for stabilization of atlantoaxial pathology in three toy breed dogs," *Veterinary and Comparative Orthopaedics and Traumatology*, vol. 24, no. 3, pp. 246–251, 2011.

[9] S. Marbacher, A. Lukes, I. Vajtai, and C. Ozdoba, "Surgical approach for synovial cyst of the atlantoaxial joint: a case report and review of the literature," *Spine*, vol. 34, no. 15, pp. E528–E533, 2009.

[10] J. J. Van Gompel, J. M. Morris, J. L. Kasperbauer, D. E. Graner, and W. E. Krauss, "Cystic deterioration of the C1-2 articulation: clinical implications and treatment outcomes," *Journal of Neurosurgery*, vol. 14, no. 4, pp. 437–443, 2011.

[11] B. D. Birch, A. G. Khandji, and P. C. McCormick, "Atlantoaxial degenerative articular cysts," *Journal of Neurosurgery*, vol. 85, no. 5, pp. 810–816, 1996.

[12] L. Mendes-Araújo, C. Rangel, R. C. Domingues, and E. L. Gasparetto, "Atlantoaxial synovial cyst causing isolated unilateral hypoglossal nerve paralysis," *British Journal of Radiology*, vol. 83, no. 986, pp. e35–e38, 2010.

[13] T. Sagiuchi, S. Shimizu, R. Tanaka, S. Tachibana, and K. Fujii, "Regression of an atlantoaxial degenerative articular cyst associated with subluxation during conservative treatment: case report and review of the literature," *Journal of Neurosurgery*, vol. 5, no. 2, pp. 161–164, 2006.

[14] S. Eustacchio, M. Trummer, F. Unger, and G. Flaschka, "Intraspinal synovial cyst at the craniocervical junction," *Zentralblatt fur Neurochirurgie*, vol. 64, no. 3, pp. 86–89, 2003.

[15] P. C. Cecchi, M. T. Peltz, P. Rizzo, A. Musumeci, G. Pinna, and A. Schwarz, "Conservative treatment of an atlantoaxial degenerative articular cyst: case report," *Spine Journal*, vol. 8, no. 4, pp. 687–690, 2008.

[16] O. Velán, A. Rabadán, L. Paganini, and L. Langhi, "Atlantoaxial joint synovial cyst: diagnosis and percutaneous treatment," *CardioVascular and Interventional Radiology*, vol. 31, no. 6, pp. 1219–1221, 2008.

32

Rapid Evaluation of Mutant Exon-11 in *c-kit* in a Recurrent MCT Case Using CD117 Immunocytofluorescence, FACS-Cell Sorting, and PCR

Dettachai Ketpun,[1,2] **Achariya Sailasuta,**[1] **Prapruddee Piyaviriyakul,**[2] **Nattawat Onlamoon,**[3] **and Kovit Pattanapanyasat**[3]

[1] *STAR, Molecular Biology Research on Animal Oncology, Department of Pathology, Faculty of Veterinary Science, Chulalongkorn University, Bangkok 10330, Thailand*
[2] *Biochemistry Unit, Department of Physiology, Faculty of Veterinary Science, Chulalongkorn University, Bangkok 10330, Thailand*
[3] *Office for Research and Development, Faculty of Medicine Siriraj Hospital, Mahidol University, Bangkok 10770, Thailand*

Correspondence should be addressed to Achariya Sailasuta; achariya.sa@chula.ac.th

Academic Editors: J. Lakritz, F. Mutinelli, and S. Stuen

A 13-year-old, poodle-mixed, male dog was referred to the oncology unit in our faculty's small animal teaching hospital with the problem of rapid recurrent MCT. The owner and the veterinarian would like to use a tyrosine kinase inhibitor (TKI) for the dog. Therefore, fine-needle aspiration (FNA) was performed to collect the MCT cells and these cells were submitted to our laboratory for the detection of internal-tandem-duplicated (ITD) mutation of exon-11 in *c-kit*, prior to the treatment. The aim of this paper is to demonstrate the use of combinatorial protocol for the rapid evaluation of ITD mutation in MCT cells harvested by FNA. However, there was no ITD-mutant exon-11 that had been observed in this case.

1. Introduction

Canine cutaneous mast cell tumors (MCT) are the second most skin tumors found in dogs. The incidence is probably medium to high in some breeds, such as boxer, bull dog, pug, poodle, labrador retriever, and golden retriever. In general, all MCT patients required an aggressive diagnosis and therapy because the progression of disease is very rapid [1]. Among obscured tumorigenesis of MCT, however, there has been much information from various studies showing that the mutation of exon-11, called internal-tandem-duplication (ITD), of proto-oncogene, *c-kit*, is involved in MCT formation. Principally, *c-kit* is a protein-coding gene responsible for KIT (CD117) formation and it is usually expressed in many cell species, such as normal mast cells, melanocytes, and Purkinje cells including MCT cells [2].

KIT is a member of the receptor-tyrosine-kinases class III (RTKs class III). It consists of three functioning domains,

extracellular (ectodomain), transmembrane (TM), and intracellular domains, respectively [3]. The intracellular domain is further separated into two subsidiary portions; juxtamembrane encoded by exon-11 and kinase domains encoded by the remaining exons. The function of KIT is triggered when the ectodomain binds to the specific ligand, *stem cell factor (SCF)*, followed by KIT dimerization and cross-autophosphorylation to tyrosine residues on the dimerized KITs. The consequence is to activate the downstream-signaling cascades, which are responsible for the growth and proliferation as well as antiapoptosis of mast cells. In case of MCT, ITD mutation of exon-11 results in the abnormally autonomous KIT dimerization without any specific ligand binding. This mechanism leads to uncontrollable autophosphorylation followed by MCT formation. Nevertheless, this type of mutation also affects MCT therapy when a tyrosine kinase inhibitor (TKI), such as SU-11654, is used [4]. Therefore, the detection of ITD-mutant exon-11 is clinically important for MCT diagnosis and therapeutic planning. However, a utilization of MCT cells collected by FNA for the detection of ITD-mutant exon-11 has not recently been reported anywhere.

The objective of this paper is to report the employment of CD117 immunocytofluorescence and FACS-cell sorting for rapid identification and isolation of MCT cells harvested by FNA. In addition, we also demonstrate the usage of these cells to diagnose ITD-mutant exon-11 by PCR in a recurrent MCT case.

2. Case Presentation

A 13-year-old, poodle-mixed, male dog was referred to the Oncology Clinic, Small Animal Teaching Hospital, Faculty of Veterinary Science, Chulalongkorn University, with the recurrent MCT-grade II (based on Patnaik histopathologic grading) at the neck and the dorsomedial of the left palmar (Figure 1). The dog was undertaken a surgical removal with prophylactic chemotherapy along the year. However, the treatment was ineffective and the progression of the disease was rapidly advanced. Finally, the owner and the responsible veterinarian planned to use a tyrosine kinase inhibitor (TKI) in this case. However, the owner was unwilling to repeat a skin biopsy for his dog. Hence, the previous tissue section was sent to our laboratory for histopathology reevaluation grounded on the novel 2-tier histopathologic grading system [5] and the veterinarian exploited FNA to aseptically collect the cell sample from the mass at the left palmar (Figure 1) for investigating ITD-mutant exon-11.

To identify MCT-cell population, a few drops of neoplastic cells from FNA were smeared on a clean silane-coated glass slide. The cells were then preserved in $4°C$ cold acetone for a minute and they were incubated by 1% bovine serum albumin (BSA) for 30 minutes at room temperature to block nonspecific proteins. The tumor cells were further incubated with PE-conjugated mouse monoclonal anti-human CD117 antibodies (Clone Y.B5.B8, Becton and Dickinson, USA) for 30 minutes at the concentration of $1:100$ at room temperature in a dark chamber. The specificity of the antibodies was already approved by our laboratory in our previous study. The MCT cells were counterstained by 4',6-Diamidino-2-Phenylindole (DAPI, Invitrogen, USA), and they were visualized under a fluorescent microscope with 575 nm light source. In this study, we also used normal mast cells and histiocytoma cells prepared by the same method, as the positive and negative controls, respectively.

For ITD-mutation assessment, the neoplastic cells were firstly purified using FACS-cell sorting. Briefly, the cells previously harvested by FNA were resuspended in $500\,\mu L$ sterile PBS. The erythrocytes were eradicated from the cell suspension by adding 10 mL of BD Facs lysing solution for 10 minutes (Becton and Dickinson, USA). Further, the cell suspension was centrifuged at $4,000\times g$ for 5 minutes and the supernatant was discarded after centrifugation. The cell pellet was then added by $500\,\mu L$ BD FacsPerm solution (Becton and Dickinson, USA) for 10 minutes to increase membrane permeability, and it was washed by PBS twice. The neoplastic

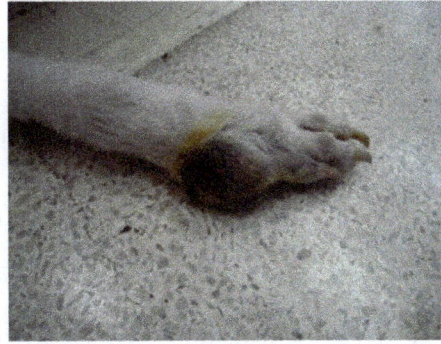

FIGURE 1: The location of MCT mass at the dorsomedial plane of the left palmar of the case in which the MCT cells were harvested from the site.

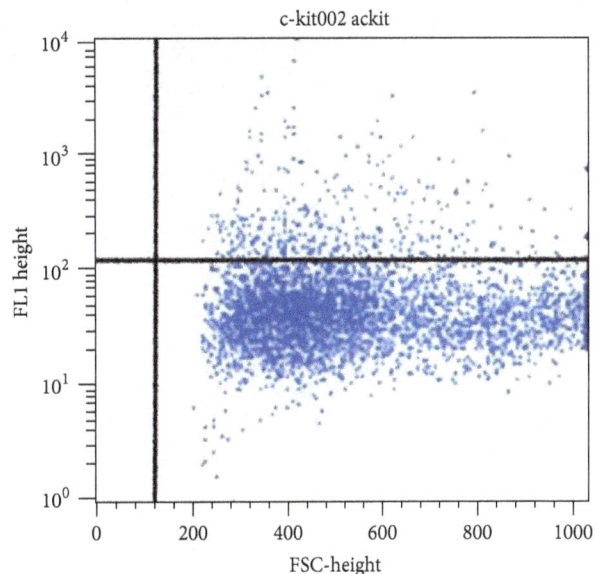

FIGURE 2: The dot plot of CD117-immunopositive MCT cells in this case was drawn back by the software. The MCT cells were gated electronically and were harvested from the cells presenting above the baseline, at the quadrant II (upper-right) of dot plot.

cells were incubated, in the dark chamber, by $100\,\mu L$ of PE directly conjugated mouse monoclonal anti-human CD117 antibodies (Clone Y.B5.B8, Becton and Dickinson, USA), at concentration of $1:200$ for 20 minutes. The cells were washed and centrifuged again at $4,000\times g$ for 5 minutes and the supernatant was then decanted. The cell sediment was resuspended in 10 mL of sterile PBS. Data acquisition was performed using BD-FACScalibur Cell Sorter with BD Cell-Sorting software system (Becton and Dickinson, USA) and the CD117-immunopositive cells were gated from the cells presenting above the threshold line, at the quadrant II of dot plot (Figure 2). The cells were sorted out and harvested into a collecting tube for PCR analysis. The monoclonal IgG was used as the isocontrol for establishing the threshold line on the dot plot.

The genomic DNA (gDNA) of FACS-sorted neoplastic cells was extracted using the commercial DNA-isolation kit (Mobio, USA) and its concentration was computed using UV-spectrophotometry. The forward and reverse primers were designed from 5′ end of exon-11 and 3′ end of intron-11 of *c-kit*, respectively [6, 7]. The sequence of forward primer was 5′-CCA TGT ATG AAG TAC AGT GGA AG-3′ and the reverse primer was 5′-GTT CCC TAA AGT CAT TGT TAC ACG-3′, respectively.

The PCR cocktail was prepared in a flat-capped PCR tube (Axygen, USA). 25 μL of PCR mixer consisted of 1.5 μL of 10X KCl buffer solution (DreamTaq, Fermantas, USA), 1.5 μL of 10X $(NH_4)_2SO_4$ buffer solution (DreamTaq, Fermantas, USA), 3 μL of 20 mM $MgCl_2$ solution (Fermantas, USA), 1 μL of 2 mM dNTP solution (Fermantas, USA), 0.5 μL of Taq polymerases (DreamTaq, Fermentas, USA), 2 μL of 10 mM forward primers solution, 2 μL of 10 mM reverse primers solution, 4 μL of purified DNA template, and 9.5 μL of nuclease-free water (Mobio, USA). The DNA template was amplified in the thermocycler (G-Storm, USA) with the batch of programmatic temperatures of 95°C for 5 minutes for initial DNA denaturation; 40 cycles of 95°C 1 minute for cyclic DNA denaturation, 57°C for 1 minute for cyclic DNA annealing, and 72°C for 1 minute for cyclic DNA extension; and 72°C for 5 minutes for complete DNA elongation [8]. DEPC water was used as the negative control in this study. Meanwhile, gDNA of non-ITD and ITD-mutant exon-11 cells prepared by College of Veterinary Medicine, Michigan State University, USA, was utilized as the normal and positive controls, respectively. In addition, we also used one positive specimen prepared by the same protocols for collating the result with this case.

Ultimately, the amplicons were separated using 2% EtBr-mixed agarose gel electrophoresis at 100 V for 40 minutes. The amplicons were visualized by the gel documentation apparatus (Bio-Rad, USA). The information was analyzed by the computerized software system, Quantity One version 4.6.9 (Bio-Rad, USA), and transformed into JPEG-imaging system using Microsoft Paint (Microsoft, USA).

Upon the study results, the histopathologic section was reclassified as the high-grade MCT. Moreover, CD117 immunocytofluorescence clearly ratified the MCT-cell population in the aspirate. All tumor cells strongly exhibited CD117 immunopositivity on their plasma membranes and cytoplasm; meanwhile, their nuclei were stained blue by DAPI, as shown in Figure 3. It is noteworthy to notice that there were some CD117-immunonegative cells presenting in the smear. These cells were not MCT cells as compared to the negative control.

In addition, approximately 400,000 FNA-MCT cells were harvested by FACS-cell sorting. The genomic DNA of these cells was extracted using the aforementioned protocol and its concentration was 156.65 μg/mL. There was no ITD mutant exon-11 of *c-kit* observed in this case (Figure 4). The single band of PCR product in this case was 191 bp compared to the positive control and the positive specimen (2 product bands at 191 bp and 250 bp, resp.) and the normal control (191-bp).

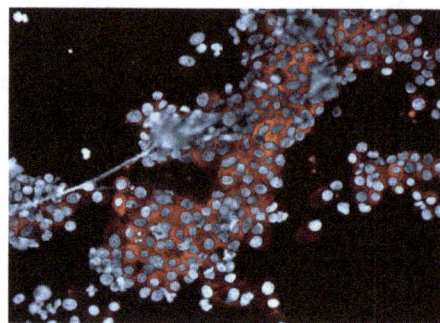

FIGURE 3: CD117 immunocytofluorescence has confirmed MCT subpopulation in the aspirate. The nuclei were stained blue by DAPI. Notably, some cells were non-MCT cells because of lack of CD117 immunopositivity in their cytoplasm and on plasma membranes.

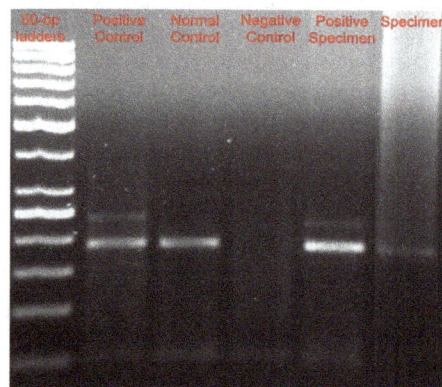

FIGURE 4: The 191 bp of PCR product in this case (in specimen lane) substantially suggested that there was no ITD-mutant exon-1, as well as in the normal control. Notably, the PCR products of the positive control and the positive specimen from the other case consisted of 2 distinct bands at 191 bp and 250 bp (ITD).

3. Discussion

The ITD-mutant exon-11 in *c-kit* is seemingly essential in MCT tumorigenesis as this mutation has been widely studied [3, 6, 8]. Moreover, the ITD-mutation of exon-11 also influences a TKI administration. Basically, MCT patients who possess ITD-exon-11, usually respond to a TKI therapy greater than nonmutational patients [4].

In this study, we have demonstrated an alternative protocol for rapid MCT diagnosis. CD117-immunocytofluorescence could enhance our ability for precise identification of MCT cells. Particularly, in high-grade MCT in which the neoplastic cells are usually pleomorphic and their morphology might mimic other neoplastic cells, such as round-cell tumor cells. Moreover, FACS-cell sorting could rapidly facilitate us to purify the MCT population. These MCT cells were a good source of cells which could be utilized to detect the ITD-mutant exon-11, at least in this case. A rapid diagnosis of ITD-mutant exon-11 may help a veterinarian to decide himself on a TKI usage.

In this case, we supposed that this case should have mutant exon-11 due to an aggressive behavior of the neoplasm. However, ITD-mutant exon-11 was not observed in this case. This might suggest that the mutant exon-11 might not associate with histopathologic grade, but it should associate with the recurrence rate. However, we strongly recommend that a further study based on our combinatorial protocol must be performed in a large population to ensure the advantage of this protocol, before this combinatorial method will be used as a standard protocol for rapid MCT diagnosis in the future.

Conflict of Interests

The authors would like to clarify that there is no conflict of interests with any financial organization regarding the materials discussed in this paper.

References

[1] M. M. Welle, C. R. Bley, J. Howard, and S. Rüfenacht, "Canine mast cell tumours: a review of the pathogenesis, clinical features, pathology and treatment," *Veterinary Dermatology*, vol. 19, no. 6, pp. 321–339, 2008.

[2] M. Morini, G. Bettini, R. Preziosi, and L. Mandrioli, "C-kit gene product (CD117) immunoreactivity in canine and feline paraffin sections," *Journal of Histochemistry and Cytochemistry*, vol. 52, no. 5, pp. 705–708, 2004.

[3] S. Letard, Y. Yang, K. Hanssens et al., "Gain-of-function mutations in the extracellular domain of KIT are common in canine mast cell tumors," *Molecular Cancer Research*, vol. 6, no. 7, pp. 1137–1145, 2008.

[4] C. A. London, P. B. Malpas, S. L. Wood-Follis et al., "Multicenter, placebo-controlled, double-blind, randomized study of oral toceranib phosphate (SU11654), a receptor tyrosine kinase inhibitor, for the treatment of dogs with recurrent (either local or distant) mast cell tumor following surgical excision," *Clinical Cancer Research*, vol. 15, no. 11, pp. 3856–3865, 2009.

[5] M. Kiupel, J. D. Webster, K. L. Bailey et al., "Proposal of a 2-tier histologic grading system for canine cutaneous mast cell tumors to more accurately predict biological behavior," *Veterinary Pathology*, vol. 48, no. 1, pp. 147–155, 2011.

[6] C. L. R. Jones, R. A. Grahn, M. B. Chien, L. A. Lyons, and C. A. London, "Detection of *c-kit* mutations in canine mast cell tumors using fluorescent polyacrylamide gel electrophoresis," *Journal of Veterinary Diagnostic Investigation*, vol. 16, no. 2, pp. 95–100, 2004.

[7] R. Zavodovskaya, M. B. Chien, and C. A. London, "Use of kit internal tandem duplications to establish mast cell tumor clonality in 2 dogs," *Journal of Veterinary Internal Medicine*, vol. 6, pp. 915–917, 2004.

[8] J. D. Webster, V. Yuzbasiyan-Gurkan, J. B. Kaneene, R. Miller, J. H. Resau, and M. Kiupel, "The role of *c-kit* in tumorigenesis: evaluation in canine cutaneous mast cell tumors," *Neoplasia*, vol. 8, no. 2, pp. 104–111, 2006.

33

Pedicled Instep Flap and Tibial Nerve Reconstruction in a Cynomolgus Monkey [*Macaca fascicularis*]

Ruth Weiss,[1] **Reto Wettstein,**[2] **Elisabeth Artemis Kappos,**[2] **Björn Jacobsen,**[3] **Daniel Kalbermatten,**[2] **and Alessandra Bergadano**[1]

[1]*Roche Pharma Research and Early Development, Pharmaceutical Sciences, Comparative Medicine, Roche Innovation Center, Basel, Switzerland*
[2]*Department of Plastic, Reconstructive, Aesthetic and Hand Surgery, University Hospital of Basel, Basel, Switzerland*
[3]*Roche Pharma Research and Early Development, Pharmaceutical Sciences, Toxicology and Pathology, Roche Innovation Center, Basel, Switzerland*

Correspondence should be addressed to Alessandra Bergadano; alessandra.bergadano@roche.com

Academic Editor: Changbaig Hyun

A male cynomolgus monkey experienced extensive soft tissue trauma to the right caudal calf area. Some weeks after complete healing of the original wounds, the monkey developed a chronic pressure sore on plantar surface of the heel of its right foot. A loss of sensitivity in the sole of the foot was hypothesized. The skin defect was closed by a medial sensate pedicled instep flap followed by counter transplantation of a full thickness graft from the interdigital webspace. The integrity of the tibial nerve was revised and reconstructed by means of the turnover flap technique. Both procedures were successful. This is an uncommon case in an exotic veterinary patient as it demonstrates a reconstructive skin flap procedure for the treatment of a chronic, denervated wound in combination with the successful reconstruction of 2.5 cm gap in the tibial nerve.

1. Introduction

A male, 6-year-old cynomolgus monkey (*Macaca fascicularis*), weighting 8.5 kg, suffered extensive soft tissue injuries to the right caudal calf secondary to a bite wound from another monkey. The injuries included the partial transection of the gastrocnemius muscle and the complete transection of the Achilles tendon. The latter remained dysfunctional after complete healing of the original wounds. Several weeks after resolution of the original lesions the monkey developed a chronic wound on the plantar surface of the heel of its right foot. The wound resisted all attempts of conservative treatment following the principles of standard wound care. Although during the course of the disease the animal temporarily demonstrated nonweight bearing lameness, the exposed wound seemed remarkably insensitive to the load of body weight. All these factors combined supported the hypothesis of a loss of sensitivity to the sole of the foot. The plantigrade locomotion in combination with the dysfunctional Achilles tendon and the resulting immobility of the

heel further aggravated the pressure on the wound. Based on the clinical finding and the evolution of the wound the following surgical procedures were planned: coverage of the heel wound with a "pedicled instep flap," exploration, and possible reconstruction of a tibial nerve injury using the "turnover flap technique."

The animal presented in this case report is part of a group of animals instrumented with telemetric implants allowing measuring hemodynamic parameters in free-moving animals for cardiovascular safety pharmacology studies. Therefore the value of the animal justified the efforts bestowed on its full recovery as well as the potential discomfort associated with the surgery and postoperative recovery phase. All animals were housed in an AAALAC accredited facility and according to the Swiss animal welfare legislation. The NHPs lived in highly hierarchized social groups of 3 to 8 individuals, exclusively indoor in big pens of concrete and metal in one air-conditioned barrier unit. Room temperature was kept constant between 22.5°C and 22.8°C and relative humidity between 50 and 60% (range 40 to 80%), with artificial and natural light. They were fed a laboratory monkey food (70–100 g/day/animal) and daily selection of fresh vegetables. Popcorn and alternatively a mix of cereals, soja, and sunflower seeds were given freely on the ground, once weekly as part of the olfactory enrichment program. Raspberry syrup in water and dry raisins, peanuts, and jelly sweets (Haribos®) were also given weekly during their training sessions as positive reinforcement. Nonchlorinated drinking water (IWB, Basel-Stadt) was available ad libitum.

A structured enrichment program was available with structural elements always present in the pen (ladders, barrels, and sand box) and hanging or free items (kongs, nut cages, puzzle feeders, paint and paper rolls, pet-bottles, and surprise boxes) as auditive (TV) and olfactory (popcorn) elements on a rotational weekly base. The structural elements are used also as visual barriers additional to colored divisions.

Serological testing for tuberculosis, measles, cercopithecine herpes I, and simian viruses (SIV, SRV, and STLV) was performed annually while complete blood counts and clinical chemistries, diabetic markers, and bacteriological and parasitological fecal examination were performed quarterly as part of clinical health checks.

2. Case Presentation

2.1. Balanced Anesthesia and Analgesia Protocol.
After intramuscular sedation (Ketamine/Ketasol-100® and Midazolam/Dormicum®) anesthesia was induced with intravenous administration of alfaxalone (Alfaxan®); after endotracheal intubation anesthesia was maintained with sevoflurane (Sevoflurane®) a popliteal nerve block (lidocaine 2%/Xylocaine 2%) as well as fentanyl (Fentanyl®) CRI ensured perioperative analgesia. Postoperatively carprofen (Rimadyl®) and buprenorphine (Temgesic®) were administered as needed based on a numeric pain score for nonhuman primates (NHPs) developed in house.

2.2. Surgical Procedure "Pedicled Instep Flap".
The lesion was situated in the middle of the weight bearing part of the heel of the foot, about 2.5 × 3.5 cm in size (Figure 1).

Thereby it compromised nearly 90% of the weight bearing part of the animal's heel. The calcaneal bone was covered merely by nonviable granulation tissue. Radiographs revealed inflammation of the adjoining structures, that is, the soft tissues of the ankle joint as well as probable osteomyelitis in the calcaneal bone (Figure 2).

The animal was placed in a prone position. The surgical area was prepared in an aseptic manner. The heel flap operation was performed under tourniquet control. After debridement and reconditioning of the wound, the macroscopically affected part of the calcaneal bone was removed by means of bone rongeur. In the process superficial as well as deep bone biopsies were taken. Histopathologically, the removed part of the calcaneus showed a superficial massive fibrosis mixed with small vessels indicative for mature granulation tissue as well as a sparse infiltration of mononuclear inflammatory cells. A slow-release, self-dissolving gentamycin sponge (Septocoll®E 40, Biomet) was inserted into the resulting bone defect. After localization of the medial plantar artery

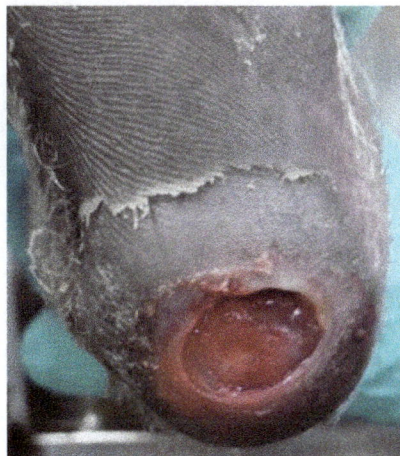

FIGURE 1: 2.5 × 3.5 cm lesion situated in the middle of the weight bearing part of the heel of the foot.

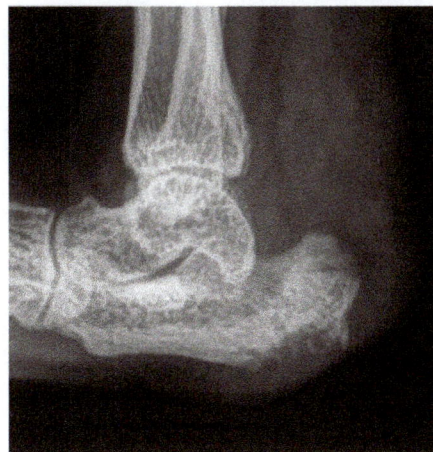

FIGURE 2: Radiographs of the animal's foot taken 26 days before the surgical intervention.

via Doppler, an adequately sized flap in relation to the animal's heel surface was dissected around the instep area, to ensure complete coverage of the heel lesion without tension. The neurovascular pedicle was preserved containing superficial branches of the median plantar artery as well as cutaneous branches of the median plantar nerve. The flap was positioned over the defect and attached to the surrounding tissue via continuous subcutaneous followed by continuous intracutaneous sutures (both Vicryl 4.0) and a cutaneous suture (Ethilon 4.0). The donor site was covered by counter transplantation of a full thickness graft from the interdigital webspace in between the digiti pedis I and digiti pedis II of the ipsilateral foot (Figure 3). The graft was fixated via simple interrupted sutures (PDS 5.0).

After surgery the affected foot was protected with a half-cast for approx. 5 weeks. Until sensitivity had recovered the foot was continuously covered with a light protection bandage.

2.3. Surgical Procedure Tibial Nerve Reconstruction.
Based on the location of the original wounds an injury to the tibial

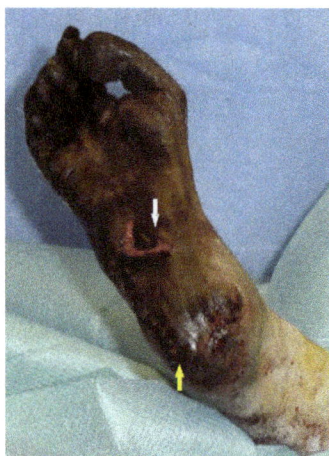

FIGURE 3: Pedicled instep flap (yellow arrow), donor site covered by counter transplantation of a full thickness graft from the interdigital webspace in between the digiti pedis I and digiti pedis II of the ipsilateral foot (white arrow).

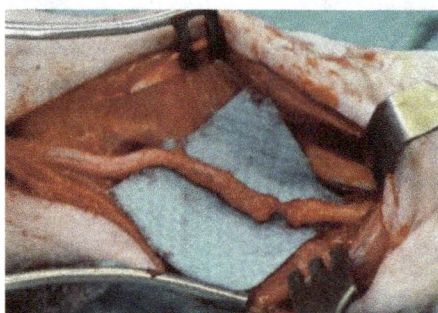

FIGURE 4: Complete transection of the tibial nerve in the midcalf area (intraoperative image).

nerve was possible in several locations. The tibial nerve was explored and eventually found severed in the midcalf area, allegedly distal to the motor branches of the nerve (Figure 4).

According to Sunderland's classification the injury corresponded to a grade V injury [1]. Histopathology confirmed the expected degeneration of the distal nerve stump consisting of mature fibrous tissue mixed with inflammatory cells. On the proximal stump, traumatic neuroma formation was suspected from macroscopic appearance. Histopathologically, loose nerval tissue with the presence of vital axons, Schwann cells, and myelin sheaths embedded in mature fibrous tissue were detected. Reconditioning of the stumps, that is, removal of scar tissue and trimming to healthy fascicular structures, resulted in a gap of approximately 25 mm. Under 2.5 magnification the tibial nerve was dissected. After careful preparation of the fascicles and splitting of the distal nerve stump a turnover flap was formed. The nerve flap was turned over to reach the proximal end of the nerve. This way the integrity of the nerve was reconstructed by means of the "fascicular turnover flap method" developed by Koshima et al. [2]. This technique allowed for tension-free bridging of the defect. Coaptation of the nerve flap was performed using epineural sutures (Nylon 8.0). The

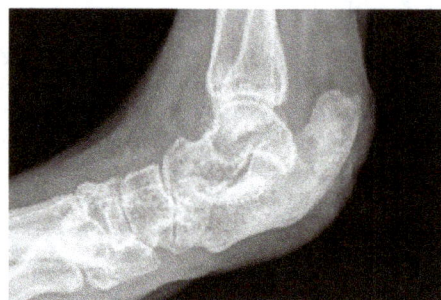

FIGURE 5: Control radiographs (33 days after surgery) illustrating the normalization of the calcaneal bone as well as the soft tissue structures around the ankle joint.

wound was closed via continuous subcutaneous followed by continuous intracutaneous sutures (both Vicryl 4.0) and a cutaneous suture (Ethilon 4.0).

2.4. Follow-Up Phase. Postoperatively the monkey received a veterinary formulation of amoxicillin/clavulanic acid (Synulox®) in total for 12 weeks based on bacteriology bone culture results. The postoperative phase of both wounds was uneventful apart from a slight delay in wound healing on the most lateral portion of the heel flap.

33 days after surgery control radiographs illustrated the normalization of the calcaneal bone structure as well as the soft tissue around the ankle joint (Figure 5).

84 days after surgery return of sensitivity to the plantar surface—in particular the flap area—could be objectively established by means of selective thermal stimulation of Aδ and C fibers. The flap area and the contralateral uninjured heel (acting as own control) were stimulated with a pen-type thermal stimulator. The hand-held pen (contact area of approx. 0.5 cm^2) was applied to the skin of the heel and the temperature gradually increased with a rate of 6.5°C/s (cut-off 55°C) until a withdrawal reflex was elicited consisting of flexion of the ankle and knee joints. Reproducible thresholds could be elicited upon stimulation of the transplanted flap area compared to the contralateral healthy heel area.

During the weeks following the bandage removal, function and load on the recovering foot gradually improved. At long-term follow-up, more than one year after the intervention the flap was visually indistinguishable from the surrounding skin and its durability and function seemed equal to that of normal plantar skin. Functionally, only a decrease in range of motion of the toes was persisting and when running the animal intermittently favored the formerly injured foot. However, most of the residual gait abnormality was due to the dysfunctional Achilles tendon. About 1 year after full recovery the animal had to be euthanized due to reasons unrelated to the injuries presented in this case report. In the autopsy the reconstructed nerve section was found to be completely healed.

3. Discussion

In the case presented here, impairment in wound healing was apparent, characterized by the lack of wound contraction and a sluggish formation of granulation tissue. This is in striking contrast to the usually excellent healing potential of traumatic injuries in NHPs. The shortcomings in wound healing were tentatively related to the denervated state of the injured skin in addition to the inauspicious conditions, that is, exposure to wear and body excretions. The absence of sensitivity to the sole of foot was confirmed later when the tibial nerve (N) was found severed. Trophic ulceration of digital pads has been described in veterinary medicine [3–5]. It is well established that in clinical practice wound healing is delayed in denervated skin areas even without additional hindering factors such as pressure and/or impaired vascularization (i.e., diabetes). There are striking features in biochemical wound characteristics that can be linked to denervation such as depleted levels of nerve growth factor, *substance P* and *calcitonin gene-related peptide* [6]. Fujiwara et al. demonstrated in a novel *in vitro* model the role of neuronal processes in the differentiation of fibroblasts to myofibroblasts and in consequence secretion of collagen fibers essential for wound contraction [7]. Animal models support these observations. In denervated wounds in rats Richards et al. demonstrated reduced neuropeptide concentration, reduced monocyte, and macrophage as well as T lymphocyte counts and in consequence reduced monocyte and macrophage chemotaxis. Delay in wound healing was illustrated by recording of delayed wound contraction [8].

The anatomic structure of the plantar surface of the primate foot as the main weight bearing body surface represents a highly specialized architecture to be able to buffer the pressure and shear forces. The glabrous epidermis and dermis are much thicker than in any other part of the body. Vertical fibrous septa extend from the dermis to the underlying fascia subdividing subcutaneous fat into discrete compartments. Reconstructions of defects to the plantar skin are technically challenging, as skin transplanted from other regions of the body is unable to withstand the strain of weight bearing. The instep area however represents the ideal donor site; while it provides the necessary anatomical characteristics, it is not needed for weight bearing [9, 10]. The medial plantar artery and parts of the N. plantaris medialis are included in the neurovascular pedicle of the flap. Neurovascular free and island flaps have been applied successfully in veterinary medicine in order to replace injured canine foot pads [3, 5, 11]. In human patients Wan et al. could demonstrate at 6 months to 1 year after sensate medial plantar flap transposition that the sensation of the recipient area retained the quality of the donor site, thereby surpassing the sensation of the contralateral normal heel [12]. Differences can be found in the quality of sensation such as temperature, pressure, and two-point discrimination [13]. Then again in a long-term comparison noninnervated free flaps (spontaneous reinnervation) have not proven to be superior to reinnervated free flaps (sensory nerve preservation or coaptation) [14]. However, in our animal patient regain of sensation as soon as possible was mandatory to prevent traumatic reinjury and therefore enhance flap durability, since the lack of sensation was likely the cause of the pathology in the first place. It was believed that, by perpetuating the continuity of sensory

nerve structure into the flap, nerve regeneration would be facilitated, even though the underlying impediment was the midcalf tibial nerve injury.

The prognosis for bridging its 25 mm defect without surgical intervention would have been poor. In order to provide a scaffold for smooth and unbranched axoplasmic migration into the Schwann cell tube of the distal stump, the continuity of the severed N. tibialis had to be reconstructed. The surgical reconstruction was performed approx. 15 weeks after the original injury had occurred. After a delay of more than 8 weeks axoplasmic recannulation may be hindered due to stromal fibrosis and narrowing of Schwann cells in the distal stump. The rather novel fascicular turnover flap technique applied in this case was first introduced by Koshima and coauthors in 2010 [2]. It allows for bridging of nerve defects over 20 mm in length using the injured nerve as its own donor nerve. As a special asset this technique results in a vascularized nerve graft. A free nerve graft has to rely on the vascularization of the recipient bed until spontaneous revascularization occurs. In veterinary medicine autologous free nerve grafting has been applied with satisfactory results [15]. However, the vascularization of nerve grafts becomes principal, where thick grafts are involved, in large defects or in cases such as ours where the graft meets up with a scarred recipient bed; the longer the gap the higher the risk of atrophy as well as fibrous ingrowth into the distal anastomosis area [16]. Vascularization of nerve grafts has been linked to suppression of fibrosis and leads to a swifter recovery and a better end result concerning sensorimotor nerve function [17, 18]. The expected speed of nerval regeneration is about 1–3 mm/day.

When the pressure sore first developed we unsuccessfully tried to test for sensibility in the affected region by means of skin pinching and/or needle picking. While being successfully applied in small animal patients such as dogs and cats, the sensitivity testing based on mechanical pinching and needle picking in this case yielded only inconclusive results. Therefore up to the surgery and the visual revision of the tibial nerve the loss of sensitivity remained a hypothesis. About 3 months after surgery, return in nociceptive sensitivity in the injured heel could be assessed using selective thermal stimulation of Aδ and C fibers which elicited a reproducible withdrawal reflex. Heat pain activates Aδ or C nociceptors depending on the intensity of the stimulus and whether the skin is heated at a rapid or a slow rate, respectively. The use of thermal stimulation is a model of phasic pain and allows for exploring the peripheral nociceptive pathways [19–21]. We can speculate that also tactile sensitivity carried by the Aβ fibers was restored anatomically and physiologically.

In addition to the systemic medication a gentamycin sponge (Septocoll E 40) was fitted into the mold in the calcaneal bone that had resulted from bone debriding. Antibiotic-impregnated beads had already been used successfully in a case of calcaneal osteomyelitis resistant to conventional medical therapy in a Rhesus Macaque [22]. However, neither histopathology nor microbiologic culture from the specimens taken at the moment of surgery was able to confirm active infection as a cause for the delay in wound healing.

4. Conclusion

This is a unique report in veterinary medicine describing the successful surgical repair of a chronic plantar defect by the "pedicled instep flap" technique and the reconstruction of the tibial nerve. It demonstrates the consequence of denervation on the development and evolution of a skin defect in the tibial nerve's autonomous zone, the sole of the foot. Thereby it brings to mind the crucial part of innervation in the process of wound healing.

Competing Interests

The authors declare that they have no competing interests.

Acknowledgments

The authors would like to express their appreciation to the following members of Comparative Medicine at Roche, Basel, for their assistance and support in the diligent care of the animal: Dr. Eva Maria Amen, Muriel Brecheisen, Michel Keller, Rafael de Carvalho, Mirjam Brönnimann, and Walter Stamm. In addition, the authors would like to express their gratitude for the contribution to the success of this case to Dr. med. vet. Cecile Werren, Professor Claudia Spadavecchia, and Dr. med. vet. Andrea Greiter-Wilke.

References

[1] S. Sunderland, "A classification of peripheral nerve injuries producing loss of function," *Brain*, vol. 74, no. 4, pp. 491–516, 1951.

[2] I. Koshima, M. Narushima, M. Mihara, G. Uchida, and M. Nakagawa, "Fascicular turnover flap for nerve gaps," *Journal of Plastic, Reconstructive & Aesthetic Surgery*, vol. 63, no. 6, pp. 1008–1014, 2010.

[3] K. C. Danielson, M. Kent, and K. Cornell, "Successful treatment of a metacarpal trophic ulcer utilizing a neurovascular island flap," *Journal of the American Animal Hospital Association*, vol. 45, no. 4, pp. 176–180, 2009.

[4] S. E. Gibbons and W. M. McKee, "Spontaneous healing of a trophic ulcer of the metatarsal pad in a dog," *Journal of Small Animal Practice*, vol. 45, no. 12, pp. 623–625, 2004.

[5] R. A. Read, "Probable trophic pad ulceration following traumatic denervation report of two cases in dogs," *Veterinary Surgery*, vol. 15, no. 1, pp. 40–44, 1986.

[6] A. R. Barker, G. D. Rosson, and A. L. Dellon, "Wound healing in denervated tissue," *Annals of Plastic Surgery*, vol. 57, no. 3, pp. 339–342, 2006.

[7] T. Fujiwara, T. Kubo, S. Kanazawa et al., "Direct contact of fibroblasts with neuronal processes promotes differentiation to myofibroblasts and induces contraction of collagen matrix in vitro," *Wound Repair and Regeneration*, vol. 21, no. 4, pp. 588–594, 2013.

[8] A. M. Richards, J. Mitsou, D. C. Floyd, G. Terenghi, and D. A. McGrouther, "Neural innervation and healing," *The Lancet*, vol. 350, no. 9074, pp. 339–340, 1997.

[9] O. Scheufler, D. Kalbermatten, and G. Pierer, "Instep free flap for plantar soft tissue reconstruction: indications and options," *Microsurgery*, vol. 27, no. 3, pp. 174–180, 2007.

[10] W. A. Morrison, D. M. Crabb, B. M. O'Brien, and A. Jenkins, "The instep of the foot as a fasciocutaneous island and as a free flap for heel defects," *Plastic and Reconstructive Surgery*, vol. 72, no. 1, pp. 56–63, 1983.

[11] A. W. P. Basher, J. D. Fowler, and C. V. A. Bowen, "Free tissue transfer of digital foot pads for reconstruction of the distal limb in the dog," *Microsurgery*, vol. 12, no. 2, pp. 118–124, 1991.

[12] D. C. Wan, J. Gabbay, B. Levi, J. B. Boyd, and J. W. Granzow, "Quality of innervation in sensate medial plantar flaps for heel reconstruction," *Plastic and Reconstructive Surgery*, vol. 127, no. 2, pp. 723–730, 2011.

[13] M. G. Burnett and E. L. Zager, "Pathophysiology of peripheral nerve injury: a brief review," *Neurosurgical Focus*, vol. 16, no. 5, p. E1, 2004.

[14] Z. Potparić and N. Rajačić, "Long-term results of weight-bearing foot reconstruction with non-innervated and reinnervated free flaps," *British Journal of Plastic Surgery*, vol. 50, no. 3, pp. 176–181, 1997.

[15] N. Granger, P. Moissonnier, L. Fanchon, A. Hidalgo, K. Gnirs, and S. Blot, "Cutaneous saphenous nerve graft for the treatment of sciatic neurotmesis in a dog," *Journal of the American Veterinary Medical Association*, vol. 229, no. 1, pp. 82–86, 2006.

[16] L. M. Wolford and E. L. Stevao, "Considerations in nerve repair," *Proceedings (Baylor University. Medical Center)*, vol. 16, no. 2, pp. 152–156, 2003.

[17] F. Kanaya, J. Firrell, T.-M. Tsai, and W. C. Breidenbach, "Functional results of vascularized versus nonvascularized nerve grafting," *Plastic and Reconstructive Surgery*, vol. 89, no. 5, pp. 924–930, 1992.

[18] K. Doi, K. Tamaru, K. Sakai, N. Kuwata, Y. Kurafuji, and S. Kawai, "A comparison of vascularized and conventional sural nerve grafts," *Journal of Hand Surgery*, vol. 17, no. 4, pp. 670–676, 1992.

[19] D. C. Yeomans, V. Pirec, and H. K. Proudfit, "Nociceptive responses to high and low rates of noxious cutaneous heating are mediated by different nociceptors in the rat: behavioral evidence," *Pain*, vol. 68, no. 1, pp. 133–140, 1996.

[20] D. C. Yeomans and H. K. Proudfit, "Nociceptive responses to high and low rates of noxious cutaneous heating are mediated by different nociceptors in the rat: electrophysiological evidence," *Pain*, vol. 68, no. 1, pp. 141–150, 1996.

[21] D. C. Yeomans and H. K. Proudfit, "Characterization of the foot withdrawal response to noxious radiant heat in the rat," *Pain*, vol. 59, no. 1, pp. 85–94, 1994.

[22] K. R. Kelly, A. R. Kapatkin, A. L. Zwingenberger, and K. L. Christe, "Efficacy of antibiotic-impregnated polymethyl-methacrylate beads in a rhesus macaque (Macaca mulatta) with osteomyelitis," *Comparative Medicine*, vol. 62, no. 4, pp. 311–315, 2012.

34

Hiccup-Like Response in a Dog Anesthetized with Isoflurane

Enzo Vettorato and Federico Corletto

Dick White Referrals, Station Farm, London Road, Six Mile Bottom, Cambridgeshire CB8 0UH, UK

Correspondence should be addressed to Enzo Vettorato; ev2@dwr.co.uk

Academic Editor: Lysimachos G. Papazoglou

An eight-year-old, female intact Golden Retriever underwent magnetic resonance imaging (MRI) for investigation of urinary and faecal incontinence. Soon after induction of general anesthesia, tracheal intubation, and isoflurane administration, hiccup-like movements were evident. These hiccup-like movements did not respond to hyperventilation and increase of anesthetic. After having ruled out pulmonary disease, the animal was reanesthetized with a similar technique; hiccup-like movements reoccurred and did not stop after discontinuation of isoflurane and commencement of a propofol infusion. Eventually, a nondepolarizing neuromuscular blocking agent was administered to stop the hiccup-like response and allow MRI to be performed. This case report describes the pathophysiology of hiccup-like response and its management in a dog.

1. Introduction

Hiccup (or hiccough) is a brief powerful inspiratory effort accompanied by closure of the glottis [1]. In cats, it results from activation of a reflex whose afferent fibres originate from the pharyngeal branch of the glossopharyngeal nerve [2], and the efferent ones from the vagal motoneuron, projecting to the phrenic nerve and laryngeal intrinsic muscles. The central pattern generator of the hiccup reflex seems to be in the reticular formation of the brainstem [3]. Hiccup can occur at any moment of the respiratory cycle, including expiration, but typically follows the inspiratory peak [1].

General anesthesia is described as one of the potential causes of hiccup in medical literature [3–5]. Even if the feline species has been extensively used to study the pathophysiology of hiccup [2, 6–8], no clinical reports are present in veterinary medicine literature describing the *singultus* manifestation in anesthetized animals.

This report describes the hiccup-like response that was encountered in a dog anesthetized with isoflurane.

2. Case Presentation

An eight-year-old, female intact Golden Retriever, weighing 27 kg, was referred for investigation of urinary and faecal incontinence, which acutely appeared following two months of chronic vaginal discharge. The latter partially responded to antibiotic treatment. After neurological consultation, the animal was scheduled for magnetic resonance imaging (MRI) of the lumbar-sacral region under general anesthesia.

On preanesthetic examination the dog appeared slightly nervous but in good physical condition (ASA II). The heart rate was 90 beats *per* minute (bpm), respiratory rate was 15 breaths *per* minute (brpm), pulse quality was good, mucous membranes were pink, and capillary refill time was less than 2 seconds. Thoracic and cardiac auscultation were unremarkable, as were the results of hematological and biochemical blood tests.

After a mild sedation was achieved administering methadone intramuscularly (0.2 mg kg^{-1}; Synastone, Auden Mckenzie Ltd., UK), anesthesia was induced intravenously 30 minutes later with fentanyl (3 μg kg^{-1}; Sublimaze, Janssen-Cilag Ltd., UK) and propofol (2.5 mg kg^{-1}; Rapinovet, Schering-plough Animal Health UK). The trachea was intubated with a cuffed tube; the cuff was inflated; intubation was unremarkable. Anesthesia was maintained with isoflurane (IsoFlo, Abbott Laboratoires, UK) in 100% oxygen, delivered through a circle system. Monitoring consisted of capnography, measurement of inspired and expired anesthetic gases and oxygen, measurement of noninvasive arterial blood pressure (Datex AS3, Helsinki, Finland), and esophageal stethoscope.

TABLE 1: Arterial blood gas collected taken from a dog with hiccup-like response while anesthetized with isoflurane in oxygen 100%. $PaCO_2$: arterial carbon dioxide partial pressure; $PE'CO_2$: end-expiratory partial pressure of carbon dioxide; PaO_2: arterial oxygen partial pressure; FiO_2: inspiratory fraction of oxygen; HCO_3^-: bicarbonate; Na^+: sodium; K^+: potassium; Cl^-: chloride.

pH	$PaCO_2$ mmHg	$PE'CO_2$ mmHg	PaO_2 mmHg	FiO_2 %	HCO_3^- mmol L^{-1}	Na^+ mmol L^{-1}	K^+ mmol L^{-1}	Cl^- mmol L^{-1}
7.49	29	22	541	89	18.7	157	3.2	118

Shortly after commencement of isoflurane administration, a gasping breathing pattern was noted, with a respiratory rate of 40–50 brpm and jerk movements of the mouth and all four limbs. Heart rate was 140 bpm. Inadequate depth of anesthesia was considered the cause of the observed movements; thus ventilation was assisted manually (15 brpm) and the vaporizer setting was increased from 2% to 3% (oxygen $3 L min^{-1}$) in order to deepen the anesthetic plane. Further, a bolus of fentanyl ($1 \mu g kg^{-1}$) was administered intravenously. At that time, end-expiratory carbon dioxide tension ($PE'CO_2$) was 22 mmHg. Because the respiratory pattern did not change during the following 10 minutes, and suspecting an underlying pulmonary disease, MRI was cancelled while thoracic radiographs and an arterial blood gases analysis were performed. Radiographs were unremarkable and alkalemia due to primary respiratory alkalosis was apparent in the arterial blood gases analysis results (Table 1). The dog was allowed to recover from general anesthesia. Once the vaporizer was turned off and the breathing system flushed with oxygen, the dog's breathing pattern improved and became normal. The recovery from general anesthesia was uneventful. MRI was rescheduled for the following day.

On day 2, preanesthetic assessment was unremarkable and similar to that obtained the previous day. Dexmedetomidine ($1.25 \mu g kg^{-1}$ Dexdomitor, Orion Pharma, Finland) and methadone ($0.25 mg kg^{-1}$) were administered slowly intravenously. The resulting sedative effect was good with the animal relaxed in lateral recumbency. Anesthesia was induced with propofol ($1.5 mg kg^{-1}$) and, after intubation of the trachea with a cuffed tube, maintained with isoflurane (vaporizer setting was 3%) in 100% oxygen at the flow of $3 L min^{-1}$, delivered through a circle system. Also in this occasion tracheal intubation was unremarkable.

As on day 1, the animal started gasping and jerking continuously as soon it was connected to the breathing system. At that point, isoflurane was immediately turned off and the breathing system flushed with pure oxygen. Anesthesia was then maintained with a constant rate infusion (CRI) of propofol ($0.3 mg kg^{-1} min^{-1}$), after slow administration of a loading dose ($0.5 mg kg^{-1}$). As the animal's breathing pattern did not improve, atracurium ($0.2 mg kg^{-1}$, Tracrium Injection, GlaxoSmithKline, UK) was administered intravenously and intermittent positive pressure ventilation (Penlon Nuffield 200 ventilator) was started to maintain eucapnia ($PE'CO_2$ 35–45 mmHg). Respiratory rate was set to 15 breathes per minute, tidal volume was 300 mL, and peak inspiratory pressure was $12 cmH_2O$. The rest of the anesthetic time was uneventful, but it was necessary to top up atracurium every 15–20 minutes, because hiccups restarted as soon as neuromuscular function started returning.

An extensive invasive sacrococcygeal neoplasia was found on MRI. The owner decided to euthanize the dog but declined postmortem examination.

3. Discussion

In contrast to eupneic breathing, hiccups combine a sudden powerful coordinated burst of the inspiratory muscles of the thorax, diaphragm, neck, accessory, and external intercostal muscles with an inhibition of the expiratory abdominal muscles, active movement of the tongue toward the roof of the mouth, and active adduction of the glottis, which occurs after the beginning of inspiratory flow and it is responsible for the peculiar sound [1]. Differently from sneezing and coughing, hiccup is not a protective reflex. In fact, during coughing and sneezing a vigorous expiratory effort is produced causing expulsion of irritants in the upper respiratory airway [9]. Moreover, hiccup has to be distinguished from reverse sneezing. The latter is a mechanosensitive aspiration reflex and consists of a paroxysmal inspiratory effort (stertor) associated with adduction of laryngeal cartilages. The negative pleural and tracheal pressure generated by the inspiration allows an increase of the inspiratory inflow once the glottis opens, resulting in potential aspiration of foreign material trapped in the nasopharynx [9].

The physiology of hiccup has been extensively studied in cats [2, 6–8]. The mechanical (cotton-tipped swab) stimulation of the dorsal aspect of the epipharynx has been associated with hiccup. The response to such stimulation is characterized by a strong inspiratory effort, large peak of negative inspiratory pressure (less then $-20 cmH_2O$), spasmodic activity of the diaphragm, no contraction of the abdominal muscles, and phasic inhibition of the abductor laryngeal muscle (posterior cricoarytenoid muscle) [7]. In particular, the electrical stimulation of the pharyngeal branch of the glossopharyngeal nerve (PB-IX) is responsible for hiccup. On the contrary, the stimulation of the main trunk of the IX cranial nerve evokes an expiratory reflex (cough), but not an inspiratory (hiccup-like) response [2]. The lower brainstem, and more precisely the reticular formation, seems to be the area where the central connection of the hiccup-like reflex is located [6]. Interestingly, the coordinating motor pattern of coughing and sneezing has been occasionally elicited by an electrical stimulation applied to area in proximity to those generating hiccup [6]. Even if PB-IX was not directly stimulated in the dog of the present report, we believe that the breathing pattern seen can be described as a hiccup-like response.

A light plane of anesthesia was initially suspected to be the reason of the abnormal breathing pattern. Fentanyl was administered as a respiratory depressant and manual IPPV was started in order to increase the alveolar ventilation and therefore the uptake of anesthetic agent. Further, the lung's inflation, activating the stretch receptors in the bronchi and bronchioles, can stimulate the Hering-Breuer reflex, which should inhibit the normal respiratory pattern and should also inhibit hiccup [10]. According to Butt Jr. et al. [3], hiccupping during anesthesia can be managed by deepening anesthesia and hyperventilation with the aim of causing apnoea and then inhibition of spontaneous ventilation. Moreover, continuous positive airway pressure seems to be an efficacious method to stop hiccup during anesthesia [11]. However, in the presence of hiccup, the decrease of arterial carbon dioxide tension ($PaCO_2$) caused by IPPV can produce the opposite effect. The frequency of hiccups seems to be inversely correlated to the $PaCO_2$: the frequency of hiccup decreases with increasing $PaCO_2$ [1], and this may be the physiological explanation for the old notion that breath-holding will stop hiccups. This could also explain why the dog did not respond to our initial treatment, which resulted in hyperventilation and respiratory alkalosis, as confirmed by arterial blood gas analysis. While in children in whom the trachea was not intubated hiccup was associated with a decrease in respiratory frequency and minute volume, oxygen desaturation, and relative bradycardia, hiccupping spells were characterized by hyperventilation and respiratory alkalosis if the trachea was intubated [12].

The lack of pulmonary disease, ruled out by thoracic radiographs, the acute onset of hiccup following commencement of isoflurane administration, and establishment of a normal breathing pattern as soon as the animal was disconnected form the breathing system were the reasons for suspecting that the hiccup was an unusual adverse reaction of the animal to the volatile anesthetic. Activation of γ-aminobutyric acid $(GABA)_A$ receptors may facilitate hiccup in humans; on the contrary, baclofen, a $GABA_B$-receptor agonist, is one of the most effective drugs for the treatment of intractable hiccup [13]. The interaction between halogenated anesthetics and GABA receptors is one of the possible mechanisms of action by which volatile anesthetics depress the central nervous system (CNS) and produce unconsciousness [14]. Isoflurane facilitates the hiccup-like reflex in cats by activating the central and peripheral $GABA_A$-receptors, but it also suppresses it by activating central and peripheral $GABA_B$-receptors [8]. However, the same study showed that the hiccup-like response is inhibited proportionally to the alveolar isoflurane concentration, thus lending support to Butt's theory [3]. In the case here reported, hiccup did not respond to hyperventilation and deepening of anesthesia, and for this reason a constant rate infusion of propofol was started. Persistence of hiccup during propofol infusion may be explained by the fact that propofol, as well as benzodiazepines and ultrashort acting barbiturates, may facilitate hiccup in humans by activating $GABA_A$ receptors [15–17].

Intubation, with consequent stimulation of the glottis seems to be a possible cause of hiccup in humans [18]. The use of supra glottis airways devices (laryngeal mask, LMA) has been advocated as a possible treatment for hiccup [19], even if 74/179 cases of hiccup after induction of anesthesia were

trigged by LMA insertion [20]. Unfortunately, a LMA was not available at the time. Total intravenous anesthesia without endotracheal intubation or any other mean of securing the airway could have potentially stopped the hiccupping episode; however as hiccup has been associated with relaxation of the lower oesophageal sphincter [21, 22] with reflux occurring in up to 40% of human beings with hiccup [23], this would not be a safe option.

Several drugs and techniques have been considered for treatment of hiccup in humans [3–5, 24]. Ketamine (0.4–0.5 $mg\,kg^{-1}$ IV) has been reported to rapidly terminate hiccup during anesthesia [25] and in the postoperative period [26] by acting centrally as well as at the spinal cord level [27]. Even if the hiccup did not stop by deepening anesthesia we cannot exclude that a more profound preanesthetic sedation would have helped in controlling such hiccup-response.

Neuromuscular blocking (NMB) agents are probably the most reliable way to stop hiccup during anesthesia, rapidly stopping diaphragmatic contractions. However, they cannot be considered as specific treatment of hiccup, because they do not remove the real cause of the *singultus* and do not affect the neuronal circuitry that produces it. In fact, when the paralysis starts to wear off, the return of the diaphragmatic activity may be associated with a new hiccup-like pattern, as in the case here reported. Furthermore, the use of NMB agents has to be judicious: if inadequate plane of anesthesia or surgical stimulation is suspected as cause of hiccup, the use of NMB agents should be avoided, and anesthesia should be deepened and/or analgesics should be administered prior to consideration of neuromuscular block.

4. Conclusion

Acute hiccup is a potential complication that can occur during sedation and general anesthesia not only in humans but also in dogs. Many interventions have been proposed to treat it, but the current literature does not suggest a single effective treatment. The administration of NMB agents can be helpful when a real cause of hiccup cannot be identified and inadequate anesthesia and analgesia have been ruled out as possible causes.

Competing Interests

The authors declare that there are no competing interests regarding the publication of this paper.

References

[1] J. N. Davis, "An experimental study of hiccup," *Brain*, vol. 93, no. 4, pp. 851–872, 1970.

[2] T. Kondo, H. Toyooka, and H. Arita, "Hiccup reflex is mediated by pharyngeal branch of glossopharyngeal nerve in cats," *Neuroscience Research*, vol. 47, no. 3, pp. 317–321, 2003.

[3] H. R. Butt Jr., W. Hamelberg, and J. Jacoby, "Hiccup: its possible cause and treatment in anesthesia," *Anesthesia & Analgesia*, vol. 40, no. 2, pp. 181–185, 1961.

[4] J. H. Lewis, "Hiccups: causes and cures," *Journal of Clinical Gastroenterology*, vol. 7, no. 6, pp. 539–552, 1985.

[5] P. Kranke, L. H. Eberhart, A. M. Morin, J. Cracknell, C.-A. Greim, and N. Roewer, "Treatment of hiccup during general anaesthesia or sedation: a qualitative systematic review," *European Journal of Anaesthesiology*, vol. 20, no. 3, pp. 239–244, 2003.

[6] H. Arita, T. Oshima, I. Kita, and M. Sakamoto, "Generation of hiccup by electrical stimulation in medulla of cats," *Neuroscience Letters*, vol. 175, no. 1-2, pp. 67–70, 1994.

[7] T. Oshima, M. Sakamoto, and H. Arita, "Hiccuplike response elicited by mechanical stimulation of dorsal epipharynx of cats," *Journal of Applied Physiology*, vol. 76, no. 5, pp. 1888–1895, 1994.

[8] T. Oshima and S. Dohi, "Isoflurane facilitates hiccup-like reflex through gamma aminobutyric acid (GABA)$_A$- and suppresses through GABA$_B$-receptors in pentobarbital-anesthetized cats," *Anesthesia & Analgesia*, vol. 98, no. 2, pp. 346–352, 2004.

[9] B. C. McKiernan, "Sneezing and nasal discharge," in *Textbook of Veterinary Internal Medicine*, S. J. Ettinger and E. C. Fieldman, Eds., pp. 79–85, WB Saunders, Philadelphia, Pa, USA, 4th edition, 1995.

[10] A. Baraka, "Inhibition of hiccup by pulmonary inflation," *Anesthesiology*, vol. 32, no. 3, pp. 271–273, 1970.

[11] C. Saitto, G. Gristina, and E. V. Cosmi, "Treatment of hiccups by continuous positive airway pressure (CPAP) in anesthetized subjects," *Anesthesiology*, vol. 57, no. 4, p. 345, 1982.

[12] R. T. Brouillette, B. T. Thach, Y. K. Abu-Osba, and S. L. Wilson, "Hiccups in infants: characteristics and effects on ventilation," *The Journal of Pediatrics*, vol. 96, no. 2, pp. 219–225, 1980.

[13] C. Guelaud, T. Similowski, J.-L. Bizec, J. Cabane, W. A. Whitelaw, and J.-P. Derenne, "Baclofen therapy for chronic hiccup," *European Respiratory Journal*, vol. 8, no. 2, pp. 235–237, 1995.

[14] K. W. Miller, "The nature of sites of general anaesthetic action," *British Journal of Anaesthesia*, vol. 89, no. 1, pp. 17–31, 2002.

[15] M. V. Jones, N. L. Harrison, D. B. Pritchett, and T. G. Hales, "Modulation of the GABA$_A$ receptor by propofol is independent of the γ subunit," *Journal of Pharmacology and Experimental Therapeutics*, vol. 274, no. 2, pp. 962–968, 1995.

[16] D. B. Pritchett, H. Sontheimer, B. D. Shivers et al., "Importance of a novel GABA$_A$ receptor subunit for benzodiazepine pharmacology," *Nature*, vol. 338, no. 6216, pp. 582–585, 1989.

[17] R. L. MacDonald, C. J. Rogers, and R. E. Twyman, "Barbiturate regulation of kinetic properties of the GABA(A) receptor channel of mouse spinal neurones in culture," *Journal of Physiology*, vol. 417, pp. 483–500, 1989.

[18] C. W. Mayo, "Hiccup," *The Journal of Surgery, Gynecology, and Obstetrics*, vol. 55, pp. 700–708, 1932.

[19] A. Baraka, "Inhibition of hiccups by the laryngeal mask airway," *Anaesthesia*, vol. 59, no. 9, p. 926, 2004.

[20] J. Brimacombe and C. Keller, "Inhibition of hiccups by the laryngeal mask airway is ineffective," *Anaesthesia*, vol. 59, no. 11, p. 1144, 2004.

[21] H. J. Skinner, B. Y. M. Ho, and R. P. Mahajan, "Gastro-oesophageal reflux with the laryngeal mask during day-case gynaecological laparoscopy," *British Journal of Anaesthesia*, vol. 80, no. 5, pp. 675–676, 1998.

[22] C. J. Roberts and N. W. Goodman, "Gastro-oesophageal reflux during elective laparoscopy," *Anaesthesia*, vol. 45, no. 12, pp. 1009–1011, 1990.

[23] R. G. Vanner, "Gastro-oesophageal reflex and hiccup during anaesthesia," *Anaesthesia*, vol. 48, no. 1, pp. 92–93, 1993.

[24] S. Launois, J. L. Bizec, W. A. Whitelaw, J. Cabane, and J. P. Derenne, "Hiccup in adults: an overview," *European Respiratory Journal*, vol. 6, no. 4, pp. 563–575, 1993.

[25] M. Tavakoli and G. Corssen, "Control of hiccups by ketamine: a preliminary report," *Alabama Journal of Medical Sciences*, vol. 11, no. 3, pp. 229–230, 1974.

[26] J. Teodorowicz and M. Zimny, "The effect of ketamine in patients with refractory hiccups in the postoperative period: preliminary report," *Anaesthesia Resuscitation and Intensive Therapy Journal*, vol. 3, no. 3, pp. 271–272, 1975.

[27] T. R. Shantha, "Ketamine for the treatment of hiccups during and following anesthesia: a preliminary report," *Anesthesia & Analgesia*, vol. 52, no. 5, pp. 822–824, 1973.

35

Coinfection with *Tritrichomonas foetus* and *Giardia duodenalis* in Two Cats with Chronic Diarrhea

Sergio A. Zanzani,[1] Alessia L. Gazzonis,[1] Paola Scarpa,[1] Emanuela Olivieri,[2] Hans-Jörg Balzer,[3] and Maria Teresa Manfredi[1]

[1]*Department of Veterinary Medicine, Università degli Studi di Milano, Milano, Italy*
[2]*Department of Veterinary Medicine, Università degli Studi di Perugia, Perugia, Italy*
[3]*IDEXX Laboratories, Ludwigsburg, Germany*

Correspondence should be addressed to Sergio A. Zanzani; sergio.zanzani@unimi.it

Academic Editor: Changbaig Hyun

A *Tritrichomonas foetus* and *Giardia duodenalis* mixed infection was diagnosed in two Maine Coon cats aged six months. One of them presented a history of chronic liquid diarrhea and of several unsuccessful treatments. In both cats, *G. duodenalis* and trichomonads were detected in fecal smears from freshly voided feces; the presence of *T. foetus* was confirmed by a real-time PCR assay. The cats completely recovered after treatment with ronidazole. In a refrigerated fecal sample collected from the cat with chronic diarrhea, drop-shaped trichomonad pseudocysts smaller than *G. duodenalis* cysts were detected. They appeared brownish or light-bluish when stained with Lugol's solution or with Giemsa stain, respectively, and their morphological features were similar to those expressed by bovine *T. foetus* pseudocysts *in vitro*. Existence of pseudocysts even in feline trichomonads is noteworthy as they could represent a form of protozoan resistance due to unfavorable conditions whose detection in refrigerated feces can be a useful clue for clinicians.

1. Introduction

Tritrichomonas foetus, agent of bovine trichomonosis, was recently recognized as a primary cause of feline trichomoniasis, a large bowel disease characterized by intermittent or chronic diarrhea mainly occurring in multihoused cats from catteries or shelters [1–3]. The infection was frequently diagnosed in cats younger than 1 year with worldwide distribution [4]. Similar to other trichomonads, for example, those infecting humans, *T. foetus* presents only a trophozoite stage although a pseudocyst stage was described for the bovine isolate [5, 6]. *Giardia duodenalis* is an intestinal protozoan with a large diffusion and prevalence values highly variable in domestic cats [7–9]. Several surveys showed that cats host specific or zoonotic *Giardia* assemblages [7, 9, 10]. *Giardia* has often been found in the feces of diarrheic cats singly or in coinfection with *T. foetus* [11]. However, reports of coinfection with both of these enteropathogens are limited, and no pseudocyst stage of *T. foetus* in cat feces was previously reported [5]. Further, ronidazole was documented to be effective for the control of *Tritrichomonas* infection in cats whereas its efficacy against *Giardia* was demonstrated only in dogs [12]. This article reports a coinfection with *T. foetus* and *G. duodenalis* in two owned cats and the pseudocyst stage of *T. foetus* in feline feces with its morphology.

2. Case Presentation

Two littermate Maine Coon females aged six months underwent examination by the referring veterinarian as one of them presented a 3-month history of liquid malodorous diarrhea. A previous diagnosis following coprological analyses in both cats had indicated an infection sustained by ascarids and the animals had been treated by practitioners with milbemycine oxime and praziquantel (2 mg/kg bw and 5 mg/kg bw, resp., PO, single administration). Due to persistent diarrhea, in the affected cat coprological analyses were repeated to verify both effectiveness of treatment against ascarids and a possible infection with *Giardia*. The cat resulted in being positive for *Giardia* coproantigens (IDEXX SNAP® *Giardia* Test, IDEXX Laboratories, Hoofddorp, Netherlands) and was treated with fenbendazole (50 mg/kg bw, PO, SID) for 5 days, obtaining only a moderate and transient improvement of feces consistence. As some weeks after this treatment liquid diarrhea continued, another fecal test was performed revealing the persistence of *Giardia* coproantigens. A treatment with spiramycin and metronidazole (75000 IU/kg bw 12.5 mg/kg bw, PO, SID) followed for 10 days. The feces became formed and no longer malodorous, but few days after treatment signs recurred. In the meantime, the two cats still continued to use the same litter and even the one whose feces had always been formed began to present mucous diarrhea. Thus, fecal samples collected from the two animals were submitted to the Veterinary Parasitology Laboratory of University of Milan for parasitological evaluation. Overall, parasitological analysis was performed on two fecal samples for each cat. The first two samples were analyzed after refrigeration in the same day, whereas the following samples were analyzed fresh having them delivered within almost 30 minutes after defecation. Centrifugation-flotation technique by NaNO$_3$ solution (s.g. 1200 g/L), fresh fecal smears stained with Lugol's solution, and *Giardia* and *Cryptosporidium* coproantigens detection by an available commercial kit (RIDA®QUICK *Cryptosporidium/Giardia* Combi, R-Biopharm AG, Darmstadt, Germany) were performed.

No protozoan cysts or trophozoites and no ova of helminths were detected by centrifugation-flotation technique in both cats, whereas they were positives to *Giardia*-coproantigens. However, in the fecal smear stained with Lugol's solution obtained from the refrigerated sample of the cat with chronic liquid diarrhea, several cysts and trophozoites of *G. duodenalis* and unidentified elements were found. The latter appeared smaller (length: average 8.18 μm, min–max 6.98–8.88 μm; width: average 6.35 μm, min–max 6.06–6.83 μm) than cysts and trophozoites of *G. duodenalis*, were drop-shaped and brownish in color. An additional Giemsa stained fecal smear confirmed the presence of the unidentified drop-shaped elements (DSE) together with *G. duodenalis* cysts and trophozoites (Figure 1) and detected other elements showing clear morphological features of trichomonads trophozoites (Figure 2). At Giemsa staining, DSE appeared stained light-bluish; they presented a partially smooth surface, an undulated portion, and an internal curved linear structure, pink-violet stained, resembling the curved costa observed in bovine *T. foetus* living pseudocysts. In addition, some of DSE in the fecal smear stained with Lugol's solution presented an internal oval structure (Figure 3) [6, 13]. According to the morphological features of the parasitic elements, an infection sustained by *T. foetus* or by *Pentatrichomonas hominis* was then hypothesized. Analysis of the second fecal samples by saline solution-diluted fresh fecal smear confirmed only presence of trophozoites belonging to *T. foetus/P. hominis* showing an undulating membrane, the flagella, and a rapid forward motion (Figure 4). The fecal samples were processed for molecular analysis by a real-time PCR targeting *T. foetus* 5.8S rRNA gene (AF339736) that was performed at IDEXX Laboratories, Vet Med Labor

GmbH, as previously described [11]. Molecular analyses of extracted nucleic acid from the fecal samples of the two cats confirmed the organism to be *T. foetus*. The diagnosis was mixed intestinal infection with *T. foetus* and *G. duodenalis* in both cats. Following the results of the latest parasitological analysis and, primarily, the diagnosis of *T. foetus* infection, the two animals were treated with ronidazole (30 mg/kg bw, PO, SID) for 14 days. Before suspending therapy, parasitological analyses and PCR assays were performed and the fecal samples tested negative. Six weeks after treatment, the owner reported that the two cats had formed feces and they still tested negative for parasitological analysis.

3. Discussion

T. foetus and *G. duodenalis* are both causative agents of diarrhea in cats, and their observed prevalence is extremely variable in owned cats. In a recent study, 0.7% of cats presented to a cat clinic were shedding *T. foetus*, whereas it in cat shows the prevalence of *T. foetus* infection exceeded 30% [2]. Prevalence of *G. duodenalis* in owned cats, estimated using detection of coproantigens, showed a high variability [7, 9, 14]. *T. foetus* and *G. duodenalis* mixed infection in purebred cat is likely quite a common condition (prevalence = 4.35% to 22.72%) [15, 16]. Diagnosis of *T. foetus* from fecal samples can be performed by different methods such as copromicroscopic examination, fecal cultures (InPouch TF-Feline), and PCR. Cultures and PCR have been considered methods with high sensitivity; however, cultures need a long time of incubation (12 days) before a sample can be considered negative or positive for *T. foetus*. Further, in microscopic analysis of fecal smears or cultures aimed at searching for *T. foetus* trophozoites, the examined fecal samples should be from fresh voided feces or rectal swabs in which live trophozoites are more easily recognized. More recently, low specificity of cultures was demonstrated and a possible misdiagnosis of tritrichomonosis in cats using InPouchTM TF-Feline medium might occur [17]. In cats, *T. foetus* is considered trichomonads with no existing cyst form; nevertheless, formation of pseudocysts or of true cysts has been already observed in several trichomonads, probably as a response to environmental stress [18]. Pseudocysts with internalization of flagella were usually observed in *T. foetus* isolated from cattle both *in vitro* and *in vivo* [13, 18]. *In vitro*, a large number of pseudocysts of bovine *T. foetus* can be obtained from cultures grown at 37°C when cooled to 4°C for 4 h [5]. DSE isolated in the feces of diarrheic cats had morphological features similar to those observed in bovine *T. foetus* living pseudocysts obtained *in vitro*. Particularly, they presented an internal oval structure resembling the nucleus and some undulations due to the movement of the internalized recurrent flagellum inside the cells of bovine *T. foetus* living pseudocysts recorded by differential interference contrast microscopy [5]. Even though further investigations should be performed under experimental conditions, DSE found in feline feces could be reasonably considered *T. foetus* pseudocysts. Moreover, their detection in fecal smears stained with Lugol's solution or Giemsa stain obtained from a refrigerated sample could be of particular interest for clinicians as positive control

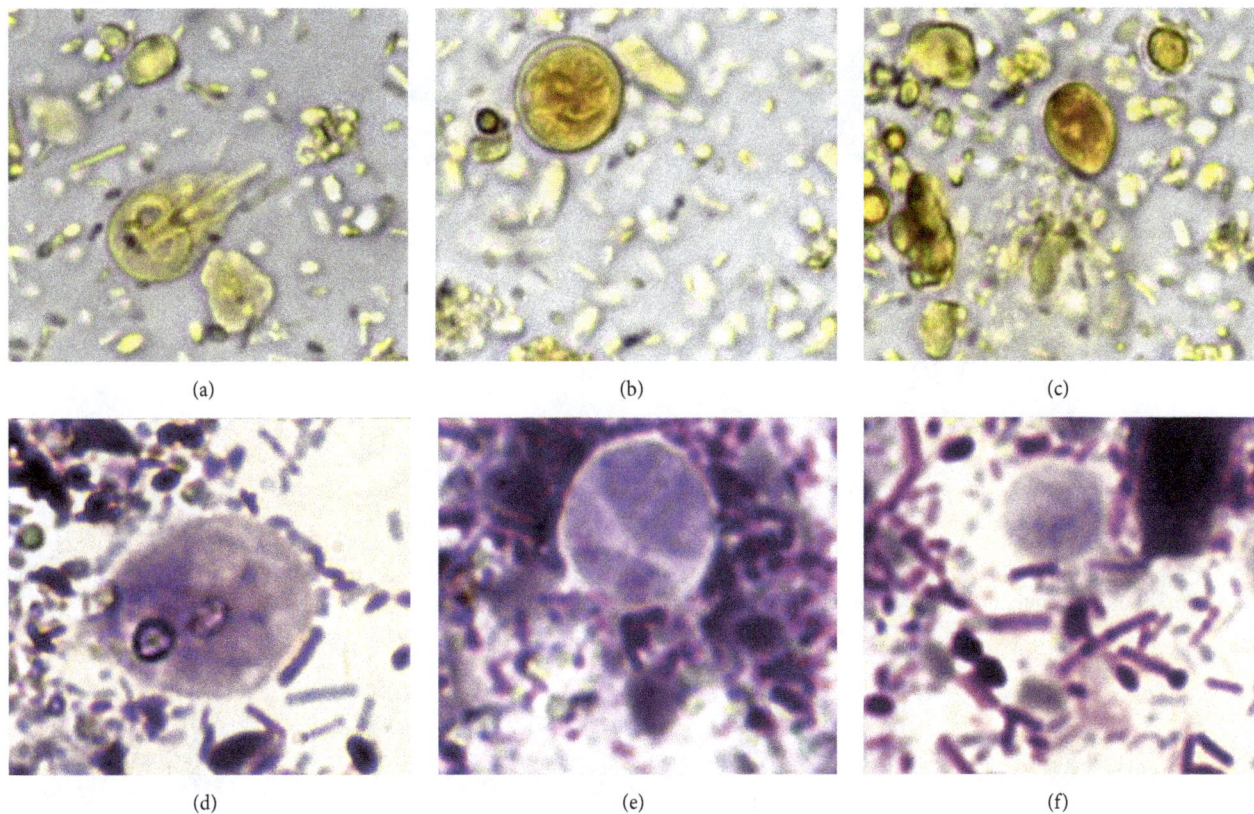

FIGURE 1: Fecal smears from a 6-month-old female Maine Coon cat with chronic liquid diarrhea stained with Lugol's solution (a–c) and Giemsa stain (d–f); (a) and (d) showed *Giardia duodenalis* trophozoite; (b) and (e) showed a *Giardia duodenalis* cyst; (c) and (f) showed drop-shaped trichomonads (630x).

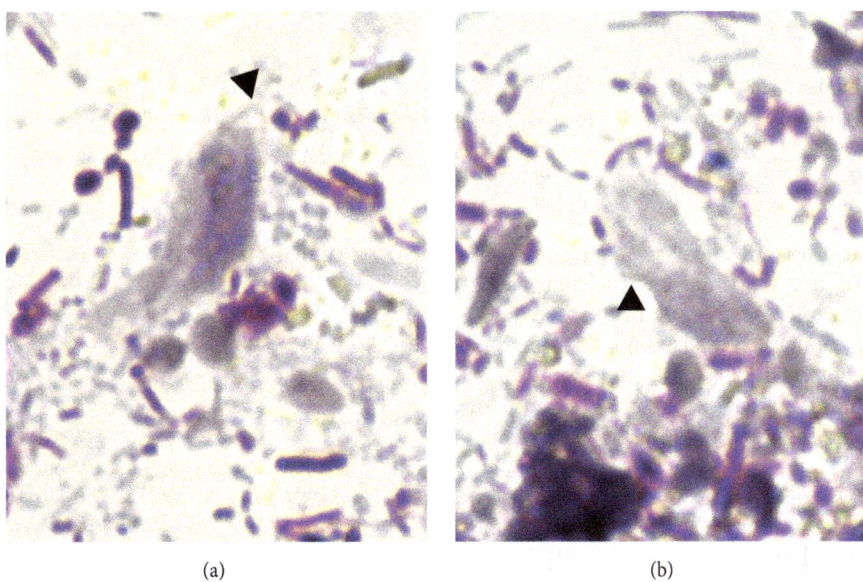

FIGURE 2: Trichomonads in fecal smear from the cat with diarrhea. Arrow heads in (a) indicate anterior flagella emerging from the trophozoite, while arrow heads in (b) indicate undulating membrane (1000x).

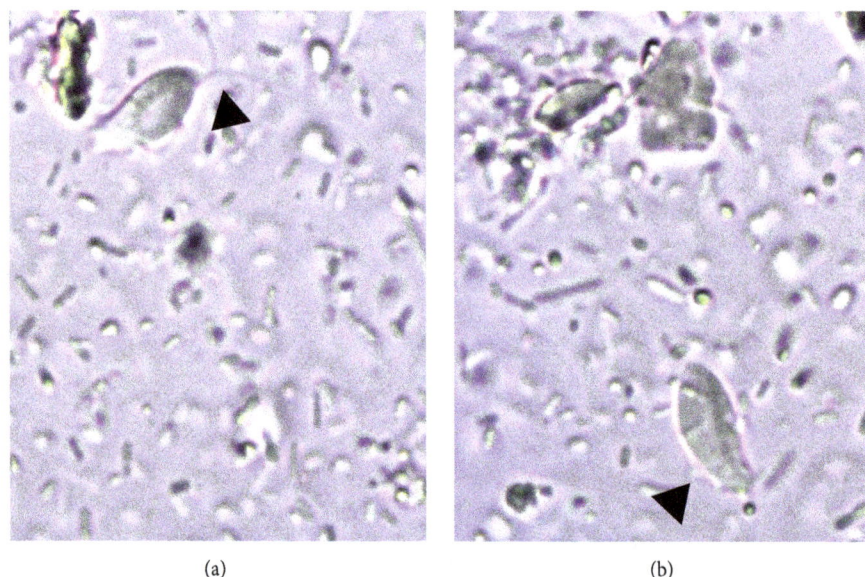

FIGURE 3: Typical morphology of trichomonads observed in saline solution-diluted fresh fecal smear from the cat with diarrhea. Arrow heads in (a) and in (b) indicate anterior flagella and undulating membrane, respectively (630x).

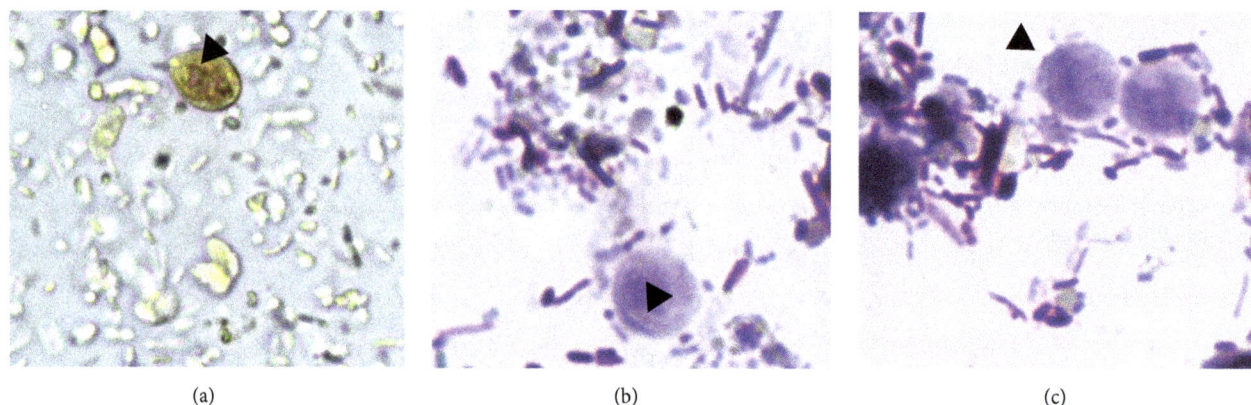

FIGURE 4: Drop-shaped unidentified elements in fecal smears stained with Lugol's solution (a) and Giemsa stain (b-c). Arrow heads in (a) indicate an internal oval structure (400x). Arrow heads in (b) indicate a curved linear structure (1000x). Arrow heads in (c) indicate an undulated portion of the surface (1000x).

with supporting the diagnosis of *T. foetus* infections in cats and catteries [11, 19]. To date, the presence of trichomonads can be detected via light microscopy only in freshly voided feces [4]. Moreover, pseudocysts could represent a form of parasite resistance developing under unfavorable conditions, explaining both the observed environmental resilience of feline *T. foetus* in feces at room temperature and at +4°C after 24 h storage and their diffusion among feline hosts in shelters or catteries [20]. As for *Giardia*, the infection is usually treated with fenbendazole and metronidazole, whereas ronidazole is currently the treatment of choice against *T. foetus* [21]. In this case report, ronidazole was effective against both *T. foetus* and *G. duodenalis*. In addition, this is the first report showing the effectiveness of ronidazole against *G. duodenalis* in cats, as this medication had been previously successfully used against this agent only in kennel dogs [12].

Competing Interests

Authors declare that there is no conflict of interests regarding the publication of this paper.

References

[1] M. G. Levy, J. L. Gookin, M. Poore, A. J. Birkenheuer, M. J. Dykstra, and R. W. Litaker, "*Tritrichomonas foetus* and not *Pentatrichomonas hominis* is the etiologic agent of feline trichomonal diarrhea," *Journal of Parasitology*, vol. 89, no. 1, pp. 99–104, 2003.

[2] A. Hosein, S. A. Kruth, D. L. Pearl et al., "Isolation of *Tritrichomonas foetus* from cats sampled at a cat clinic, cat shows and a humane society in southern Ontario," *Journal of Feline Medicine and Surgery*, vol. 15, no. 8, pp. 706–711, 2013.

[3] C. Profizi, A. Cian, D. Meloni et al., "Prevalence of *Tritrichomonas foetus* infections in French catteries," *Veterinary Parasitology*, vol. 196, no. 1-2, pp. 50–55, 2013.

[4] C. Yao and L. S. Köster, "*Tritrichomonas foetus* infection, a cause of chronic diarrhea in the domestic cat," *Veterinary Research*, vol. 46, article 35, 2015.

[5] M. Benchimol, "Trichomonads under microscopy," *Microscopy and Microanalysis*, vol. 10, no. 5, pp. 528–550, 2004.

[6] R. Meyer Mariante, L. Coutinho Lopes, and M. Benchimol, "*Tritrichomonas foetus* pseudocysts adhere to vaginal epithelial cells in a contact-dependent manner," *Parasitology Research*, vol. 92, no. 4, pp. 303–312, 2004.

[7] C. Epe, G. Rehkter, T. Schnieder, L. Lorentzen, and L. Kreienbrock, "*Giardia* in symptomatic dogs and cats in Europe—results of a European study," *Veterinary Parasitology*, vol. 173, no. 1-2, pp. 32–38, 2010.

[8] N. Itoh, H. Ikegami, M. Takagi et al., "Prevalence of intestinal parasites in private-household cats in Japan," *Journal of Feline Medicine and Surgery*, vol. 14, no. 6, pp. 436–439, 2012.

[9] S. A. Zanzani, A. L. Gazzonis, P. Scarpa, F. Berrilli, and M. T. Manfredi, "Intestinal parasites of owned dogs and cats from metropolitan and micropolitan areas: prevalence, zoonotic risks, and pet owner awareness in northern Italy," *BioMed Research International*, vol. 2014, Article ID 696508, 10 pages, 2014.

[10] U. Ryan and S. M. Cacciò, "Zoonotic potential of *Giardia*," *International Journal for Parasitology*, vol. 43, no. 12-13, pp. 943–956, 2013.

[11] J. K. Paris, S. Wills, H.-J. Balzer, D. J. Shaw, and D. A. Gunn-Moore, "Enteropathogen co-infection in UK cats with diarrhoea," *BMC Veterinary Research*, vol. 10, article 13, 2014.

[12] R. Fiechter, P. Deplazes, and M. Schnyder, "Control of *Giardia* infections with ronidazole and intensive hygiene management in a dog kennel," *Veterinary Parasitology*, vol. 187, no. 1-2, pp. 93–98, 2012.

[13] A. Pereira-Neves, C. M. Campero, A. Martínez, and M. Benchimol, "Identification of *Tritrichomonas foetus* pseudocysts in fresh preputial secretion samples from bulls," *Veterinary Parasitology*, vol. 175, no. 1-2, pp. 1–8, 2011.

[14] F. Riggio, R. Mannella, G. Ariti, and S. Perrucci, "Intestinal and lung parasites in owned dogs and cats from central Italy," *Veterinary Parasitology*, vol. 193, no. 1–3, pp. 78–84, 2013.

[15] D. D. Kingsbury, S. L. Marks, N. J. Cave, and R. A. Grahn, "Identification of *Tritrichomonas foetus* and *Giardia* spp. infection in pedigree show cats in New Zealand," *New Zealand Veterinary Journal*, vol. 58, no. 1, pp. 6–10, 2010.

[16] K. A. Kuehner, S. L. Marks, P. H. Kass et al., "*Tritrichomonas foetus* infection in purebred cats in Germany: prevalence of clinical signs and the role of co-infection with other enteroparasites," *Journal of Feline Medicine and Surgery*, vol. 13, no. 4, pp. 251–258, 2011.

[17] V. Ceplecha, M. Svoboda, I. Čepička, R. Husník, K. Horáčková, and V. Svobodová, "InPouch[6] TF-Feline medium is not specific for *Tritrichomonas foetus*," *Veterinary Parasitology*, vol. 196, no. 3-4, pp. 503–505, 2013.

[18] A. Pereira-Neves, K. C. Ribeiro, and M. Benchimol, "Pseudocysts in trichomonads—new insights," *Protist*, vol. 154, no. 3-4, pp. 313–329, 2003.

[19] T. Gruffydd-Jones, D. Addie, S. Belák et al., "Giardiasis in cats: ABCD guidelines on prevention and management," *Journal of Feline Medicine and Surgery*, vol. 15, no. 7, pp. 650–652, 2013.

[20] S. Hale, J. M. Norris, and J. Šlapeta, "Prolonged resilience of *Tritrichomonas foetus* in cat faeces at ambient temperature," *Veterinary Parasitology*, vol. 166, no. 1-2, pp. 60–65, 2009.

[21] J. L. Gookin, C. N. Copple, M. G. Papich et al., "Efficacy of ronidazole for treatment of feline *Tritrichomonas foetus* infection," *Journal of Veterinary Internal Medicine*, vol. 20, no. 3, pp. 536–543, 2006.

36

Long-Term Outcome of *En Bloc* Extensive Resection of the Penis and Prepuce Associated with a Permanent Perineal Urethrostomy in a Gelding Affected by Squamous Cell Carcinoma

Paola Straticò, Vincenzo Varasano, Gianluca Celani, Riccardo Suriano, and Lucio Petrizzi

Faculty of Veterinary Medicine, University of Teramo, OVUD, Località Piano D'Accio, 64100 Teramo, Italy

Correspondence should be addressed to Paola Straticò; pstratico80@gmail.com

Academic Editor: Carlos Gutiérrez

A 15-year-old gelding was referred for a florid, cauliflower-like ulcerated mass, enclosing penis and prepuce together with penile urethra showing a malodorous purulent and blood-stained discharge and larvae infestation. *En bloc* extensive resection of the penis and prepuce, without penile retroversion or pexy to ventral abdomen associated with a permanent perineal urethrostomy, was performed. Histology of the mass revealed a squamous cell carcinoma of penis and prepuce. The surgical technique that was adopted is a modified version of that already described that allows a more proximal resection of the penile body and is a valid option for treating advanced SCC lesions involving the penis. Early postsurgical complications (mild strangury, haemorrhage from the urethrostomy site and its partial dehiscence, and infection of the abdominal wound) were managed with a medical treatment and resolved within 5 to 12 days. Three years after surgery the horse is in good body condition and does not show any sign of recurrence or disorders related to the surgery.

1. Introduction

Penile and preputial tumours are among the most common neoplasms in the horse, accounting for 6–10% of all neoplastic disorders in this species [1], with squamous cell carcinomas (SCC) being the most common [2]. It may arise *de novo* or from a malignant transformation of a squamous papilloma [2, 3]. It commonly occurs on the glans and internal lamina of the prepuce. It is locally invasive and has a low grade of malignancy [2, 4].

Suggested treatments of small and not complicated SCC of penis and prepuce are cryotherapy [5, 6] and chemotherapy [7, 8].

For extensive SCC surgical excision is recommended. Segmental posthectomy (reefing) and partial phallectomy [9–12] are indicated if only the distal portion of the penis is involved and the remaining free part of the penis can extend beyond the preputial orifice during urination. If penis, prepuce, and regional lymph nodes are extensively involved,

surgical options are *en bloc* resection with or without penile retroversion [13–15] or penile transection just distal to a perineal urethrostomy [16, 17].

In a long-term follow-up study, 9 cases of SCC infiltrating the penile body were described with a survival rate of 55% (5/9) after penile amputation and urethrostomy [2]. Mair et al. described *en bloc* resection of penis and prepuce and superficial inguinal lymph nodes with penile retroversion in 4 horses affected by SCC with 100% survival rate in 1-year follow-up without recurrences [4]. Penile amputation and sheath ablation without penile retroversion were first described by Doles et al. [14] in 25 geldings, with a positive long-term outcome in 8 horses. In the case series by Archer and Edwards [15], 5 geldings undergoing *en bloc* resection of the penis for SCC had a positive long-term follow-up without recurrences; in one case urine scalding due to lateral deviation of the urinary flow was reported. Another retrospective study by Van den Top et al. [1] reported that *en bloc* resection of penis and prepuce was performed in 13 out of 77 horses

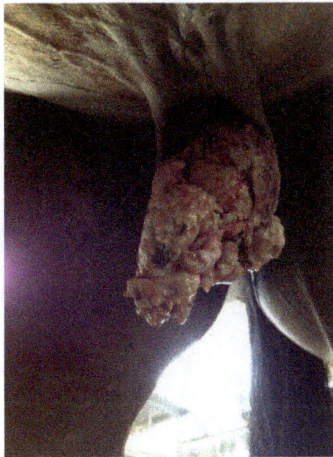

FIGURE 1: Macroscopic appearance of the penile mass at admission showing a florid, cauliflower-like ulcerated mass disrupting the normal anatomy of penis and prepuce.

affected by SCC with lymph node enlargement and extensive genital involvement. Eight horses were available for follow-up and only one suffered neoplastic recurrence within 18 months [1]. Wylie and Payne described a modified surgical technique consisting in subischial urethrostomy and penile amputation with preputial ablation, for the treatment of different severe pathologies (SCC, melanomas, chronic preputial discharge, and paraphimosis) in 15 horses. Median follow-up time was 25.1 months, survival rate 18 months after surgery was 65%, and 6 out of 15 patients were euthanized, 4 of which for reasons related to the procedure [18].

Short- and long-term complication associated with the surgical procedures consisted in cystitis, mild to severe haemorrhage [13–15], wound swelling and infection, urine scalding, second-intention healing of urethral stoma after dehiscence of the suture line, and recurrence of neoplasia [1].

This case report describes the successful treatment of a penile SCC in a gelding with *en bloc* extensive resection of penis and prepuce without penile retroversion, together with a permanent perineal urethrostomy, after a 3-year follow-up period, adding information about long-term clinical outcome after surgical treatment.

2. Case Presentation

A 15-year-old Argentinian Warmblood gelding was referred for treatment of a long-standing penile lesion affected by myiasis.

At referral the main complaint was a florid, cauliflower-like ulcerated mass, measuring 10 cm in diameter that enclosed the *glans penis* together with penile urethra (Figure 1) with malodorous purulent and blood-stained discharge together with areas of necrosis. The mass was infested by *muscae* spp. larvae. Poor body condition score (BCS 4/9) and strangury were also present.

Once penis prolapse was obtained by intravenous administration with acepromazine 30 μg/kg, palpation of the penis revealed a diffuse thickening of the penile shaft with multiple

ulcerations involving the inner and outer laminae of the preputial fold. Due to the regional anatomical alterations related to the mass (phlegmon and oedema), inguinal lymph nodes were not palpable. For the same reason ultrasonographic examination of external genitalia and regional lymph nodes was not conclusive. Transrectal examination was unremarkable.

Urine analysis revealed the presence of leukocytes and nitrites, consistent with urinary tract inflammation. As the clinical condition of the horse and the primary lesion were severe, suggesting complete excision in any case, fine needle aspiration or excisional biopsies were not attempted; therefore surgical removal was combined with harvesting material for histopathological examination.

Based on clinical findings differential diagnoses were SCC of the penis and prepuce and/or habronemiasis. Due to the infiltrating pattern and the diffusion of the disorder and to the presence of multiple nonhealing lesions, leading, respectively, to difficulty at micturition and local infection, an *en bloc* resection of the penis and prepuce was decided; the eventuality of a penile retroversion or a permanent perineal urethrostomy was considered according to the intraoperatory findings and the degree of infiltration of the penis body [14]. Systemic NSAIDS (flunixin meglumine, 1.1. mg/kg i.v. q24 h) and antibiotic (sulfadiazine-trimethoprim, 30 kg/kg p.o. q24 h) therapies were initiated before surgery.

Surgery was performed under general anaesthesia with isoflurane with the horse in dorsal recumbence. For the *en bloc* resection, a fusiform 40 cm long skin incision starting at the umbilicus was made along the midline. It extended caudally encircling the preputial orifice. Blunt dissection of subcutaneous tissue was performed around the penis until the abdominal fascia was reached and the body of the penis was released from its anatomic and vascular connections. Haemorrhage was controlled with electrocauterization and ligation of the major vessels (dorsal penis arteries and veins). The dissection plane was extended to both the external inguinal rings and the external pudendal arteries and vein were ligated. The superficial inguinal lymph nodes appeared enlarged and therefore were excised. At palpation the penile body was extensively thickened suggesting amputation as proximal as possible: so penile retroversion was excluded and perineal urethrostomy was performed. To this aim, a tourniquet was applied proximally to the shaft of the penis and an extensive resection was performed close to the ischiatic arch, dividing the suspensory ligament of penis. The proximal stump showed a normal macroscopic appearance and was sutured with double transfixing sutures (2 USP absorbable multifilament) placed through the penile body in a dorsoventral direction, to obtain adequate haemostasis. Once urethral lumen was clearly visible a urinary catheter was placed. The outer perimeter of the tunica albuginea was apposed in a simple interrupted pattern with a 2/0 USP monofilament absorbable suture.

For permanent urethrostomy a 8 cm skin incision was created on the perineal raphe starting about 7-8 cm below the anus, ending at the level of the ischiatic arch. Blunt dissection of subcutis, penis retractor muscles, and bulbospongiosus muscles was achieved until the urethra was visualized. The

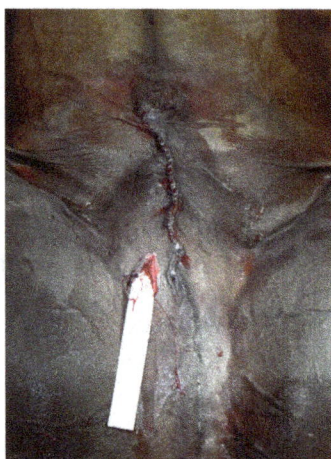

FIGURE 2: Abdominal wall suture and a multitubular drain applied at the scrotal region.

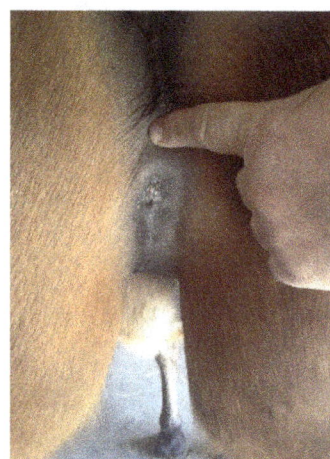

FIGURE 3: Macroscopic appearance of the perineal urinary meatus 3 years after surgery: urethral stoma underwent a progressive contraction until stabilization, allowing normal urination without urine scalding.

penis retractor muscles were sutured to the subcutis in a simple continuous pattern, using a 0 USP monofilament absorbable material. Then the urethral wall was incised longitudinally for about 6 cm and the mucosa sutured to the skin in a simple interrupted pattern with a 2/0 USP monofilament nonabsorbable material.

The subcutis of the abdominal wound was sutured with a 0 USP monofilament absorbable suture material in a simple continuous pattern and the skin was sutured with metallic staples. A multitubular drain was applied laterally to the midline to the abdominal wall suture at the scrotal region (Figure 2).

After recovery from anaesthesia the horse showed a moderate haemorrhage from the urethrostomy, which was particularly evident at the end of urination, leading after 48 h to a marked reduction of PCV (15%) and TP (4,5 g/dL). As the haemorrhage seemed to come from the corpus spongiosum penis and surgical haemostasis was not feasible, it was successfully managed by the administration of tranexamic acid (15 mg/kg i.v. q12 h) for 2 days. Oral support with vitamin B complex and folic and pantothenic acid was given for 10 days until PCV and TP reached, respectively, 30% and 6.8 g/dL.

Strangury but not pollakiuria was observed 3 days after surgery.

Three days after surgery, the horse showed a serosanguineous collection above the abdominal wound and a moderate purulent discharge from the skin incision that were managed with daily manual massage and local disinfection. Five days after surgery, the urinary catheter and the multitubular drain were removed without complications.

On day 12 standing surgical revision of the urethrostomy was required to remove some necrotic urethral mucosa leading to a partial dehiscence of the wound.

Histopathology of the lesions confirmed the presumptive diagnosis of SCC of the penis and prepuce invading the subcutaneous tissue, not the albuginea. Lymphocytic and neutrophilic infiltration of the corpus cavernosum suggested

chronic balanitis; moderate subcutaneous eosinophilic infiltration was also detected but no evidence of Habronema spp. infestation was found. The margins of the excised tissues were free of neoplastic cells, and the regional lymph nodes were inflamed but not affected by the neoplastic process.

After skin staples removal 14 days after surgery, the horse was discharged. Urination was unremarkable from the perineal stoma. No urine scalding or subcutaneous infiltration could be observed. PCV and TP values were back to preoperatory values.

A clinical follow-up performed 2 months after surgery revealed reduction of the urethrostomy to a diameter of about 1.5/2 cm. Anyhow urination was unaffected with a mare attitude and no urine scalding was detected.

A 3-year follow-up showed no recurrence of the neoplasm with normal urination. Urethrostomy did not show any further stricture as well as no urine scalding (Figure 3).

3. Discussion

In this case report the long-term (3 years) successful treatment of a SCC of the penis body and prepuce in a gelding is described. The surgical treatment of the disorder was achieved with an en bloc extensive resection of penis and prepuce without penile retroversion as previously described [14] associated with a permanent perineal urethrostomy.

Differential diagnoses in presence of preputial masses, oedema, and discharge, difficulty at urinating, and phimosis are other neoplastic disorders (squamous papilloma, fibrosarcoma, adenocarcinoma, neurofibroma, basal cell carcinoma, and melanoma) [1, 2] and nonneoplastic pathologies such as epithelial hyperplasia, cutaneous infection with Habronema spp., Halicephalobus spp., or Draschia megastoma, and coital exanthema by EHV-3 [2, 19, 20]. Although for antemortem diagnosis results of microscopic examination of cutaneous biopsy specimens or possibly aspirate samples of the lesion are useful [21] these were not undertaken because of the degree of swelling, abscessation, and ulceration at the penis and prepuce causing dysuria and systemic illness. Therefore a surgical approach was chosen to remove the mass and restore normal urinary function as a salvage procedure.

En bloc resection of penis and prepuce is indicated in cases where external genitalia are extensively affected by the neoplasia. It allows removal of the penis as far proximal as possible until healthy tissue is recognized. Despite invasiveness and postoperatory complications, this technique allows a high rate of success for the cases described in the literature with long-term survival and few tumour recurrences [1, 2, 4, 13, 15].

En bloc resection of penis and prepuce is usually associated with penile retroversion and suture of the penile stump to a subischial skin incision to create a new urinary meatus [13]. In the case series of Archer and Edwards the original technique of Markel was slightly modified to achieve an urethrostomy stoma in subischial position, about 20 cm below the anus, accomplished through a penile stump retroversion [15].

According to Van Harreveld et al. an option is to transect the penis just distal to the site typical of a routine perineal urethrostomy. The corpus cavernosum penis is closed and secured to local fascia and subcutaneous tissue, and a permanent perineal urethrostomy is performed. To our knowledge, no published reports of the long-term outcome of this surgical technique in the horse exist; the authors remark that this technique has worked well and appears to avoid the creation of a flexure in the penis [16].

Recently Wylie and Payne reported 15 cases of extensive penile disorders treated with a subischial urethrostomy and penile amputation with preputial ablation performed under general anaesthesia in dorsal recumbence. Eleven SCC, 2 melanomas, 1 chronic preputial discharge without neoplasia, and 1 paraphimosis secondary to sedation were included. They describe a median survival time of 25.1 months, with 64.3% (9/14 cases) surviving >18 months [18].

In the case described here, to find a normal macroscopic aspect of penile shaft and be consistently sure of the absence of neoplastic tissue left, the penile amputation had to be made very close to the ischiatic arch. To remove all the affected tissue the penile body was excised extensively, more proximally than in the position described by Archer and Edwards [15]; for this reason not enough penile tissue was left to perform a retroversion. So the urinary flow was diverted through a permanent perineal urethrostomy. Differently from the paper of Wylie and Payne, a permanent urinary meatus was created in the perineum after penile amputation, as distal as possible from the anus to avoid faecal contamination and urine scalding. Performing penile amputation before urethrostomy allows the surgeon to evaluate intraoperatively the degree of infiltration of the penile body giving the opportunity to adjust the extension of the amputation.

Although penile retroversion allows the surgeon to direct urinary outflow more caudally than does penile amputation without retroversion [13], no problems due to dysuria or misdirection of the urinary flow and consequent urine scalding were encountered.

In order to reduce ascending infections from the external urinary meatus, the ventral retractor penis muscles were sutured to the subcutis at the urethrostomy site, hypothesizing that their contraction could act as an external urinary sphincter closing the external opening of the stoma at the end of urination, avoiding bacteria ingress, urine dripping, and secondary scalding. The suture of the muscles to the subcutis ensured also a secure fixation of the penis stump, avoiding subcutaneous infiltration of urine.

The complications after surgery encountered in this case were not different from those already described, particularly haemorrhage from the corpus spongiosum at the end of urination, infection of the abdominal wound, and partial dehiscence of the urethral mucosa sutured to the perineum [13, 22, 23].

Postoperative haemorrhage was managed with the administration of tranexamic acid until bleeding stopped. Although haemorrhage is a well described major complication associated with this surgery, the preemptive use of antifibrinolytic agents was not attempted because of the concern about a possible increase in the risk of thromboembolic complications, such as deep vein thrombosis and acute myocardial infarction, related to the use of these drugs in human medicine [24, 25]. Furthermore there are only few refereed studies validating the use of these drugs in the horse. Failure of response to procoagulant agents could have been managed through blood transfusion.

Infection of the abdominal wound was managed by local daily disinfection and use of antimicrobial without other sequelae.

The dehiscence of a permanent urethrostomy can be due to the excessive manipulation of urethral tissue [26] or to excessive tension on the sutures; in our case the haematic infiltration of the subcutaneous tissue consequent to the bleeding from the corpus spongiosum could have increased tension on the urethrostomy sutures leading to a partial dehiscence.

Even though stricture formation can be a complication in 1/3 of perineal urethrostomy cases during early postoperative period and after removal of the urinary catheter [23–26], we did not observe dysuria due to urethral stricture. Two months after surgery a relative stenosis of the urethrostomy occurred, not affecting urinary emission.

The advantages of the *en bloc* extensive resection of the penis and prepuce without penile retroversion associated with a permanent urethrostomy were the removal of as much penile body as possible, minimizing recurrence and avoiding tension related to phallopexy, and the possibility to create a urinary meatus which is functional and cosmetically similar to the mare's.

Postoperative histopathology revealed an infiltration of neoplastic cells in the subcutaneous tissue close to the albuginea, but not in the *corpus cavernosum penis*, which was affected by chronic balanitis, worsened by the presence of myiasis; the chronic balanitis probably contributed to the palpable thickening of the body of the penis, simulating neoplastic infiltration. Although macroscopically enlarged, inguinal lymph nodes did not contain neoplastic cell, but, consistently with literature [1], only marked signs of regional inflammation and lymphoid hyperplasia. Whenever phlegmon and inflammation of the inguinal tissues are present, the sensibility and specificity of ultrasonographic examination and fine needle aspiration of inguinal lymph nodes are reduced [1]. So in order to avoid recurrences extensive surgery was recommended.

The lack of a standardized approach to follow-up evaluation and the definition of clinical success limit an objective consideration about the efficacy of the treatment itself and its prognostic value. Since most of the surgical treatments for penile and preputial disorders are considered as salvage procedures, compromising reproductive and original anatomy, it is essential to the clinician to perform a detailed evaluation of each clinical case and the appropriate treatment.

In this case report the *en bloc* extensive resection of the penis and prepuce without penile retroversion and permanent urethrostomy allowed the successful treatment of a locally invasive SCC of penis and prepuce in a gelding without recurrence after a 3-year follow-up time. Although short- and long-term complications occurred, they were managed and did not compromise the clinical outcome.

Competing Interests

The authors declare that there are no competing interests regarding the publication of this paper.

References

[1] J. G. B. Van den Top, N. de Heer, W. R. Klein, and J. M. Ensink, "Penile and preputial tumours in the horse: a retrospective study of 114 affected horses," *Equine Veterinary Journal*, vol. 40, no. 6, pp. 528–532, 2008.

[2] S. Howarth, V. M. Lucke, and H. Pearson, "Squamous cell carcinoma of the equine external genitalia: a review and assessment of penile amputation and urethrostomy as a surgical treatment," *Equine Veterinary Journal*, vol. 23, no. 1, pp. 53–58, 1991.

[3] R. E. Junge, J. P. Sundberg, and W. D. Lancaster, "Papillomas and squamous cell carcinomas of horses," *Journal of the American Veterinary Medical Association*, vol. 185, no. 6, pp. 656–659, 1984.

[4] T. S. Mair, J. P. Walmsley, and T. J. Phillips, "Surgical treatment of 45 horses affected by squamous cell carcinoma of the penis and prepuce," *Equine Veterinary Journal*, vol. 32, no. 5, pp. 406–410, 2000.

[5] J. R. Joyce, "Cryosurgical treatment of tumors of horses and cattle," *Journal of American Veterinary Medicine Association*, vol. 168, no. 3, pp. 226–229, 1976.

[6] J. A. Stick and R. E. Hoffer, "Results of cryosurgical treatment of equine penile neoplasms," *Journal of Equine Medicine and Surgery*, vol. 2, pp. 505–507, 1978.

[7] A. P. Theon, J. R. Pascoe, G. P. Carlson, and D. N. Krag, "Intratumoral chemotherapy with cisplatin in oily emulsion in horses," *Journal of the American Veterinary Medical Association*, vol. 202, no. 2, pp. 261–267, 1993.

[8] L. A. Fortier and M. A. MacHarg, "Topical use of 5-fluorouracil for treatment of squamous cell carcinoma of the external genitalia of horses: 11 cases (1988–1992)," *Journal of the American Veterinary Medical Association*, vol. 205, no. 8, pp. 1183–1185, 1994.

[9] W. Williams, "Tumours of the penis, prepuce and sheath," in *The Diseases of the Genital Organs of Domestic Animals*, W. Williams and W. L. Williams, Eds., p. 219, W.L. Williams, 3rd edition, 1943.

[10] E. Frank, "Affection of the tail, anus, rectum, vagina and penis," in *Veterinary Surgery*, E. Frank, Ed., p. 277, Burgess Publishing, 7th edition, 1964.

[11] E. A. Scott, "A technique for amputation of equine penis," *Journal of American Veterinary Medicine Association*, vol. 168, no. 11, pp. 1047–1051, 1976.

[12] J. D. Perkins, J. Schumacher, R. W. Waguespack, and M. Hanrath, "Penile retroversion and partial phallectomy performed in a standing horse," *Veterinary Record*, vol. 153, no. 6, pp. 184–185, 2003.

[13] M. D. Markel, J. D. Wheat, and K. Jones, "Genital neoplasms treated by en bloc resection and penile retroversion in horses: 10 cases (1977–1986)," *Journal of the American Veterinary Medical Association*, vol. 192, no. 3, pp. 396–400, 1988.

[14] J. Doles, J. W. Williams, and T. B. Yarbrough, "Penile amputation and sheath ablation in the horse," *Veterinary Surgery*, vol. 30, no. 4, pp. 327–331, 2001.

[15] D. C. Archer and G. B. Edwards, "*En bloc* resection of the penis in five geldings," *Equine Veterinary Education*, vol. 16, no. 1, pp. 12–19, 2004.

[16] P. D. Van Harreveld, P. D. Gaughan, and J. D. Lillich, "Penile surgery in horses," *The Compendium for Continuing Education of the Practicing Veterinarian*, vol. 20, no. 8, pp. 947–954, 1998.

[17] J. G. B. Van den Top, "Squamous cell carcinoma of the penis and prepuce," in *Robinson's Current Therapy in Equine Medicine*, K. A. Sprayberry and N. E. Robinson, Eds., p. 418, Saunders Elsevier, 7th edition, 2014.

[18] C. E. Wylie and R. J. Payne, "A modified surgical technique for penile amputation and preputial ablation in the horse," *Equine Veterinary Education*, vol. 28, no. 5, pp. 269–275, 2016.

[19] A. C. Strafuss, "Squamous cell carcinoma in horses," *Journal of the American Veterinary Medical Association*, vol. 168, no. 1, pp. 61–62, 1976.

[20] D. D. Varner and J. Schumacher, "Diseases of the penis," in *Equine Medicine and Surgery*, P. T. Colahan, I. G. Mayhew, A. M. Merritt et al., Eds., p. 1061, American Veterinary Publication Incorporated, 5th edition, 1999.

[21] S. D. Cramer, M. A. Breshears, and H. J. Qualls, "Pathology in practice," *Journal of the American Veterinary Medical Association*, vol. 238, no. 5, pp. 581–583, 2011.

[22] J. Schumacher, "Penis and prepuce," in *Equine Surgery*, J. A. Auer and J. A. Stick, Eds., p. 811, Saunders Elsevier, 3rd edition, 2006.

[23] I. Kilcoyne and J. Dechant, "Complications associated with perineal urethrotomy in 27 equids," *Veterinary Surgery*, vol. 43, no. 6, pp. 691–696, 2014.

[24] C. J. Dunn and K. L. Goa, "Tranexamic acid: a review of its use in surgery and other indications," *Drugs*, vol. 57, no. 6, pp. 1005–1032, 1999.

[25] J. R. Brown, N. J. O. Birkmeyer, and G. T. O'Connor, "Meta-analysis comparing the effectiveness and adverse outcomes of antifibrinolytic agents in cardiac surgery," *Circulation*, vol. 115, no. 22, pp. 2801–2813, 2007.

[26] D. E. Bjorling, "Urethra," in *Trattato di Chirurgia dei Piccoli Animali*, D. Slatter, Ed., p. 1638, Antonio Delfino Editore, 1st edition, 2005.

PERMISSIONS

All chapters in this book were first published in CRIVM, by Hindawi Publishing Corporation; hereby published with permission under the Creative Commons Attribution License or equivalent. Every chapter published in this book has been scrutinized by our experts. Their significance has been extensively debated. The topics covered herein carry significant findings which will fuel the growth of the discipline. They may even be implemented as practical applications or may be referred to as a beginning point for another development.

The contributors of this book come from diverse backgrounds, making this book a truly international effort. This book will bring forth new frontiers with its revolutionizing research information and detailed analysis of the nascent developments around the world.

We would like to thank all the contributing authors for lending their expertise to make the book truly unique. They have played a crucial role in the development of this book. Without their invaluable contributions this book wouldn't have been possible. They have made vital efforts to compile up to date information on the varied aspects of this subject to make this book a valuable addition to the collection of many professionals and students.

This book was conceptualized with the vision of imparting up-to-date information and advanced data in this field. To ensure the same, a matchless editorial board was set up. Every individual on the board went through rigorous rounds of assessment to prove their worth. After which they invested a large part of their time researching and compiling the most relevant data for our readers.

The editorial board has been involved in producing this book since its inception. They have spent rigorous hours researching and exploring the diverse topics which have resulted in the successful publishing of this book. They have passed on their knowledge of decades through this book. To expedite this challenging task, the publisher supported the team at every step. A small team of assistant editors was also appointed to further simplify the editing procedure and attain best results for the readers.

Apart from the editorial board, the designing team has also invested a significant amount of their time in understanding the subject and creating the most relevant covers. They scrutinized every image to scout for the most suitable representation of the subject and create an appropriate cover for the book.

The publishing team has been an ardent support to the editorial, designing and production team. Their endless efforts to recruit the best for this project, has resulted in the accomplishment of this book. They are a veteran in the field of academics and their pool of knowledge is as vast as their experience in printing. Their expertise and guidance has proved useful at every step. Their uncompromising quality standards have made this book an exceptional effort. Their encouragement from time to time has been an inspiration for everyone.

The publisher and the editorial board hope that this book will prove to be a valuable piece of knowledge for researchers, students, practitioners and scholars across the globe.

LIST OF CONTRIBUTORS

Masaki Michishita, Junki Yasui, Rei Nakahira, Hisashi Yoshimura and Kimimasa Takahashi
Department of Veterinary Pathology, Nippon Veterinary and Life Science University, 1-7-1 Musashino, Kyounan-cho, Tokyo 180-8602, Japan

K. Hamilton, S. Langley-Hobbs, C. Warren-Smith and K. Parsons
Langford Veterinary Services, University of Bristol, Langford BS40 5DU, UK

Marian A. Taulescu, Laura FãrcaG and Cornel Cstoi
Pathology Department, Faculty of Veterinary Medicine, University of Agricultural Sciences and Veterinary Medicine, 3-5 Calea Mãnãştur Street, 400372 Cluj-Napoca, Romania

Irina Amorim and Fatima Gärtner
Department of Pathology and Molecular Immunology of the Institute of Biomedical Sciences Abel Salazar (ICBAS), University of Porto, Rua Jorge Viterbo Ferreira Nr. 228, 4050 313 Porto, Portugal

Mircea V. Mircean
Department of Internal Medicine, Faculty of Veterinary Medicine, University of Agricultural Sciences and Veterinary Medicine, 3-5 Calea Mãnãştur Street, 400372 Cluj-Napoca, Romania

Devorah Marks Stowe, Kevin L. Anderson, James S. Guy, Keith E. Linder and Carol B. Grindem
North Carolina State University College of Veterinary Medicine, 1060 William Moore Drive, Raleigh, NC 27607, USA

Amy W. Hodshon
Department of Small Animal Clinical Sciences, College of Veterinary Medicine, The University of Tennessee, 2407 River Drive, Knoxville, TN 37996, USA

Jill Narak
Department of Clinical Sciences, Auburn University, Auburn, AL 36849, USA

Linden E. Craig
Department of Biomedical and Diagnostic Sciences, College of Veterinary Medicine, The University of Tennessee, 2407 River Drive, Knoxville, TN 37996, USA

Andrea Matthews
Antech Imaging Services, Charlottetown, PE, Canada C1A 1B6

Mark E. Robarge, Stephen D. Lenz and William L. Wigle
Department of Comparative Pathobiology and Indiana Animal Disease Diagnostic Laboratory, Purdue University, 406 S. University Street, West Lafayette, IN 47907, USA

Jonathan E. Beever
Department of Animal Sciences, University of Illinois, 1207West Gregory Drive, Urbana, IL 61801, USA

Christopher J. Lynch
Department of Cellular and Molecular Physiology, Penn State University College of Medicine, 500 University Drive, Hershey, PA 17033, USA

Arvind Sharma, Adarsh Kumar and Sheikh Imran
Department of Veterinary Surgery and Radiology, College of Veterinary and Animal Sciences, CSK HP Agriculture University, Himachal Pradesh, Palampur 176062, India

Pankaj Sood
Department of Veterinary Gynaecology and Obstetrics, College of Veterinary and Animal Sciences, CSK HP Agriculture University, Himachal Pradesh, Palampur 176062, India

Rajesh Kumar Asrani
Department of Veterinary Pathology, College of Veterinary and Animal Sciences, CSK HP Agriculture University, Himachal Pradesh, Palampur 176062, India

Nora Nogradi and Amanda L. Koehne
William R. Pritchard Veterinary Medical Teaching Hospital, University of California, Davis, One Shield Avenue, Davis, CA 95616, USA

F. Charles Mohr and Sean D. Owens
Department of Pathology, Microbiology and Immunology, School of Veterinary Medicine, University of California Davis, Davis, One Shield Avenue, Davis, CA 95616, USA

Meera C. Heller
Department of Medicine and Epidemiology, School of Veterinary Medicine, University of California Davis, Davis, One Shield Avenue, Davis, CA 95616, USA
Department of Veterinary Medicine and Surgery, University of Missouri, 900 East Campus Drive, Columbia, MO65211, USA

Ashley Malmlov, Craig Miller and Colleen Duncan
Department of Microbiology, Immunology and Pathology, Colorado State University, Fort Collins, 200West Lake Street, 1644 CampusDelivery, Fort Collins, CO 80523, USA

Terry Campbell and Eric Monnet
Veterinary Teaching Hospital, Colorado State University, Fort Collins, CO 80523, USA

Becca Miceli
The Wild Animal Sanctuary, Keenesburg, CO 80643, USA

Amanda Whiton, Juergen Schumacher, Erika E. Evans and Edward Ramsay
Department of Small Animal Clinical Sciences, College of Veterinary Medicine, University of Tennessee, 2407 River Drive, Knoxville, TN 37996, USA

Janelle M. Novak and Robert Donnell
Department of Biomedical and Diagnostic Sciences, College of Veterinary Medicine, University of Tennessee, Knoxville, TN 37996, USA

Amanda Crews
Department of Biomedical and Diagnostic Sciences, College of Veterinary Medicine, University of Tennessee, Knoxville, TN 37996, USA
Professional Veterinary Pathology Services, Columbia, SC 29203, USA

Lori J. Best, Shelley J. Newman, Daniel A. Ward and Diane V. H. Hendrix
University of Tennessee, 2407 River Drive, Knoxville, TN 37919, USA

Mohamed M. Elhanafy and Dennis D. French
Department of Veterinary Clinical Medicine, Rural Animal Health Management, 1008 W. Hazelwood Drive, 223 Large Animal Clinic, Urbana, IL 61802, USA

Silke Hecht, April M. Durant,William H. Adams and Gordon A. Conklin
Department of Small Animal Clinical Sciences, C247 Veterinary Medical Center, University of Tennessee College of Veterinary Medicine, 2407 River Dr., Knoxville, TN 37996, USA

Gwynne E. Kinley, Connie W. Schmitt and Julie Stephens-Devalle
Veterinary Services Program,Walter Reed Army Institute of Research/Naval Medical Research Center, 511 Robert Grant Avenue, Silver Spring, MD 20910, USA

Angelo Pasquale Giannuzzi, Antonio De Simone,Mario Ricciardi and Floriana Gernone
"Pingry" Veterinary Hospital, Via Medaglie d'Oro 5, 70126 Bari, Italy

Karolin Schoellhorn, Bernhard Schoellhorn and Ulrich Rytz
Division of Small Animal Surgery and Orthopedics, Department of Clinical Veterinary Medicine, Vetsuisse Faculty, University of Berne, Laenggassstrasse 128, 3012 Berne, Switzerland

Corinne Gurtner and Maja M. Suter
Institute of Animal Pathology, Vetsuisse Faculty, University of Berne, Laenggassstrasse 122, 3012 Berne, Switzerland

Katrin Timm and Petra J. Roosje
Division of Clinical Dermatology, Department of Clinical Veterinary Medicine, Vetsuisse Faculty, University of Berne, Laenggassstrasse 128, 3012 Berne, Switzerland

Daniela Proverbio, Eva Spada, Giada Bagnagatti De Giorgi, and Roberta Perego
Dipartimento di Scienze Veterinarie per la Salute, la Produzione Animale e la Sicurezza Alimentare, Università degli Studi di Milano, Via G. Celoria, 10-20133 Milano, Italy

Carl Bradbrook and Louise Clark
Davies Veterinary Specialists, Manor Farm Business Park, Higham Gobion, Hitchin SG5 3HR, UK

Martina Mosing
Department of Anaesthesia, Vetsuisse Faculty, University of Zurich, Winterthurerstrasse 260, 8057 Zurich, Switzerland

Trisha J. Oura
Tufts Veterinary Emergency Treatment and Specialties, 525 South Street, Walpole, MA 02081, USA

Peter J. Early, Samuel H. Jennings, Melissa J. Lewis and Jeremy R. Tobias
North Carolina State University Veterinary Teaching Hospital, 1052William Moore Drive, Raleigh, NC 27607, USA

Donald E. Thrall
Associate Dean for Research, Ross University School of Veterinary Medicine, P.O. Box 334, Basseterre, Saint Kitts, USA

Jill Narak and D. Michael Tillson
Department of Clinical Sciences, Auburn University College of Veterinary Medicine, Auburn, AL 36849, USA

Emily C. Graff
Department of Pathobiology, Auburn University College of Veterinary Medicine, Auburn, AL 36849, USA

Katrin Saile
Department of Clinical Sciences, Auburn University College of Veterinary Medicine, Auburn, AL 36849, USA
Pittsburgh Veterinary Specialty and Emergency Center, 807 Camp Horne Road, Pittsburgh, PA 15237, USA

Isamu Kanemoto
Chayagasaka Animal Hospital, 1-1-5 Shinnishi, Chikusa, Nagoya, Aichi 464-0003, Japan

Daisuke Taguchi
Chayagasaka Animal Hospital, 1-1-5 Shinnishi, Chikusa, Nagoya, Aichi 464-0003, Japan
Green Animal Hospital, 179 Tamakake-maeda, Nanbu, Sannohe, Aomori 039-0101, Japan

Satoko Yokoyama
Chayagasaka Animal Hospital, 1-1-5 Shinnishi, Chikusa, Nagoya, Aichi 464-0003, Japan
Miyashita Animal Hospital, 5-8-29 Keigoya, Kure, Hiroshima 737-0012, Japan

Masashi Mizuno
Chayagasaka Animal Hospital, 1-1-5 Shinnishi, Chikusa, Nagoya, Aichi 464-0003, Japan
4Veterinary Internal Medicine of Nihon University, 1866 Kameino, Fujisawa, Kanagawa 252-8510, Japan

Makoto Washizu
Animal Teaching Hospital of Gihu University, 1-1 Yanagido, Gifu 501-1193, Japan

Jennifer N. Niemuth and James R. Flowers
College of Veterinary Medicine, North Carolina State University, 1060William Moore Drive,
Raleigh, NC 27607, USA

Joni V. Allgood
College of Veterinary Medicine, North Carolina State University, 1060William Moore Drive,
Raleigh, NC 27607, USA
Happy Tails Veterinary Emergency Clinic, Greensboro, NC 27418, USA

Ryan S. De Voe and Brigid V. Troan
College of Veterinary Medicine, North Carolina State University, 1060William Moore Drive, Raleigh, NC 27607, USA

North Carolina Zoological Park, 4401 Zoo Parkway, Asheboro, NC 27205, USA

Geoffrey A. Wood
Department of Pathobiology, Ontario Veterinary College, University of Guelph, Guelph, ON, Canada N1G 2W1

Hibret A. Adissu
Department of Pathobiology, Ontario Veterinary College, University of Guelph, Guelph, ON, Canada N1G 2W1
Centre for Modeling Human Disease, Toronto Centre for Phenogenomics, 25 Orde Street, Toronto, ON, Canada M5T 3H7

John D. Baird
Department of Clinical Studies, Ontario Veterinary College, University of Guelph, Guelph, ON, Canada N1G 2W1

Ashley Hanna, Susanne M. Stieger-Vanegas, Melissa Esser, John Schlipf and Jacob Mecham
Department of Clinical Sciences, College of Veterinary Medicine, Oregon State University, Magruder Hall, Corvallis, OR 97331, USA

Jerry R. Heidel
Department of Biomedical Sciences, College of Veterinary Medicine, Oregon State University, Magruder Hall, Corvallis, OR 97331, USA

Eli B. Cohen
Departments of Clinical and Molecular Biomedical Sciences, College of Veterinary Medicine, North Carolina State University, 1060William Moore Drive, Raleigh, NC 27607, USA

Jenessa L. Gjeltema
Departments of Clinical and Molecular Biomedical Sciences, College of Veterinary Medicine, North Carolina State University, 1060William Moore Drive, Raleigh, NC 27607, USA
North Carolina Zoo, Asheboro, NC 27205, USA
Environmental Medicine Consortium, College of Veterinary Medicine, North Carolina State University, Raleigh, NC 27207, USA

Robert A. MacLean
Environmental Medicine Consortium, College of Veterinary Medicine, North Carolina State University, Raleigh, NC 27207, USA
Audubon Nature Institute, 6500 Magazine Street, New Orleans, LA 70118, USA

Ryan S. De Voe
Environmental Medicine Consortium, College of Veterinary Medicine, North Carolina State University, Raleigh, NC 27207, USA
Disney's Animal Kingdom, Orlando, FL 32830, USA

Gwendolyna Romkes and Johanna Corinna Eule
Small Animal Clinic, Faculty of Veterinary Medicine, Freie Universit'at Berlin, Oertzenweg 19b, 14163 Berlin, Germany

Julia V. Coutin and Otto I. Lanz
Department of Small Animal Clinical Sciences, Virginia-Maryland Regional College of VeterinaryMedicine, Blacksburg, VA 24061, USA

Jeremy L. Shomper
Department of Small Animal Clinical Sciences, Virginia-Maryland Regional College of VeterinaryMedicine, Blacksburg, VA 24061, USA
University of Missouri, College of Veterinary Medicine, Columbia, MO 65211, USA

Emmanouil I. Papadogiannakis
Department of Veterinary Public Health, National School of Public Health, 115 21 Athens, Greece
Small Animal Dermatology Clinic, Alimos, 174 55 Athens, Greece

Emmanouil N. Velonakis
Department of Applied Microbiology and Immunology, National School of Public Health, 115 21 Athens, Greece

Gregory K. Spanakos
Department of Parasitology, Entomology and Tropical Diseases, National School of Public Health, 115 21 Athens, Greece

Alexander F. Koutinas
Quality Veterinary Practice, 383 33 Volos, Greece

Carlos Eduardo Fonseca-Alves and Aline Gonçalves Corrêa
Department of Veterinary Clinic, School of Veterinary Medicine and Animal Science, Universidade Estadual Paulista, Botucatu, SP, Brazil

Fabiana Elias
Department of Veterinary Medicine, Federal University of Southern Border, Realeza, PR, Brazil

Sabryna Gouveia Calazans
Department of Veterinary Medicine, University of Franca, Franca, SP, Brazil

Margaret Cohn-Urbach and Annie Chen
Department of Veterinary Clinical Sciences, College of Veterinary Medicine,Washington State University, P.O. Box 647010, Pullman,WA 99164-7010, USA

Gary Haldorson
Department of Veterinary Microbiology and Pathology, College of Veterinary Medicine,Washington State University, P.O. Box 647040, Pullman,WA 99164-7040, USA

Stephanie Thomovsky
Department of Veterinary Clinical Sciences, College of Veterinary Medicine, Purdue University, 625 Harrison Street, West Lafayette, IN 47907-2026, USA

Franck Forterre
Small Animal Clinic, Department of Clinical Veterinary Medicine, Vetsuisse Faculty, University of Berne, 3012 Berne, Switzerland
Department of Neurosurgery, Vetsuisse Faculty, University of Berne, Länggassstrasse 128, 3012 Berne, Switzerland

Núria Vizcaino Reves
Small Animal Clinic, Department of Clinical Veterinary Medicine, Vetsuisse Faculty, University of Berne, 3012 Berne, Switzerland
Department of Surgery, Vetsuisse Faculty, University of Berne, Länggassstrasse 128, 3012 Berne, Switzerland

Christina Stahl and Karine Gendron
Small Animal Clinic, Department of Clinical Veterinary Medicine, Vetsuisse Faculty, University of Berne, 3012 Berne, Switzerland
Department of Radiology, Vetsuisse Faculty, University of Berne, Länggassstrasse 128, 3012 Berne, Switzerland

Stephan Rupp
Tierklinik Hofheim, Im Langgewann 9, am Taunus, 65719 Hofheim, Germany

Achariya Sailasuta
STAR, Molecular Biology Research on Animal Oncology, Department of Pathology, Faculty of Veterinary Science, Chulalongkorn University, Bangkok 10330,Thailand

Dettachai Ketpun
STAR, Molecular Biology Research on Animal Oncology, Department of Pathology, Faculty of Veterinary Science, Chulalongkorn University, Bangkok 10330,Thailand
Biochemistry Unit, Department of Physiology, Faculty of Veterinary Science, Chulalongkorn University, Bangkok 10330,Thailand

Prapruddee Piyaviriyakul
Biochemistry Unit, Department of Physiology, Faculty of Veterinary Science, Chulalongkorn University, Bangkok 10330,Thailand

Nattawat Onlamoon and Kovit Pattanapanyasat
Office for Research and Development, Faculty of Medicine Siriraj Hospital, Mahidol University, Bangkok 10770, Thailand

Ruth Weiss and Alessandra Bergadano
Roche Pharma Research and Early Development, Pharmaceutical Sciences, Comparative Medicine, Roche Innovation Center, Basel, Switzerland

Reto Wettstein, Elisabeth Artemis Kappos and Daniel Kalbermatten
Department of Plastic, Reconstructive, Aesthetic and Hand Surgery, University Hospital of Basel, Basel, Switzerland

Björn Jacobsen
Roche Pharma Research and Early Development, Pharmaceutical Sciences, Toxicology and Pathology, Roche Innovation Center, Basel, Switzerland

Enzo Vettorato and Federico Corletto
Dick White Referrals, Station Farm, London Road, Six Mile Bottom, Cambridgeshire CB8 0UH, UK

Sergio A. Zanzani, Alessia L. Gazzonis, Paola Scarpa and Maria Teresa Manfredi
Department of Veterinary Medicine, Università degli Studi di Milano,Milano, Italy

Emanuela Olivieri
Department of Veterinary Medicine, Università degli Studi di Perugia, Perugia, Italy

Hans-Jörg Balzer
IDEXX Laboratories, Ludwigsburg, Germany

Paola Straticò, Vincenzo Varasano, Gianluca Celani, Riccardo Suriano and Lucio Petrizzi
Faculty of Veterinary Medicine, University of Teramo, OVUD, Località Piano D'Accio, 64100 Teramo, Italy

Index

www.ingramcontent.com/pod-product-compliance
Lightning Source LLC
Chambersburg PA
CBHW050450200326
41458CB00014B/5123